THE DEVELOPMENT OF SHYNESS
AND SOCIAL WITHDRAWAL

SOCIAL, EMOTIONAL, AND PERSONALITY DEVELOPMENT IN CONTEXT

Kenneth H. Rubin, *Series Editor*

Handbook of Peer Interactions, Relationships, and Groups
Edited by Kenneth H. Rubin, William M. Bukowski, and Brett Laursen

The Development of Shyness and Social Withdrawal
Edited by Kenneth H. Rubin and Robert J. Coplan

The Development
of Shyness
and Social Withdrawal

Edited by
KENNETH H. RUBIN
ROBERT J. COPLAN

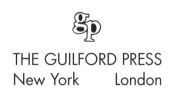

THE GUILFORD PRESS
New York   London

© 2010 The Guilford Press
A Division of Guilford Publications, Inc.
72 Spring Street, New York, NY 10012
www.guilford.com

Printed in the United States of America

This book is printed on acid-free paper.

Last digit is print number: 9 8 7 6 5 4 3 2 1

Library of Congress Cataloging-in-Publication Data
is available from the Publisher.

ISBN 978-1-60623-522-5 (hardcover)

To our sociable and well-regulated children,
Amy and Joshua Rubin and Adam and Jaimie Coplan,

and to our grandchildren, Julius and Isabella Rubin
and Jonah-Bear Rubin Flett

About the Editors

Kenneth H. Rubin, PhD, is Professor of Human Development and Director of the Center for Children, Relationships, and Culture at the University of Maryland. His research interests include children's peer and family relationships and their social and emotional development. Dr. Rubin is the recipient of a Killam Research Fellowship (Canada Council) and an Ontario Mental Health Senior Research Fellowship, is past president of the International Society for the Study of Behavioral Development, and has published 11 books and over 240 peer-reviewed chapters and articles. He is a Fellow of the Canadian and American Psychological Associations and the Association for Psychological Science.

Robert J. Coplan, PhD, is a developmental psychologist and Professor of Psychology at Carleton University in Ottawa, Canada. His research interests concern the overlap between children's social–emotional functioning and developmental psychopathology, with a primary focus on the development of shyness and social anxiety in childhood. Dr. Coplan is Editor of the journal *Social Development* and the author of the forthcoming books *What Teachers Need to Know about Shyness* and *Social Development in Childhood and Adolescence: A Contemporary Reader.*

Contributors

Yair Amichai-Hamburger, PhD, Sammy Ofer School of Communications, Interdisciplinary Center, Herzliya, Israel

Jens B. Asendorpf, PhD, Department of Psychology, Humboldt University, Berlin, Germany

Julie Bowker, PhD, Department of Psychology, University at Buffalo, The State University of New York, Buffalo, New York

Arnold H. Buss, PhD, Department of Psychology, University of Texas at Austin, Austin, Texas

Charissa S. L. Cheah, PhD, University of Maryland, Baltimore County, Baltimore, Maryland

Xinyin Chen, PhD, Department of Psychology, University of Western Ontario, London, Ontario, Canada

Jeremy S. Cohen, MA, Department of Psychology, Temple University, Philadelphia, Pennsylvania

Robert J. Coplan, PhD, Department of Psychology, Carleton University, Ottawa, Ontario, Canada

Sarah A. Crawley, MA, Department of Psychology, Temple University, Philadelphia, Pennsylvania

W. Ray Crozier, PhD, School of Social Work and Psychology, University of East Anglia, Norwich, United Kingdom

Julie M. Edmunds, MA, Department of Psychology, Temple University, Philadelphia, Pennsylvania

Mary Ann Evans, PhD, Department of Psychology, University of Guelph, Guelph, Ontario, Canada

Nathan A. Fox, PhD, Department of Human Development, University of Maryland, College Park, College Park, Maryland

Heidi Gazelle, PhD, Department of Psychology, University of North Carolina at Greensboro, Greensboro, North Carolina

Paul D. Hastings, PhD, Department of Psychology, University of California at Davis, Davis, California

Kathleen Hughes, PhD, Department of Psychology, Carleton University, Ottawa, Ontario, Canada

Philip C. Kendall, PhD, Department of Psychology, Temple University, Philadelphia, Pennsylvania

Matthew P. Mychailyszyn, MA, Department of Psychology, Temple University, Philadelphia, Pennsylvania

Jacob N. Nuselovici, PhD, Department of Psychology, Concordia University, Montreal, Quebec, Canada

Ronald M. Rapee, PhD, Department of Psychology, Macquarie University, Sydney, Australia

Bethany C. Reeb-Sutherland, PhD, Department of Human Development, University of Maryland, College Park, College Park, Maryland

Hilary Claire Rowsell, BA, Department of Psychology, Carleton University, Ottawa, Ontario, Canada

Kenneth H. Rubin, PhD, Center for Children, Relationships, and Culture, and Department of Human Development, University of Maryland, College Park, College Park, Maryland

Louis A. Schmidt, PhD, Department of Psychology, Neuroscience and Behaviour, McMaster University, Hamilton, Ontario, Canada

Barry H. Schneider, PhD, Department of Psychology, University of Ottawa, Ottawa, Ontario, Canada

Murray Weeks, MA, Department of Psychology, Carleton University, Ottawa, Ontario, Canada

Contents

xi

III. PERSONAL AND
INTERPERSONAL PROCESSES

IV. CONTEXTS

V. CLINICAL RESEARCH, PRACTICE, AND TREATMENT

THE DEVELOPMENT OF SHYNESS
AND SOCIAL WITHDRAWAL

PART I

INTRODUCTION

1

Social Withdrawal
and Shyness in Childhood

History, Theories,
Definitions, and Assessments

ROBERT J. COPLAN
KENNETH H. RUBIN

A casual observer of preschoolers' free play in the company of peers is likely to witness many distinct patterns of interrelations among the children. For example, some children would be interacting in small groups, perhaps engaged in sociodramatic play or taking turns playing a rule-governed game. Other children would be playing next to each other, drawing pictures or building with blocks, periodically monitoring what others are doing. Finally, still other children would be playing quietly alone or just watching their peers play, without trying to join in.

Historically, researchers have been more interested in children's peer interactions and in children who display socially competent behavior than in those who, for whatever reason, refrain from engaging in peer interaction. However, as the chapters in this volume demonstrate, in recent years there has been a veritable explosion of research into the construct of *social withdrawal* in childhood. In this introductory chapter, we describe the history of the study of social withdrawal, provide definitions and a conceptual overview of the phenomenon, briefly outline relevant methodological issues, and preview the contents of the chapters in this volume.

HISTORICAL OVERVIEW

The origins of the psychological study of social withdrawal can be traced back to three relatively distinct "branches" of historical research. To begin with, well over 100 years ago, a small group of theorists and researchers began to emphasize the importance of studying children's peer relations and interaction. Cooley (1902) was among the first to suggest that peer interaction made a significant contribution to children's socialization. In their early work, Piaget (e.g., 1926) and Mead (1934) also argued that peer interaction provides a critical context for learning about the self and others. A few years later, Sullivan (1953) proposed that the experience of peer relationships is essential for the child's development of the concepts of mutual respect, equality, and reciprocity. These theorists have had a lasting and profound influence on the contemporary study of children's peer relationships (Rubin, Bukowski, & Parker, 2006). However, by highlighting the importance peer relations in the development of children, they also drew attention to the notion that it might be important to consider children who do *not* frequently engage in interactions with peers.

A second branch of research emerged in the 1920s, when some of the first observational studies of children's social participation with peers were undertaken. This led to the development of various taxonomies for delineating different types of social interaction in play groups (e.g., Bott, 1928; Verry, 1923). Lehman (1926; Lehman & Anderson, 1928) was particularly interested in children who frequently played alone in the presence of peers. He characterized the differences between solitary and social play as they related to measures of sociability and other character traits. Most well known of this research was the work of Parten (1932), who observed preschool children during free play in a nursery school setting over a 9-month period. In her taxonomy of social participation were several types of socially withdrawn behaviors, including remaining unoccupied, onlooking (i.e., observing others but not joining in) and engaging in solitary play (in the presence of peers). This behavioral taxonomy went on to form the building blocks for the later study of multiple forms of children's nonsocial play and social withdrawal (e.g., Coplan, Rubin, Fox, Calkins, & Stewart, 1994; Rubin, 1982).

Finally, also starting in the early 1920s, a small group of education researchers began to suggest that shy children might require extra attention from educators in the school setting (e.g., Craig, 1922). Dealy (1923) reported the case histories of 38 "problem children" in kindergarten to grade 2 who were "destined to cost the state some money" (p. 128). Roughly half of these children were characterized by extreme sensitivity or timidity. A few years later, Lowenstein and Svendsen (1938) conducted what was likely the first intervention program for shy and withdrawn children. They selected 13 boys (ages 6–8 years) characterized as shy or withdrawn and sent them to a small farm camp, where other children were present for a period of 6–8 weeks. Follow-up assessments demonstrated improvement in 10 of the 13 children, allowing the authors to conclude that "considerable modification of the behavior of shy children can be affected" (p. 652).

Notwithstanding these pockets of early interest, social withdrawal was long considered to be of limited developmental significance, particularly within the clinical literature. For example, Morris, Soroker, and Burruss (1954) conducted a follow-back study of a group of 54 adults who had been admitted to a child guidance clinic as shy or withdrawn 16–27 years previously. They concluded that these adults were "on the whole getting along quite well" that "one has the impression that most … turn out to be average/normal people in most respects" and that we are quite likely "overconcerned about these personality characteristics" (p. 753). Subsequent (and often-cited) review articles suggested that social withdrawal in childhood was relatively unstable and not significantly predictive of maladjustment during the adolescent and adult periods (Kohlberg, LaCrosse, & Ricks, 1972; Robins, 1966).

In the 1980s, Jerome Kagan and colleagues brought increased attention to the temperamental trait of *behavioral inhibition* (Garcia-Coll, Kagan, & Reznick, 1984; Kagan, Reznick, Clarke, Snidman, & Garcia-Coll, 1984; Kagan, Reznick, & Snidman, 1988; Reznick et al., 1986). Kagan described extremely inhibited children as wary and reserved in the face of novelty, and argued that such children possessed a lower threshold for psychophysiological arousal. This seminal work was among the first to emphasize the biological substrates of shyness, as well as its stability from infancy to later childhood (particularly among extreme groups).

Also in the 1980s, Rubin and colleagues began reporting results from the Waterloo Longitudinal Study (e.g., Rubin, 1985; Rubin & Both, 1989; Rubin, Hymel, & Mills, 1989; Rubin, Chen, & Hymel, 1993). One of the first comprehensive longitudinal studies to focus specifically on the construct of social withdrawal, this study followed children from preschool to adolescence. The results of this research provided some of strongest evidence to date that social withdrawal was a relatively stable phenomenon that was contemporaneously and predictively associated with a host of negative outcomes, including negative self-worth, loneliness, depressive symptoms, internalizing problems, and peer rejection.

The wider dissemination of research into development and inhibition, shyness, and social withdrawal likely contributed to increased attention from a clinical perspective. For example, by the early 1990s results from a number of both retrospective and longitudinal studies demonstrated empirical links between behavioral inhibition in early childhood and the development of anxiety disorders (particularly social phobia) in later childhood, adolescence, and adulthood (Biederman et al., 1990, 1993; Hirschfeld et al., 1992; Rosenbaum et al., 1988; Rosenbaum, Biederman, Hirshfeld, Bolduc, & Chaloff, 1991). Empirical links also emerged between social withdrawal and the etiology of childhood depression (e.g., Bell-Dolan, Reaven, & Peterson, 1993; Mullins, Peterson, Wonderlich, & Reaven, 1986). Perhaps as a result, social withdrawal also began to be more widely cited as evidence of an internalizing problem (Achenbach & Edelbrock, 1981) or overcontrolled disorder (e.g., Lewis & Miller, 1990).

In 1993, Rubin and Asendorpf published the first edited volume specifically related to the study of social withdrawal in childhood. This book collected and reviewed the research conducted up to that date and called for increased attention in the future to the study of social withdrawal. In many ways, this current volume can be viewed as a logical follow-up to this 1993 book, wherein we examine the veritable explosion of research in the study of shyness and social withdrawal in the intervening 20 years.

NOMENCLATURE, DEFINITIONS, AND CONCEPTUALIZATIONS

Discussions of the study of shyness, inhibition, and social withdrawal have often begun with the proviso that this research area is plagued by a lack of conceptual clarity. Contributing to this confusion has been a plethora of terms that are defined inconsistently. Moreover, at various times, these terms have been employed (often interchangeably) to refer to temperamental and personality traits, motivational and interpersonal processes, and/or observable behaviors. A (likely incomplete!) list of these terms is provided in Table 1.1.

Rubin and Asendorpf (e.g., Asendorpf, 1990; Rubin, 1982; Rubin & Asendorpf, 1993) were the first to attempt to organize these varied constructs in a psychologically meaningful manner. Their conceptual and definitional model provided the "theoretical backbone" for this research area. Herein we restate the core components of this conceptual taxonomy, while updating various components to reflect the current state of theoretical and empirical knowledge (Rubin, Coplan, & Bowker, 2009). A model of our updated *taxonomy of solitude* is displayed in Figure 1.1.

We begin with the broad notion of behavioral "solitude," which encompasses all instances of children spending time "alone" (i.e., a lack of social interaction) in the presence of peers (i.e., potential play partners). Rubin (1982) originally proposed the distinction between two causal processes that may underlie children's lack of social interaction. The first is "active isolation," which denotes the process whereby some children spend time

TABLE 1.1. Terms Previously Employed in the Literature Pertaining to "Solitude"

- *Constructs related to the processes that may contribute to solitude*
  - active isolation
  - passive withdrawal
  - peer exclusion
  - peer neglect
  - peer rejection
  - social withdrawal

- *Constructs related to inhibition, shyness, and anxiety*
  - inhibition
    —behavioral inhibition (BI)
    —behavioral inhibition system (BIS)
    —social inhibition

  - shyness
    —(low) approach
    —conflicted shyness
    —fearful shyness
    —self-conscious shyness
    —social fear
    —slow to warm up

  - anxiety
    —anxious withdrawal
    —anxious solitude
    —reticence
    —social anxiety
    —social avoidance
    —social phobia
    —social wariness

- *Constructs related to a preference for solitude*
  - introverted
  - solitary–passive
  - (low) sociability
  - social disinterest
  - (low) sociotropy
  - solitropy
  - unsociability

alone (in the presence of available play partners) because they are actively excluded, rejected, and/or isolated by their peers. There is a large and growing literature related to a wide range of factors that may lead to active isolation by peers, with perhaps the most attention paid to the display of non-normative, socially unskilled, and/or socially unacceptable behaviors (e.g., aggression, impulsivity, social immaturity) (see Rubin, Bukowski, et al., 2006, for a recent review). The second is "social withdrawal" (which was originally labeled as passive withdrawal), and refers to the child's removing him- or herself *from* the peer group (for whatever reason). In this regard, social withdrawal is viewed as emanating from factors internal to the child (Rubin & Asendorpf, 1993).

In more recent years, a potentially complex relation between these two processes has been delineated. It now seems clear that whereas some children may initially remove themselves from social interaction (i.e., socially withdraw), they also come to be excluded by peers. Indeed, the two processes likely become increasingly related through transactional influences over time (Rubin et al., 2009). We maintain that it is of important conceptual interest to distinguish between social withdrawal and active isolation. Notwithstanding, the joint and interactive contributions of both of these processes should be considered over time.

We have come to construe "social withdrawal" itself as an umbrella term to describe removing oneself from peer interaction for a variety of different "motivations" (Rubin & Coplan, 2004). As depicted in Figure 1.1, researchers have focused primarily on two broadly defined "reasons" why children may withdraw from social interaction. The first reason concerns aspects of emotional dysregulation specifically related to fear and anxiety, whereas the second reason relates to a nonfearful preference for solitary activities. This latter construct has only recently begun to receive attention.

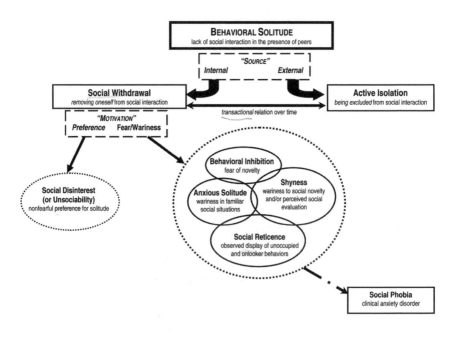

FIGURE 1.1. A taxonomy of solitude.

in the developmental literature; it has become increasingly apparent that some children engage in less social interaction because they are "socially disinterested" (or unsociable) and may simply prefer to play alone (Asendorpf, 1990; Coplan, Prakash, O'Neil, & Armer, 2004; Coplan, Girardi, Findlay, & Frohlick, 2007). Among adults, the preference for solitude has been referred to as a "solitropic orientation" (Leary, Herbst, & McCrary, 2003). However, the developmental implications of this construct are not well understood (for a detailed discussion of this construct, see Coplan & Weeks, Chapter 4, this volume).

In contrast, considerable research attention has been paid to children who withdraw from social interaction because they are afraid or anxious. In this regard, several related constructs have emerged (see Table 1.1). From one perspective, Kagan, Fox, and colleagues (e.g., Fox, Henderson, Marshall, Nichols, & Ghera, 2005; Kagan et al., 1984; Kagan, Snidman, Kahn, & Towsley, 2007) have used the term "behavioral inhibition" (*BI*) to describe biologically based wariness during exposure to novel people, things, and places. In later work, Rubin and colleagues (e.g., Rubin, Hastings, Stewart, Henderson, & Chen, 1997) focused more specifically on "social inhibition," which they referred to as *BI* in the company of unfamiliar *peers*.

From a somewhat different perspective, "shyness" has been conceptualized as (temperamental) wariness in the face of social novelty and/or self-conscious behavior in situations of perceived social evaluation (Asendorpf, 1991; Cheek & Buss, 1981; Crozier, 1995; Zimbardo, 1977). It has been suggested that shyness arises from an "approach–avoidance" conflict (e.g., Asenforpf, 1990), sometimes also referred to as conflicted shyness (e.g., Coplan et al., 2004), whereby a child's desire to interact socially with peers (i.e., a social approach motivation) is at odds with a simultaneous desire to avoid social contact (i.e., a social avoidance motivation) because of social fear and anxiety.

Relatedly, "social reticence" represents a behavioral construct that comprises the frequently observed display of onlooking (i.e., watching of others but not joining in) and remaining unoccupied in social company (Coplan et al., 1994). These behaviors appear to be a marker for social fear and anxiety in the presence of both unfamiliar and familiar peers (Coplan & Arbeau, 2008). Similarly, the term "anxious solitude" has been used to denote social wariness displayed specifically in familiar peer contexts (e.g., Gazelle & Ladd, 2003; Gazelle & Rudolph, 2004).

Finally, there is a conceptual similarity between these constructs (prevalent in the developmental psychology literature) and the term "social phobia" (sometimes also labeled "social anxiety disorder"), a clinically diagnosed anxiety disorder characterized by "a marked and persistent fear of social or performance situations in which embarrassment may occur" (American Psychiatric Association, 1994, p. 411). Social phobia and extreme shyness (or BI) share many characteristics in childhood (Degnan & Fox, 2007; Rapee & Coplan, in press). Indeed, Rapee, Kennedy, Ingram, Edwards, and Sweeney (2005) have reported that 90% of "extremely shy" preschool-age children meet criteria for an anxiety disorder. As well, empirical links between BI in early childhood and the later development of anxiety disorders (particularly social phobia) continue to emerge (e.g., Biederman et al., 2001; Schwartz, Snidman, & Kagan, 1999). There also remains a continued debate as to whether social phobia may actually represent an extreme form of shyness in children and adults (e.g., Chavira, Stein, & Malcarne, 2002; Rapee & Coplan, in press).

All of these terms describe various iterations of the process of withdrawal from social interactions because of underlying fear, anxiety, and social wariness. Is it possible to reconcile these somewhat different (but clearly overlapping) constructs? One approach is to integrate these constructs within a developmental perspective. In this regard, we present a version of this model, albeit simplified, herein.

Approximately 15% of infants come into the world with an inherent biologically based predisposition to respond with wariness and distress in the face of novelty (i.e., BI). In early childhood these wary responses become particularly pronounced in the context of meeting new people (i.e., "fearful shyness"). With the further development of the self-system and perspective-taking skills, this social wariness extends to include feelings of embarrassment and concern in the face of perceived social evaluation (i.e., "self-conscious shyness"). As such, and with the onset of formal schooling (and its increasing social stresses), many shy children continue to feel socially ill at ease even after the school environment becomes more familiar. As a result, these children withdraw from social interactions and display overt signs of anxiety with peers at school (i.e., "social reticence" or "anxious solitude"). For a smaller proportion of these children (perhaps at the most extreme end of the distribution), these feelings of anxiety continue to escalate over time and become a debilitating psychological disorder (i.e., "social phobia") in later childhood or early adolescence.

From a theoretical perspective, we certainly acknowledge that it may be conceptually useful to offer "fine-grained" distinctions among these different terms. However, it is also important to assess the practical utility of distinguishing between behavioral inhibition, shyness, and anxious solitude. For example, in a sample of preschool-age children, consider the implications of empirically identifying "extreme groups" of inhibited, fearfully shy, self-consciously shy, and anxious solitary children. Employing this person-oriented approach, would we not expect a significant amount of overlap in the membership of these various groups? Indeed, we find it difficult to envision many instances where these extreme groups would *not* coalesce. If this is the case, does the field require the use of these different terms? In this regard, it is also important to consider issues related to the differential *assessment* of these different constructs.

MEASURES AND ASSESSMENT ISSUES

Accompanying the plethora of constructs and terms related to social withdrawal is a wide range of assessments and methodological approaches. These measures include behavioral observations, parent and teacher ratings, and peer and self-reports. Indeed, many of the terms defined in the taxonomy of social withdrawal and related constructs are supported by their own associated measures.

One set of measures comprises the general assessments of broadly defined constructs related to social withdrawal. For example, in the Revised Class Play (RCP; Masten, Morison, & Pellegrini, 1985), a widely used peer rating procedure, children nominate peers who fit various behavioral descriptors. The sensitivity/isolation factor has been used to identify children who do not frequently interact with peers, and includes items related to both shyness/withdrawal (e.g., "someone who is shy," "someone whose feelings get hurt easily") and social isolation/exclusion (e.g., "a person who is often left out," "a person who can't get others to listen"). Subsequently, researchers have suggested dropping items related to active isolation from this factor (e.g., Rubin & Mills, 1988) in order to provide a "purer" assessment of social withdrawal. Most recently, Rubin, Wojslawowicz, Rose-Krasnor, Booth-LaForce, and Burgess (2006) added items to this measure to create an Extended Class Play, which was designed to further distinguish between peer rejection/isolation/victimization (e.g., "someone who is hit or kicked by others") and shyness/social withdrawal (e.g., "someone who gets nervous about participating in class discussions").

Behavioral observations have also been employed (e.g., the *Play Observation Scale*; Rubin, 2001) to assess different forms of solitude in the presence of both unfamiliar peers in the laboratory playroom (Coplan et al., 1994; Rubin, Coplan, Fox, & Calkins, 1995) as well as familiar classmates at school (Coplan et al., 2008; Rubin, 1982). Behavioral observations have the advantage of "face validity" in terms of the broad-based assessment of behavioral solitude. There is also some evidence to suggest that subtypes of nonsocial play may be marker variables for different forms of social withdrawal. For example, displaying "onlooking" behaviors (e.g., watching others but not joining in) and remaining unoccupied in the presence of peers (labeled "reticent" behavior) appear to be indicative of social fear and anxiety (e.g., Coplan et al., 1994, 2004; Coplan et al., 2008). In contrast, the frequent display of solitary-functional (e.g., sensorimotor) and solitary–dramatic (e.g., playing make-believe by oneself) behaviors in the presence of peers (labeled "solitary–active" behaviors) has been linked to social immaturity, impulsivity, and externalizing problems (e.g., Coplan, Wichmann, & Lagacé-Séguin, 2001; Rubin, 1982; Rubin & Mills, 1988). This form of nonsocial play appears to be more closely linked with the construct of active isolation.

Finally, the frequent display of solitary–constructive and solitary–explorative activities (labeled "solitary–passive" behavior) was originally thought to represent a comparatively benign form of nonsocial play linked to the construct of unsociability (Coplan et al., 1994; Rubin, 1982; Rubin & Asendorpf, 1993). However, results from more recent studies have called these assumptions into question (e.g., Coplan et al., 2004; Harrist, Zaia, Bates, Dodge, & Pettit, 1997; Spangler & Gazelle, in press; Spinrad et al., 2004).

Numerous other measures have been developed to specifically assess the various terms and constructs previously described. For example, BI is typically assessed in an observational paradigm developed by Kagan and colleagues (1988); toddlers and preschoolers are presented with a series of novel events (including adult strangers). Inhibition is indicated by measures such as latency to approach the adult stranger, latency to offer the first spontaneous utterance, and proximity to mother.

Shyness in childhood is typically assessed with parent ratings of younger children (e.g., Colorado Child Temperament Inventory, Rowe & Plomin, 1977; Child Social Preference Scale, Coplan et al., 2004) and self-reports for older children and adolescents (e.g., Revised Cheek–Buss Shyness Scale, Cheek & Buss, 1981; Children's Shyness Questionnaire, Crozier, 1995). Finally, Gazelle and colleagues (e.g., Gazelle & Ladd, 2003) employ teacher ratings to assess children's anxious solitude at school (Child Behavior Scale, Ladd & Profilet, 1996).

There is moderate agreement between sources of assessment with regards to measures of BI, shyness, and social withdrawal (Bishop et al., 2003; Coplan et al., 2008; Spangler & Gazelle, 2009; Ladd & Profilet, 1996). However, the *discriminant* validity of these measures remains unclear; that is, whether these different assessments would provide an *empirical* distinction between some of these constructs (e.g., inhibition vs. shyness vs. anxious solitude) is a largely unanswered question. Studies assessing several of these constructs with several of these measures in the sample are required to address these issues. Ultimately, the outcome of these future studies will determine the degree to which it is "useful" to make the conceptually driven distinctions we have just described.

OVERVIEW OF THE CURRENT VOLUME

The chapters in this volume provide the reader with an excellent review of the "state of the art" in the study of shyness and social withdrawal. As delineated in this introductory chapter, the study of shyness and social withdrawal has involved multiple and complex theoretical approaches and conceptual distinctions. Indeed, the expression of behavioral solitude appears to be a multidimensional phenomenon, involving different motivational, emotional, personal, and interpersonal processes. Moreover, different types of solitary endeavors have different meanings and are associated with decidedly different outcomes.

Accordingly, Part II of this volume includes several chapters that more closely consider conceptual distinctions and theoretical approaches in the study of social withdrawal. Two of these chapters focus on the development of different types of *shyness*. Schmidt and Buss (Chapter 2) provide a historical and conceptual overview of the study of shyness. They consider key research questions regarding how shyness is conceptualized and distinguished from other, related constructs. Crozier (Chapter 3) focuses more specifically on the development of self-consciousness and embarrassment, and how these emotions are related (and distinct) from shyness. From a different perspective, Coplan and Weeks (Chapter 4) consider the construct of "unsociability," distinguishing nonfearful preference for solitude from shyness and exploring the implications of this form of social withdrawal in childhood, adolescence, and adulthood.

As well, it has now become clear that there are substantial biological and physiological underpinnings of social withdrawal. Toddlers and preschoolers who express fear when in the company of unfamiliar adults and children differ from their uninhibited counterparts in ways that imply variability in the threshold of excitability of the amygdala and its projections to the cortex, hypothalamus, sympathetic nervous system, corpus striatum, and central gray. In their chapter, Fox and Reeb-Sutherland (Chapter 5) describe the most recent links established between biology, temperamental inhibition, and social withdrawal.

Despite increasing evidence of biological contributions to the development of shyness and social withdrawal, it is also clear that interpersonal processes play a critical role. Part III of this book includes chapters that explore the importance of interactions, relationships, and groups in the study of social withdrawal. To begin with, there is a growing literature indicating that parents exert considerable influence of the developmental pathways of socially withdrawn children. In their chapter, Hastings, Nuselovici, Rubin, and Cheah (Chapter 6) describe the latest findings on the topic of parenting and social withdrawal, including a discussion of parent–child attachment, parenting beliefs, parenting behaviors, and broader parenting styles. Shy and socially withdrawn children also tend to experience considerable social difficulty among their friends and in the larger peer group (including exclusion, rejection, and victimization). In their chapter, Rubin, Bowker, and Gazelle (Chapter 7) discuss the various peer relationship domains within which socially withdrawn children find themselves. To complete this section, Asendorpf (Chapter 8) considers how interpersonal processes (including romantic relationships) impact the long-term adulthood implications of childhood shyness.

With the increased amount of recent research in this area, additional consideration has been paid to how social withdrawal might be differently manifested and expressed across different domains and environments. Part IV of this volume comprises chapters devoted to the exploration of the meanings and implications of shyness and social withdrawal in some newly considered contexts. For example, previous research has focused primarily on the social and emotional correlates of shyness and social withdrawal in childhood. In her chapter, Evans (Chapter 9) reviews the links between shyness, language, and academic functioning, with a particular focus on the role of shyness in school contexts. Recent years have also witnessed a large increase in the studies of shyness and withdrawal outside of Western cultures. Put simply, shyness appears to have quite different meanings and implications in different places around the world. Chen (Chapter 10) reviews the extant cross-cultural research.

Fifteen years ago, researchers would not have considered the Internet as a "context" for children's social and emotional development. However, the explosion of new technologies related to electronic communications have made online interactions common place, even for younger children. In their chapter, Schneider and Amichai-Hamburger (Chapter 11) consider the nature and implications of shyness "online." However, notwithstanding the seemingly limitless availability of Web-based information, many parents still turn to more traditional forms of media when interacting with their young children. In this regard, Coplan, Hughes, and Rowsell (Chapter 12) close this section by examining how shy characters are depicted and portrayed in young children's storybooks.

In Part V of this book, the most recent clinical perspectives on shyness and social anxiety are considered. Most developmental models of anxiety now include a focus on temperamental contributions. In Chapter 13, Rapee reviews the role of temperamental traits (including BI and negative emotionality) in the etiology of social phobia. Despite the increasing evidence linking social withdrawal to contemporaneous and longitudinal socioemotional difficulties, research related to intervention and prevention appears to have *declined* during this same time period. There has been some increased attention to the treatment of social anxiety and social phobia with older children and adolescents, but much less so with younger children. In the final chapter, Mychailyszyn, Cohen, Edmunds, Crawley, and Kendall (Chapter 14) describe recent innovations in the treatment of social anxiety in children and youth.

CONCLUSIONS

In their 1993 book, Rubin and Asendorpf began by describing the contents of two unsolicited letters that were received after an interview with author Rubin was reprinted in the news media. The first letter was from a concerned mother of a young socially withdrawn child and highlighted some of the ongoing research issues involved in the psychological study of this phenomenon, including questions about biological disposition ("I feel that my daughter was born this way"), parenting ("I gave up my career to do special things with her and we oftentimes clash"), extrafamilial relationships ("She would oftentimes say things like 'Susie isn't nice to me!'"), and longer-term implications ("We have real need to help our daughter, because I feel it will get much worse for her when she's in school").

In the second letter, a shy adult wrote to express his gratitude that research was now beginning to be done in this area. He lamented the previous lack of attention that he perceived was paid to difficulties experienced by socially withdrawn children ("I wish, oh how I wish, something had been done about my isolation at the tender age of 7 or 8. ... It has been a long, lonely road") but concluded that he was "so very, very happy, that help is in store for the self-isolated child."

It is our hope that after reading this book, the authors of those earlier letters might feel comfort in the amount of progress made in addressing some of the unanswered questions about social withdrawal in childhood—and that there is indeed lots of "help in store for the self-isolated child." Notwithstanding, there is still much work to be done and many more questions to address—as evidenced by this excerpt from an unsolicited e-mail received by author Coplan just this last year:

> Hi. I read your article on the internet. I don't know if you usually get letters like this or not but I have never heard speak of helping shy children until now. I'm a parent of a five year old who is extremely shy. He is exactly like me.
>
> I'm worried about him feeling the same pain and having the same problems I had as a child. I am about to graduate from university as a teacher and I plan to put into practice some of the ideas I read in your article. I'm concerned about my son though. He is about to start kindergarten and I'm afraid he going to end up with a negative attitude towards school. He went to daycare and started Pre-Kindergarten and then began refusing to go. When I arrived to pick him up everyday he was usually

playing by himself despite his constant attempts to play with the other children. I also believe the shy kid gets ignored because they are quiet and don't usually misbehave. People that aren't shy don't usually view this behavior as a problem that's hurting the children. He is currently staying at home with me, I try constantly to find playmates by going to the park or Sunday school but nothing seems to work. I was wondering if you had any suggestions on how to help him find friends to play with, help him adjust in kindergarten, and help his teacher be active in getting involved with the other kids.

Thanks for reading this. I hope to hear from you. Also if you have any suggestions for me as a teacher let me know. Thanks.

REFERENCES

Achenbach, T. M., & Edelbrock, C. (1981). Behavioral problems and competencies reported by parents of normal and disturbed children aged 4–16. *Monographs of the Society for Research in Child Development, 46* (Serial No. 1887), 88.

American Psychiatric Association. (1994). *Diagnostic and statistical manual of mental disorders* (4th ed.). Washington, DC: Author.

Asendorpf, J. (1990). Beyond social withdrawal: Shyness, unsociability and peer avoidance. *Human Development, 33,* 250–259.

Asendorpf, J. B. (1991). Development of inhibited children's coping with unfamiliarity. *Child Development, 62,* 1460–1474.

Bell-Dolan, D. J., Reaven, N., & Peterson, L. (1993). Child depression and social functioning: A multidimensional study of the linkages. *Journal of Clinical Child Psychology, 22,* 306–315.

Biederman, J., Rosenbaum, J. F., Hirshfeld, D. R., Faraone, S. V., Bolduc, E. A., Gersten, M., et al. (1990). Psychiatric correlates of behavioral inhibition in young children of parents with and without psychiatric disorders. *Archives of General Psychiatry, 47,* 21–26.

Biederman, J., Hirshfeld-Becker, D. R., Rosenbaum, J. F., Herot, C., Friedman, D., Snidman, N., et al. (2001). Further evidence of association between behavioral inhibition and social anxiety in children. *American Journal of Psychiatry, 158,* 1673–1679.

Biederman, J., Rosenbaum, J. F., Bolduc-Murphy, E. A., Faraone, S. V., Chaloff, J., Hirshfeld, D. R., et al. (1993). A 3-year follow-up of children with and without behavioral inhibition. *Journal of the American Academy of Child and Adolescent Psychiatry, 32,* 814–821.

Bott, H. (1928). Observation of play activities of three-year-old children. *Genetic Psychology Monographs, 4,* 44–88.

Chavira, D. A., Stein, M. B., & Malcarne, V. L. (2002). Scrutinizing the relationship between shyness and social phobia. *Journal of Anxiety Disorders, 16,* 585–598.

Cheek, J. M., & Buss, A. H. (1981). Shyness and sociability. *Journal of Personality and Social Psychology, 41,* 330–339.

Cooley, C. H. (1902). *Human nature and the social order.* New York: Scribner.

Coplan, R. J., & Arbeau, K. A. (2008). The stresses of a brave new world: Shyness and adjustment in kindergarten. *Journal of Research in Childhood Education, 22,* 377–389.

Coplan, R. J., Arbeau, K. A., & Armer, M. (2008). Don't fret, be supportive: Maternal characteristics linking child shyness to psychosocial and school adjustment in kindergarten. *Journal of Abnormal Child Psychology, 36,* 359–371.

Coplan, R. J., Girardi, A., Findlay, L. C., & Frohlick, S. L. (2007). Understanding solitude: Young children's attitudes and responses towards hypothetical socially-withdrawn peers. *Social Development, 16,* 390–409.

Coplan, R. J., Prakash, K., O'Neil, K., & Armer, M. (2004). Do you "want " to play?: Distinguishing between conflicted-shyness and social disinterest in early childhood. *Developmental Psychology, 40,* 244–258.

Coplan, R. J., Rubin, K. H., Fox, N. A., Calkins, S. D., & Stewart, S. (1994). Being alone, playing alone, and acting alone: Distinguishing among reticence and passive and active solitude in young children. *Child Development, 65,* 129–137.

Coplan, R. J., Wichmann, C., & Lagacé-Séguin, D. (2001). Solitary–active play: A marker variable for maladjustment in the preschool? *Journal of Research in Childhood Education, 15,* 164–172.

Craig, M. (1922). Some aspects of education and training in relation to mental disorder. *Journal of Mental Science, 68,* 209–228.

Crozier, W. R. (1995). Shyness and self-esteem in middle childhood. *British Journal of Educational Psychology, 65,* 85–95.

Dealy, C. E. (1923). Problem children in the early school grades. *Journal of Abnormal Psychology and Social Psychology, 18,* 125–136.

Degnan, K. A., & Fox, N. A. (2007). Behavioral inhibition and anxiety disorders: Multiple levels of a resilience process. *Development and Psychopathology, 19,* 729–746.

Fox, N. A., Henderson, H. A., Marshall P. J., Nichols, K. E., & Ghera, M. M. (2005). Behavioral inhibition: Linking biology and behavior within a developmental framework. *Annual Review of Psychology, 56,* 235–262.

Garcia-Coll, C., Kagan, J., & Reznick, J. S. (1984). Behavioral inhibition in young children. *Child Development, 55,* 1005–1019.

Gazelle, H., & Ladd, G. W. (2003). Anxious solitude and peer exclusion: A diathesis–stress model of internalizing trajectories in childhood. *Child Development, 74,* 257–278.

Gazelle, H., & Rudolph, K. D. (2004). Moving toward and away from the world: Social approach and avoidance trajectories in anxious solitary youth. *Child Development, 75,* 829–849.

Harrist, A. W., Zaia, A. F., Bates, J. E., Dodge, K. A., & Pettit, G. S. (1997). Subtypes of social withdrawal in early childhood: Sociometric status and social-cognitive differences across four years. *Child Development, 68,* 278–294.

Hirshfeld, D. R., Rosenbaum, J. F., Biederman, J., Bolduc, E. A., Faraone, S. V., Snidman, N., et al. (1992). Stable behavioral inhibition and its association with anxiety disorder. *Journal of the American Academy of Child and Adolescent Psychiatry, 31,* 103–111.

Kagan, J., Reznick, J. S., Clarke, C., Snidman, N., & Garcia-Coll, C. (1984). Behavioral inhibition to the unfamiliar. *Child Development, 55,* 2212–2225.

Kagan, J., Reznick, J. S., & Snidman, N. (1988). Biological bases of childhood shyness. *Science, 240,* 167–171.

Kagan, J., Snidman, N., Kahn, V., & Towsley, S. (2007). The preservation of two infant temperaments into adolescence. *Monographs of the Society for Research in Child Development, 72* (Serial No. 287), 6–80.

Kohlberg, L., LaCrosse, J., & Ricks, D. (1972). The predictability of adult mental health from childhood behavior. In B. B. Wolman (Ed.), *Manual of child psychopathology* (pp. 1217–1284). New York: McGraw-Hill.

Ladd, G. W., & Profilet, S. M. (1996). The Child Behavior Scale: A teacher report measure of young children's aggressive, withdrawn, and prosocial behaviors. *Developmental Psychology, 32,* 1008–1024.

Leary, M. R., Herbst, K. C., & McCrary, F. (2003). Finding pleasure in solitary activities: Desire for aloneness or disinterest in social contact? *Personality and Individual Differences, 35,* 59–68.

Lehman, H. C. (1926). The play activities of persons of different ages, and growth stages in play behavior. *Pedagogical Seminary, 33,* 250–272.

Lehman, H. C., & Anderson, T. H. (1928). Social participation vs. solitariness in play. *Pedagogical Seminary, 34,* 279–289.

Lewis, M., & Miller, S. M. (1990). *Handbook of developmental psychopathology.* New York: Plenum Press.

Lowenstein, P., & Svendsen, M. (1938). Experimental modification of the behavior of a selected group of shy and withdrawn children. *American Journal of Orthopsychiatry, 8,* 639–654.

Masten, A. S., Morison, P., & Pellegrini, D. S. (1985). A Revised Class Play method of peer assessment. *Developmental Psychology, 3,* 523–533.

Mead, G. H. (1934). *Mind, self, and society.* Chicago: University of Chicago Press.

Morris, D. P., Soroker, E., & Burruss, G. (1954). Follow-up studies of shy, withdrawn children: I. Evaluation of later adjustment. *American Journal of Orthopsychiatry, 24,* 743–754.

Mullins, L. L., Peterson, L., Wonderlich, S. A., & Reaven, N. M. (1986). The influence of depressive symptomatology in children on the social responses and perceptions of adults. *Journal of Child Clinical Psychology, 15,* 233–240.

Parten, M. B. (1932). Social participation among preschool children. *Journal of Abnormal Psychology, 27,* 243–269.

Piaget, J. (1926). *The language and thought of the child.* London: Routlege & Kegan Paul.

Rapee, R., & Coplan, R. J. (in press). Conceptual relations between behavioral inhibition and anxiety disorders in preschool children. *New Directions in Child Development.*

Rapee, R., Kennedy, S., Ingram, M., Edwards, S., & Sweeney, L. (2005). Prevention and early intervention of anxiety disorders in inhibited preschool children. *Journal of Consulting and Clinical Psychology, 73,* 488–497.

Reznick, J. S., Kagan, J., Snidman, N., Gersten, M., Baak, K., & Rosenberg, A. (1986). Inhibited and uninhibited children: A follow-up study. *Child Development, 57,* 660–680.

Robins, L. N. (1966). *Deviant children grown up*. Baltimore: Williams & Wilkins.

Rosenbaum, J. F., Biederman, J., Gersten, M., Hirshfeld, D. R., Meminger, S. R., Herman, J. B., et al. (1988). Behavioral inhibition in children of parents with panic disorder and agoraphobia: A controlled study. *Archives of General Psychiatry, 45,* 463–470.

Rosenbaum, J. F., Biederman, J., Hirshfeld, D. R., Bolduc, E. A., & Chaloff, J. (1991). Behavioral inhibition in children: A possible precursor to panic disorder or social phobia. *Journal of Clinical Psychiatry, 52,* 5–9.

Rowe, D. C., & Plomin, R. (1977). Temperament in early childhood. *Journal of Personality Assessment, 41,* 150–156.

Rubin, K. H. (1982). Non-social play in preschoolers: Necessary evil? *Child Development, 53,* 651–657.

Rubin, K. H. (1985). Socially withdrawn children: An "at risk" population? In B. Schneider, K. H. Rubin, & J. Ledingham (Eds.), *Children's peer relations: Issues in assessment and intervention* (pp. 125–139). New York: Springer-Verlag.

Rubin, K. H. (2001). *The Play Observation Scale (POS)*. Waterloo, Canada: University of Waterloo.

Rubin, K. H., & Asendorpf, J. B. (1993). Social withdrawal, inhibition, and shyness in childhood: Conceptual and definitional issues. *Social withdrawal, inhibition, and shyness in childhood* (pp. 3–17). Hillsdale, NJ: Erlbaum.

Rubin, K. H., & Both, L. (1989). Iris pigmentation and sociability in childhood: A re-examination. *Developmental Psychology, 22,* 717–726.

Rubin, K. H., Bukowski, W. M., & Parker, J. G. (2006). Peer interactions, relationships and groups. In N. Eisenberg (Ed.), *The handbook of child psychology* (6th ed., pp. 571–645). New York: Wiley.

Rubin, K. H., Chen, X., & Hymel, S. (1993). Socioemotional characteristics of withdrawn and aggressive children. *Merrill–Palmer Quarterly, 39,* 518–534.

Rubin, K. H., & Coplan, R. J. (2004). Paying attention to and not neglecting social withdrawal and social isolation. *Merrill–Palmer Quarterly, 50,* 506–534.

Rubin, K. H., Coplan, R. J., & Bowker, J. (2009). Social withdrawal in childhood. *Annual Review of Psychology, 60,* 11.1–11.31.

Rubin, K. H., Coplan, R. J., Fox, N. A., & Calkins, S. D. (1995). Emotionality, emotion regulation, and preschoolers' social adaptation. *Development and Psychopathology, 7,* 49–62.

Rubin, K. H., Hastings, P. D., Stewart, S. L., Henderson, H. A., & Chen, X. (1997). The consistency and concomitants of inhibition: Some of the children, all of the time. *Child Development, 68,* 467– 483.

Rubin, K. H., Hymel, S., & Mills, R. S. L. (1989). Sociability and social withdrawal in childhood: Stability and outcomes. *Journal of Personality, 57,* 238–255.

Rubin, K. H., & Mills, R. S. L. 1988. The many faces of social isolation in childhood. *Journal of Consulting and Clinical Psychology, 56,*(6), 916–924.

Rubin K. H., Wojslawowicz, J. C., Rose-Krasnor, L., Booth-LaForce, C. L., & Burgess, K. B. (2006). The best friendships of shy/withdrawn children: Prevalence, stability, and relationship quality. *Journal of Abnormal Child Psychology, 34,* 139–153.

Schwartz, C. E., Snidman, N., & Kagan, J. (1999). Adolescent social anxiety as an outcome of inhibited temperament in childhood. *Journal of the American Academy of Child and Adolescent Psychiatry, 38,* 1008–1015.

Spangler, T., & Gazelle, H. (2009). Anxious solitude, unsociability, and peer exclusion in middle childhood: A multitrait–multimethod matrix. *Social Development, 18,* 833–856.

Spinrad, T. L., Eisenberg, N., Harris, E., Hanish, L., Fabes, R. A., Kupanoff, K., et al. (2004). The relation of children's everyday nonsocial peer play behavior to their emotionality, regulation, and social functioning. *Developmental Psychology, 40,* 67–80.

Sullivan, H. S. (1953). *The interpersonal theory of psychiatry.* New York: Norton.

Verry, E. E. (1923). *A study of mental and social attitudes in the free play of preschool children.* Thesis for Master's degree, State University of Iowa, Iowa City.

Zimbardo, P. G. (1977). *Shyness: What is it and what to do about it.* New York: Symphony Press.

PART II

CONSTRUCTS AND CONCEPTUAL APPROACHES

2

Understanding Shyness
Four Questions and
Four Decades of Research

LOUIS A. SCHMIDT
ARNOLD H. BUSS

Although the study of shyness has a long and rich history (for reviews see Carducci, 1999; Hampton, 1927; Jones, Briggs, & Smith, 1986; Jones, Cheek, & Briggs, 1986; Lewinsky, 1941; Rubin & Asendorpf, 1993a; Schmidt & Schulkin, 1999; Zimbardo, 1977), there has been a burgeoning interest in the phenomenon over the last four decades, as evidenced by the many chapters in this volume. Much of the contemporary work on shyness was spawned by a shift in the *Zeitgeist* in how mainstream psychology viewed behavior that ultimately trickled down to the field of socioemotional development; that is, there was a movement away from traditional learning (Skinner, 1938) and attachment (Bowlby, 1969) models positing the importance of environmental influences, which dominated much of the early views on socioemotional development prior to, and immediately following, World War II, toward the idea that characteristics within the individual, such as temperament, play a critical role in shaping behavior. Temperament perspectives then set the stage for the contemporary study of shyness over the next several decades, as embodied in the work of two psychologists: Arnold Buss (1980, 1984, 1986; Buss & Plomin, 1975, 1984) and Jerome Kagan (1994, 1999; Kagan, Reznick, Clarke, Snidman, & Garcia-Coll, 1984; Kagan, Reznick, & Snidman, 1987, 1988), and their respective colleagues. Today, issues of whether one school of thought within developmental psychology and its respective research questions help to explain more of the variance in understanding childhood shyness has become moot. Theoretical and methodological advances in the field of neuroscience have shed new light on human ontogeny and silenced the divisions within many facets of psychology. The discipline of developmental psychology has benefited from the knowledge established in its neighboring fields to understand the complex origins of human shyness. For example, we now know that the brain is not fixed after preschool, that gene expression is plastic, and environmental influences on gene expression and biological systems play a critical role in shaping brain development. Accordingly, how shyness develops is largely embodied in an interactionist perspective involving genes, biology, and environmental interactions (Fox et al., 2005; Schmidt, Polak, & Spooner, 2005).

Human shyness is a ubiquitous phenomenon that over 90% of the population have reported experiencing at some point in their lives (Zimbardo, 1977). Shyness is thought to reflect a preoccupation of the self during real or imagined social situations (Cheek et al., 1986) and is accompanied by feelings of negative self-worth (Crozier, 1981). Some have argued that shyness reflects an emotion elicited by feelings of shame and embarrassment that lead to social inhibition (e.g., Crozier, 1999), whereas others have viewed shyness from a trait perspective, with shyness serving as a dimension of personality (e.g., Cheek & Krasnoperova, 1999; Crozier, 1979) linked to temperamental and biological origins (Buss & Plomin, 1984; Kagan, 1994). There are, in addition, a number of measurable correlates of shyness: behavioral (e.g., reduction in speech, gaze aversion; Pilkonis, 1977a, 1977b), cognitive/affective (e.g., low self-esteem, anxious thoughts; Ashbaugh, Antony, McCabe, Schmidt, & Swinson, 2005; Brunet & Schmidt, 2007, 2008; Crozier, 1981; Schmidt & Fox, 1995), and psychophysiological (e.g., right frontal electroencephalographic (EEG) asymmetry, high heart rate, high salivary cortisol levels; Addison & Schmidt, 1999; Beaton et al., 2006; Beaton, Schmidt, Ashbaugh, et al., 2008; Fox et al., 1995; Fox, Henderson, Rubin, Calkins, & Schmidt, 2001; Schmidt, 1999; Schmidt & Fox, 1994; Schmidt et al., 1997; Schmidt, Fox, Schulkin, & Gold, 1999; Schmidt, Santesso, Schulkin, & Segalowitz, 2007; Theall-Honey & Schmidt, 2006). These multiple correlates are evidenced in children and adults who are shy (see Schmidt & Schulkin, 1999, for a review). Early childhood shyness is also a known risk factor for later behavioral problems from middle childhood to adolescence (Oh, Rubin, Bowker, Booth-LaForce, Rose-Krasnor, & Laursen, 2008; Rubin, 1993; Rubin, Burgess, Kennedy, & Stewart, 2003; Rubin, Hymel, Mills, & Rose-Krasnor, 1991) and through to emerging adulthood (Beidel & Turner, 1998; Caspi, Elder, & Bem, 1988).

Although there has been considerable work devoted to the study of human shyness, and many advances due to revolutions in neuroscience that have helped us to understand shyness, since the publication of the initial volume 15 years ago (Rubin & Asendorpf, 1993a), several conceptual issues related to shyness have yet to be adequately resolved. Shyness is, for example, a construct that has been used interchangeably in studies of children and adults, with numerous terms including, but not limited to, the following: "behavioral inhibition," "social inhibition," "social wariness," "social reticence," "social withdrawal," "social anxiety," "social phobia," "timidity," "introversion," and "low sociability." The lack of conceptual clarity and the language that we use to understand shyness continues to limit scientific inquiry.

Our purpose in this chapter is to address four basic questions related to the conceptualization of shyness that continue to concern researchers, and to review empirical studies related to these four questions, conducted primarily over the last four decades. They are as follows:

1. Is shyness nothing more than low sociability?
2. Is there a distinction between shyness and behavioral inhibition?
3. Is anxious shyness different from self-conscious shyness?
4. Is shyness continuous with social phobia?

The chapter is divided among four major sections that address each of the basic questions. We conclude with some additional questions and suggestions for future research in the area.

IS SHYNESS NOTHING MORE THAN LOW SOCIABILITY?

At one time, no one asked this question, probably because the concept of introversion dominated our thinking. Introverts tend to be reticent with strangers and casual acquaintances, probably for two reasons: They prefer their own company to that of others (low sociability), and at least some of them are tense and inhibited when with others (shyness). The link between shyness and (low) sociability was assumed without question, so that, for example, on the Sociability scale of the EASI (Emotionality, Activity, Sociability, and Impulsivity) Temperament Survey (Buss & Plomin, 1975), the following item was included: "I tend to be shy." However, several years later, we questioned whether shyness was equivalent to low sociability, which meant devising separate measures of them (Cheek & Buss, 1981). Items were written separately for inhibition, tension, and awkwardness when with people (shyness) and the motivation to be with people (sociability).

Cheek and Buss (1981) administered the questionnaires to 947 college students, and a factor analysis yielded the two factors (i.e., shyness and sociability). The correlation between the shyness and sociability scales was

–.30 in the original study. A later study yielded a slightly higher correlation, –.35 (Perry & Buss, 1990). Cheek (1983) added four items to the Shyness scale. This revised Shyness scale correlated still higher with sociability: –.43 (Jones, Briggs, et al., 1986), –.47 (Bruch, Gorsky, Collins & Berger, 1989), and –.49 (Schmidt & Fox, 1994). More recently, Coplan, Prakash, O'Neil, and Mandana (2004) reported a correlation of .29 between child shyness and unsociability (as rated by parents) in a sample of 246 preschoolers, similar to the original study by Cheek and Buss (1981).

There is no obvious explanation why adding several items to the Shyness scale increases its relation with sociability. Even if we accept the higher correlations, however, it is clear that though shyness and (low) sociability are related, they are distinguishable. This conclusion was strengthened by several lines of research.

First, the shyness and sociability questionnaires were correlated with questionnaires tapping several other personality traits (Perry & Buss, 1990). Shyness correlated strongly and positively with fear, and emotional loneliness (missing a close relationship), and negatively with self-esteem and optimism. Sociability correlated moderately and negatively with social loneliness and positively with self-esteem, weakly with optimism, and not at all with fear. This pattern of correlations was another reason for distinguishing between shyness and sociability.

Second, other researchers constructed a questionnaire comprised solely of items tapping low sociability, for example, "It's not important to me that I spend a lot of time with other people" and "I usually prefer to do things alone" (Eisenberg, Fabes, & Murphy, 1995), and found evidence for the independence of shyness and sociability. The Low Sociability scale correlated only .13 with a questionnaire on shyness, which itself correlated .65 with the Cheek and Buss (1981) Shyness Questionnaire. Thus, there are other self-report questionnaires that yield findings on the orthogonality of shyness and sociability.

Third, still other studies noted distinct biological and behavioral correlates of shyness and sociability, suggesting that the two constructs are distinguishable across different levels of analysis. For example, using a design identical to that reported by Cheek and Buss (1981), Schmidt and his colleagues found that shyness and sociability were distinguishable across multiple biological and behavioral measures. For example, Beaton, Schmidt, Schulkin, et al. (2008) recently noted that shy adults exhibit greater bilateral activation in the amygdala (a brain region involved in fear modulation) in response to the presentation of unfamiliar neutral faces using functional magnetic resonance imaging (fMRI), whereas sociable adults display greater bilateral activation in the nucleus accumbens (a brain area involved in reward) in response to the presentation of the same facial stimuli using fMRI measures. Schmidt (1999) earlier found that although high-shy/high-sociable (i.e., the "conflicted" subtype) and high-shy/low-sociable (i.e., the "avoidant" subtype) undergraduates both exhibited a pattern of greater relative right frontal EEG activity at rest, which is a marker of fear dysregulation (Davidson, 2000), the two subtypes were, however, distinguishable based upon only the pattern of activity in the left, but not the right, frontal area. High-shy/high-sociable (i.e., the "conflicted" subtype) participants exhibited significantly greater activity in the left frontal EEG site than high-shy/low-sociable (i.e., the "avoidant" subtype) participants. Still earlier, it was noted that high-shy/high-sociable (i.e., the "conflicted" subtype) undergraduates exhibited a significantly faster and more stable heart rate compared with high-shy/low-sociable (i.e., the "avoidant" subtype) participants in response to an anticipated unfamiliar social situation (Schmidt & Fox, 1994).

A similar conceptualization of shy subtypes was articulated earlier by Asendorpf (1990), who argued that high and low social approach and social avoidance lead to different combinations of social behavior. For example, individuals who score high on social approach and social avoidance are described by Asendorpf as shy [Schmidt's (1999) "conflicted" group]; those who score low on social approach and high on social avoidance are described as avoidant; those who score low on social approach and low on social avoidance are introverts; and those who score high on social approach and low on social avoidance are sociable. And Eisenberg et al. (1995) reported that shyness was associated with high physiological reactivity, negative emotional intensity, dispositional negative affect, and personal distress, whereas sociability was not.

Additional studies have reported that shyness and sociability are distinguishable on a behavioral level in children and adults. For example, Page (1990) argued that shyness and sociability are a "dangerous" combination for illicit drug use among adolescents. Page reported that adolescents who scored high on measures of shyness *and* sociability were more likely to use and abuse illicit substances compared with other adolescents who scored high and low on shyness and sociability, respectively. A similar finding between shyness and sociability, and substance use and abuse among U.S. and Canadian samples of undergraduates was recently reported (Santesso, Schmidt, & Fox, 2004). More recently, the Cheek and Buss model was used to understand adaptive functioning in young adults and eating behaviors in a nonclinical sample of shy and sociable young women (Miller, Schmidt, & Vaillancourt, 2008). Shy women were more likely to have lower self-esteem and more problems with disordered eating than were their sociable counterparts. Shy *and* social children are also presumed to be on a developmental trajectory to behavioral problems (see Schmidt, 2003), although more longitudinal empirical work with children needs to be conducted on the topic (for exceptions see Coplan et al., 2004; Schmidt & Fox, 1999).

Fourth, there are studies demonstrating the independence of shyness and sociability across different cultures in children (Asendorpf & Meier, 1993) and adults (Czeschlik & Nurk, 1995; Neto, 1996). In a study with German children (Asendorpf & Meier, 1993), parents were asked about their children's shyness (e.g., "Your child is shy with strangers") and sociability (e.g., "Your child prefers to play with other children rather than alone"). The shyness–sociability correlation was –.35. The children's social behavior was then observed. Compared to unsociable children, sociable children spent more time in group play with friends outside the home. Shy children spoke less than did unshy children in unfamiliar situations.

In a comparable study with American children, parents' ratings of their children's social inhibition were related to the children's wariness in the face of social novelty, whereas teachers' ratings were related to the quality of the children's interactions (Eisenberg, Shepard, Fabes, Murphy, & Guthrie, 1998). These findings parallel those with German children on shyness and sociability.

Fifth, the distinction between shyness and sociability is also underscored by current understanding of the concept of *social withdrawal* (Rubin, Coplan, & Bowker, 2009), which includes two kinds of children. The first kind engages in solitary play and would just as soon be with toys or books as with other children (unsociable).

> A second type of withdrawn child is one who would like to engage others in interaction but for some reason is compelled to avoid them, especially in novel settings. This approach–avoidance conflict may lead to behavioral compromises such as observing others from afar or hovering along the margins of ongoing play groups. Thus, the solitary behavior of these internally conflicted children is not characterized by passive disinterest and solitary-constructiveness, but rather by social wariness. (Rubin & Asendorpf, 1993b, p. 13)

In summary, several facts have emerged from these various studies: (1) Shyness and sociability are negatively related; (2) the strength of the relation varies with the instruments used to measure these two traits; and (3) though the two are inversely related, evidence derived from varying biological and behavioral methods and measures of study demonstrates the importance of keeping the two traits separate. Sociability refers to the *motive,* strong or weak, of wanting to be with others, whereas shyness refers to *behavior* when with others, inhibited or uninhibited, as well as feelings of tension and discomfort.

We are now in a position to understand why shyness and sociability are (negatively) correlated. Unsociable people, by definition, have a relatively weak tendency to associate with others. They are in fewer social situations and are therefore less likely to habituate to novel situations, which are known to exacerbate shyness. Furthermore, those who score low in sociability, having less contact with others, may be less likely to acquire the social skills that might make them feel confident with others. From a developmental-theoretical perspective (e.g., Piaget, 1932), not interacting with others may lead to deficits in social cognition and therefore, eventually, to socially skilled behavior (Rubin et al., 2003).

What is the benefit of treating shyness and sociability as distinct constructs? One advantage of keeping the concepts separate is that we can better understand the two kinds of people who score in the middle of an introversion–extraversion scale: those who want to be with others but are inhibited when with them (sociable and shy), and those who would just as soon be alone (i.e., introverts), but are talkative and outgoing (i.e., extraverts). Interestingly, this idea has a long history in personality theory (e.g., Briggs, 1988; Eysenck, 1956).

IS THERE A DISTINCTION BETWEEN SHYNESS AND BEHAVIORAL INHIBITION?

The concept of behavioral inhibition, which first appeared in an article by Garcia-Coll, Kagan, and Reznick (1984), refers to children's shutting down their behavior in the face of uncertainty about how to handle unfamiliar stimuli. Children were exposed to the following situations: "initial meeting with an unfamiliar examiner, an encounter with an unfamiliar set of toys, a woman model displaying a trio of acts that were difficult to remember, an interaction with another female stranger, exposure to a large and odd-looking robot, and temporary separation from the mother" (Kagan et al., 1984, p. 2213). Children first seen at 21 months and classified as inhibited or uninhibited were subsequently observed at age 4 years. At the later age, the inhibited children were more cautious, had more fears, and had a higher heart rate and more heart rate variability than the uninhibited children. These trends continued into the sixth year of life (Kagan et al., 1987, 1988).

Notice that behavioral inhibition includes both social and nonsocial wariness and inhibition. Thus, Kagan and his colleagues (1984, 1987, 1988; Garcia-Coll et al., 1984) appear to have studied fear, not shyness, and we should not be surprised that fearful children might have higher and more variable heart rates than uninhibited children when confronted with unfamiliar situations.

If Kagan and his colleagues (1984, 1987, 1988; Garcia-Coll et al.,

1984) had continued to use the term "behavioral inhibition" the way it was operationally defined, there would be no problem. However, in two publications, "behavioral inhibition" and "shyness" were used synonymously. In a chapter titled "Shyness and Temperament," Kagan and Reznick (1986) reviewed their longitudinal research, sometimes using the term "behavioral inhibition" and at other times, "shyness." They repeated this usage in an article titled "Biological Basis of Childhood Shyness" (Kagan et al., 1988). Unfortunately, the confounding of shyness with fear has spread to researchers who focus specifically on *social* inhibition (shyness), not the more generalized fear of both social and nonsocial unfamiliarity. An important example is the research by Asendorpf (1989, 1990), who studied shyness but referred to it as "behavioral inhibition."

What difference does it make? How important is it to distinguish between behavioral inhibition and shyness? First, we attain conceptual clarity and do not confuse fear with shyness, which is specifically social. Thus, children who display stranger anxiety are not necessarily afraid of unfamiliar toys. Second, we can make sense of the finding that shy children do not have a higher or more variable heart rate (Asendorpf & Meier, 1993). Third, it might help us understand the different types and reasons for social and nonsocial inhibition (see, e.g., Coplan, Rubin, Fox, Calkins, & Stewart, 1994; Rubin & Mills, 1988).

For example, there is the research of Kochanska (1991), who observed children between the ages of 1½ and 3½ years. The children and their mothers first entered an unfamiliar apartment, and then an unfamiliar woman entered the room and eventually approached the child. Two patterns emerged: (1) children retreated from the stranger, and were wary and timid in response to her (social inhibition); and (2) there was little or no exploratory behavior in the apartment (nonsocial inhibition).

In a follow-up study, the children were observed again at the age of 5 years, this time interacting with an unfamiliar peer (Kochanska & Radke-Yarrow, 1992). A shyness factor, which consisted of staring, looking but not interacting, being unoccupied, and not conversing with the peer, was strongly predicted by the social inhibition (shyness) observed in the earlier study. The second factor, quality of group play, was predicted by the *non*social inhibition first identified in the earlier study: "The present findings confirm the empirical and conceptual validity of a more differentiated conceptualization of children's inhibition to the unfamiliar" (p. 332). Put another way, the shyness displayed by young children was different from nonsocial inhibition. Still further evidence of this distinction is found in the work of Rubin and his colleagues.

In a series of studies, Rubin and colleagues (Rubin, Hastings, Stewart, Henderson, & Chen, 1997; Rubin, Burgess, & Hastings, 2002) found virtually no overlap between the behavioral inhibition construct described by

Kagan and inhibition of toddlers in the company of a toddler peer. The latter was a stronger predictor of reticence 2 years later than the former. Other work by Rubin's group has noted a distinction between shyness and fear, and their longitudinal relations with parenting (see Rubin, Nelson, Hastings, & Asendorpf, 1999).

Kagan and Reznick (1986) appear to have accepted the distinction drawn here, for in a large-scale study of children, there is this quotation: "Shyness is also indexed by a fearful or avoidant reaction by the child, but differs from behavioral inhibition in that it refers strictly to responding to an unfamiliar person" (Emde et al., 1992, p. 1443).

In conclusion, the literature over the last two decades has been replete with examples of studies equating behavioral inhibition and shyness (see Schmidt & Schulkin, 1999, for a review). But are the two constructs really the same? The two are often highly related empirically. For example, Schmidt and colleagues (e.g., Fox et al., 2005; Schmidt et al., 1997) previously noted in separate studies an empirical relation between measures of behavioral inhibition from direct observation based on Kagan's definition and maternal report of shyness, as measured by the Colorado Child Temperament Inventory (Buss & Plomin, 1984; Rowe & Plomin, 1977). But are they conceptually the same? Although they share similar features, behavioral inhibition is fear based, and reflects fear and anxiety in response to social and nonsocial stimuli, whereas shyness reflects anxious self-consciousness in response to social situations and perhaps embodies more of the cognitive elements of self and self-awareness than does behavioral inhibition.

IS ANXIOUS SHYNESS DIFFERENT FROM SELF-CONSCIOUS SHYNESS?

The first psychological questionnaire on shyness appeared over 30 years ago (Pilkonis, 1977a, 1977b). A few years later it was suggested that shyness is not a unitary construct (Crozier, 1981). Buss (1986) shortly thereafter described two types of shyness: One was an "anxious shyness" (also sometimes referred to as "fearful shyness"), an early-developing shyness emerging in the second half of the first year of postnatal life and associated with fear and stranger wariness. The second type was "self-conscious shyness," a later-developing shyness emerging around the ages of 3 or 4, coinciding with the development of embarrassment, self-awareness, self-conscious emotions, and perspective taking. The two types of shyness are presumed to have different developmental timetables, immediate causes, and enduring causes (see Table 2.1).

There have been several attempts to test Buss's (1986) theory, primarily with adult participants. Previous studies have found empirical evidence that

TABLE 2.1. Anxious versus Self-Conscious Shyness

	Anxious	Self-conscious
Emotion	Fear, distress	Embarrassment
Autonomic nervous system reaction (if any)	Sympathetic	Parasympathetic
First appearance	Almost a year	3–4 years
Immediate causes	Strangers Novel social role Evaluation Poor self-preservation Foolish actions	Conspicuousness Novel social setting Breach of privacy Teasing, ridicule Overpraise
Enduring causes	Heredity Chronic fear (Low) sociability Insecure attachment Isolation Poor social skills Avoidance conditioning	Excessive socialization Public self-consciousness History of teasing, ridicule Negative appearance

differences between the two shyness subtypes can be observed on several levels. For example, Bruch, Giordano, and Pearl (1986) reported that the two subtypes differ on self-report measures of somatic anxiety, behavioral inhibition, and social skills, with anxiously shy adults exhibiting more problems in these areas. Robinson (1989) reported heart rate differences between the shyness subtypes in response to a self-presentation task and found that adults classified as self-consciously shy exhibit a significantly higher heart rate in response to the task compared with anxiously shy and nonshy participants. Schmidt and Robinson (1992) subsequently noted that anxiously shy young adults reported significantly lower self-esteem compared with their self-consciously shy and nonshy counterparts.

Schmidt and his colleagues (Santesso, Lewandowski, Davis, & Schmidt, 2006) conducted a pilot study to determine whether anxious shyness and self-conscious shyness are distinguishable on regional EEG measures collected at baseline and in response to an affective challenge. Questionnaires were used to measure shyness (Cheek, 1983), public self-consciousness (Fenigstein, Scheier, & Buss, 1975), and fearfulness (Buss & Plomin, 1984). These measures were used to define anxiously shy (n = 9) and self-consciously shy (n = 9) subtypes in the manner proposed by Buss (1986): Those adults with scores either ± 1 SD above or below the mean were defined as high and low, respectively, in shyness, self-consciousness, and fearful anxiousness (Cheek & Buss, 1981). A third group of nonshy participants (n = 9) fell 1 *SD* below the mean on all of the measures. Resting EEG measures were assessed, because the pattern of resting frontal EEG activity has been suggested to be a trait-like marker of individual differences in affective style (e.g., Davidson, 2000). In addition, EEG measures were examined during affective challenge (i.e., emotions in response to music), because the maintenance of anxious shyness and related constructs may be linked to an inability to regulate negative emotion, particularly the emotion of fear (e.g., Buss, 1986; Schmidt et al., 2005; Schmidt & Schulkin, 1999). It was predicted that the anxiously shy subtype would exhibit significantly more activity in the right frontal lead (a marker of fear dysregulation) compared with the self-consciously shy and nonshy groups at baseline and in response to fear-eliciting auditory stimuli, given that the anxiously shy group theoretically scores higher on avoidance motivation than the other two groups. Preliminary analyses revealed that the EEG patterns were in the predicted direction, although additional participants need to be tested.

The next step will be to test the Buss's (1986) theory with developmental studies of infants and children. We know that not all shy children are alike, and that these children may be on different development trajectories (Coplan et al., 1994). Conceptualizing and operationally defining different shyness subtypes may help us understand different development outcomes. For example, are children with anxious shyness at greater risk for the development of problem behaviors than children who are self-consciously shy? Do anxiously shy children develop self-conscious shyness? Is self-conscious shyness in the presence of anxious shyness a cumulative risk factor?

IS SHYNESS CONTINUOUS WITH SOCIAL PHOBIA?

Is the shyness investigated by developmental, social, and personality psychologists merely a milder form of the abnormal social behavior that comes to the attention of clinical psychologists and other mental health professionals? Or are the two kinds of social behavior qualitatively different? To answer these questions, two syndromes described in the *Diagnostic and Statistical Manual of Mental Disorders* (DSM-IV; American Psychiatric Association, 1994) require further examination.

With respect to psychiatric classification, "social phobia" is placed in the context of other anxiety reactions. It includes fear or embarrassment not only in everyday social interaction (shyness) but also when performing in front of an audience. The criteria for a diagnosis of social phobia include the following: (1) The situation provokes an immediate anxiety reaction; (2) the situation is typically avoided or, at best, endured uncomfortably; and (3) the phobia interferes with everyday functioning, or that the person is markedly upset by it. Features suggested to be associated with social phobia are special sensitivity to negative evaluation of rejection, poor self-esteem, inadequate social skills, and overt signs of anxiety.

There are two subtypes: "generalized," in which many interactive and performance situations are feared, and *"specific,"* in which just one or very few situations are feared. This distinction was made concrete in a study of clinic patients by Sternberger, Turner, Beidel, and Calhoun (1995), who classified patients as generalized

> if they feared parties (social gatherings), initiating conversations, or maintaining conversations. Patients were given a "specific" subtype diagnosis ... if they feared only circumscribed situations such as giving speeches, speaking in meetings, eating or writing in public, and/or using public restrooms. This included those who feared multiple "specific" types of situations (e.g., speeches and writing in public) but did not fear more general social situations such as parties or conversations. (p. 528)

Close examination of this distinction reveals that the generalized subtype seems equivalent to shyness: fear and avoidance of *interaction* with others. The "specific" subtype, in contrast, refers to situations in which the person may be observed by others: in a restaurant, library, or auditorium (performing). The "specific" subtype appears to be something of a catchall term. There are people who do not mind eating or writing in public but dread having to make a public speech. Indeed, surveys have revealed that fear of public speaking is so prevalent that it might be a "normal anxiety." Also, though merely being observed and performing in public probably both involve feeling conspicuous, only public performance involves evaluation by an audience.

The criteria for a diagnosis of "avoidant personality disorder" overlap but are slightly different from the criteria for generalized social phobia, the emphasis being more on avoidance: (1) avoids others at work for fear of criticism or rejection, (2) stays uninvolved unless sure of being liked or not being ridiculed, (3) is inhibited in strange social contexts, (4) feels inferior, and (5) fears being embarrassed. There is an appropriate warning that avoidant personality may be the same condition as social phobia, generalized type.

We are now in a position to add clarity to this debate by answering the question asked at the beginning of this section. Although early shyness has been linked to the development of social phobia (Heiser, Turner, & Biedel, 2003; Neal & Edelmann, 2003; Rapee & Spence, 2004), there is still some continued debate about the exact nature of the relation between shyness and social phobia. The criteria that define both generalized social phobia and avoidant personality disorder are precisely the ones that developmental, social, and personality psychologists use to define shyness. If there is any difference at all, it may be that generalized social phobia is more intense shyness, sufficient to cause people to seek help. One final point: Social phobia is too broadly defined. It includes shyness, avoidance of public places, and anxiety in the presence of an audience. These different kinds of social anxiety undoubtedly have different prevalence rates in the population. Each surely requires a different focus by therapists.

CONCLUSIONS AND FUTURE DIRECTIONS

Our goal in this chapter was to clarify our understanding of human shyness. We argued and reviewed empirical evidence that shyness is conceptually and empirically distinguishable from sociability, behavioral inhibition, and social phobia, and that there are different types of shyness. As the many chapters in this volume attest, shyness has multiple meanings across studies. Definitions of childhood shyness are often used interchangeably with definitions of adult shyness. Is shyness the same phenomenon across ages? Does shyness engender the same definition across cultures? Do these conceptual issues generalize to special populations (see, e.g., Goldberg & Schmidt, 2001; Jetha, Schmidt, & Goldberg, 2007; Schmidt, Miskovic, Boyle, & Saigal, 2008).

The lack of conceptual clarity around shyness limits scientific inquiry into the phenomenon. Work toward a unified conceptualization of shyness embodied in biological and behavioral reality is needed to facilitate basic and applied empirical research in the area. Future studies involving longitudinal, cross-culture designs would shed further light on our understanding of shyness.

ACKNOWLEDGMENTS

The writing of this chapter was supported by Operating Grants from the Social Sciences and Humanities Research Council of Canada and the Natural Sciences and Engineering Research Council of Canada awarded to Louis A. Schmidt.

REFERENCES

Addison, T. L., & Schmidt, L. A. (1999). Are women who are shy reluctant to take risks?: Behavioral and psychophysiological correlates. *Journal of Research in Personality, 33,* 352–357.

American Psychiatric Association. (1994). *Diagnostic and statistical manual of mental disorders* (4th ed.). Washington, DC: Author.

Asendorpf, J. B. (1989). Shyness as a final common pathway for two different kinds of inhibition. *Journal of Personality and Social Psychology, 57,* 481–492.

Asendorpf, J. B. (1990). Beyond social withdrawal: Shyness, unsociability, and peer avoidance. *Human Development, 33,* 250–259.

Asendorpf, J. B., & Meier, G. H. (1993). Personality effects on children's speech in everyday life: Sociability mediated exposure and shyness-mediated reactivity to social situations. *Journal of Personality and Social Psychology, 64,* 1072–1083.

Ashbaugh, A. R., Antony, M. M., McCabe, R. E., Schmidt, L. A., & Swinson, R. P. (2005). Self-evaluative biases in social anxiety. *Cognitive Therapy and Research, 29,* 387–398.

Beaton, E. A., Schmidt, L. A., Ashbaugh, A. R., Santesso, D. L., Antony, M. M., & McCabe, R. E. (2008). Resting and reactive frontal brain electrical activity (EEG) among a non-clinical sample of socially anxious adults: Does concurrent depressive mood matter? *Neuropsychiatric Disease and Treatment, 4,* 187–192.

Beaton, E. A., Schmidt, L. A., Ashbaugh, A. R., Santesso, D. L., Antony, M. M., McCabe, R. E., et al. (2006). Low salivary cortisol levels among socially anxious young adults: Preliminary evidence from a selected and a non-selected sample. *Personality and Individual Differences, 41,* 1217–1228.

Beaton, E. A., Schmidt, L. A., Schulkin, J., Antony, M. M., Swinson, R. P., & Hall, G. B. (2008). Different neural responses to stranger and personally familiar faces in shy and bold adults. *Behavioral Neuroscience, 122,* 704–709.

Beidel, D. C., & Turner, S. M. (1998). *Shy children, phobic adults.* Washington, DC: American Psychological Association.

Bowlby, J. (1969). *Attachment and loss* (Vol. 1.) New York: Basic Books.

Briggs, S. R. (1988). Shyness: Introversion or neuroticism? *Journal of Research in Personality, 22,* 290–307.

Bruch, M. A., Giordano, S., & Pearl, L. (1986). Differences between fearful and self-conscious shy subtypes in background and current adjustment. *Journal of Research in Personality, 20,* 172–186.

Bruch, M. A., Gorsky, J. M., Collins, T. M., & Berger, P. A. (1989). Shyness and sociability reexamined: A multicomponent analysis. *Journal of Personality and Social Psychology, 57,* 904–915.

Brunet, P. M., & Schmidt, L. A. (2007). Is shyness context specific?: Relation between shyness and online self-disclosure with and without a live webcam in young adults. *Journal of Research in Personality, 41,* 938–945.

Brunet, P. M., & Schmidt, L. A. (2008). Are shy adults "really" bolder online?: It depends on the context. *CyberPsychology and Behavior, 11,* 707–709.

Buss, A. H. (1980). *Self-consciousness and social anxiety.* San Francisco: Freeman.

Buss, A. H. (1984). A conception of shyness. In J. A. Daly & J. C. McCroskey (Eds.), *Avoiding communication: Shyness, reticence and communication apprehension* (pp. 39–49). Beverly Hills: Sage.

Buss, A. H. (1986). A theory of shyness. In W. H. Jones, J. M. Cheek, & S. R. Briggs (Eds.), *Shyness: Perspectives on research and treatment* (pp. 39–46). New York: Plenum Press.

Buss, A. H., & Plomin, R. (1975). *A temperament theory of personality development*. New York: Wiley-Interscience.

Buss, A. H., & Plomin, R. (1984). *Temperament: Early developing personality traits*. Hillsdale, NJ: Erlbaum.

Carducci, B. J. (1999). *Shyness: A bold new approach*. New York: HarperCollins.

Caspi, A., Elder, G. H., & Bem, D. J. (1988). Moving away from the world: Life-course patterns of shy children. *Developmental Psychology, 24*, 824–831.

Cheek, J. M. (1983). *The revised Cheek and Buss Shyness Scale*. Unpublished manuscript, Wellesley College, Wellesley, MA.

Cheek, J. M., & Buss, A. H. (1981). Shyness and sociability. *Journal of Personality and Social Psychology, 41*, 330–339.

Cheek, J. M., Carpentieri, A. M., Smith, T. G., Rierdan, J., & Koff, E. (1986). Adolescent shyness. In W. H. Jones, J. M. Cheek, & S. R. Briggs (Eds.), *Shyness: Perspectives on research and treatment* (pp. 105–115). New York: Plenum.

Cheek, J. M., & Krasnoperova, E. N. (1999). Varieties of shyness in adolescence and adulthood. In L. A. Schmidt & J. Schulkin (Eds.), *Extreme fear, shyness, and social phobia: Origins, biological mechanisms, and clinical outcomes* (pp. 224–250). New York: Oxford University Press.

Coplan, R. J., Prakash, K., O'Neil, K., & Mandana, A. (2004). Do you "want" to play?: Distinguishing between conflicted shyness and social disinterest in early childhood. *Developmental Psychology, 40*, 244–258.

Coplan, R. J., Rubin, K. H., Fox, N. A., Calkins, S. D., & Stewart, S. L. (1994). Being alone, playing alone, acting alone: Distinguishing among reticence and passive and active solitude in young children. *Child Development, 65*, 129–137.

Crozier, W. R. (1979). Shyness as a dimension of personality. *British Journal of Social and Clinical Psychology, 18*, 121–128.

Crozier, W. R. (1981). Shyness and self-esteem. *British Journal of Social Psychology, 20*, 220–222.

Crozier, W. R. (1999). Individual differences in childhood shyness: Distinguishing fearful and self-conscious shyness. In L. A. Schmidt & J. Schulkin (Eds.), *Extreme fear, shyness, and social phobia: Origins, biological mechanisms, and clinical outcomes* (pp. 14–29). New York: Oxford University Press.

Czeschlik, T., & Nurk, H. C. (1995). Shyness and sociability: Factor structure in a German sample. *European Journal of Psychological Assessment, 11*, 122–127.

Davidson, R. J. (2000). Affective style, psychopathology, and resilience: Brain mechanisms and plasticity. *American Psychologist, 55*, 1196–1214.

Eisenberg, N., Fabes, R. A., & Murphy, B. C. (1995). Relations of shyness and low sociability to regulation and emotionality. *Journal of Personality and Social Psychology, 68*, 505–517.

Eisenberg, N., Shepard, S. A., Fabes, R. A., Murphy, B. C., & Guthrie, I. K. (1998). Shyness and children's emotionality, regulation, and coping: Contemporaneous, longitudinal, and across-context relations. *Child Development, 69*, 767–790.

Emde, R. N., Plomin, R., Robinson, J. A., Corley, R., DeFries, J., Fulker, D. W., et al. (1992). Temperament, emotions, and recognition at fourteen months: The MacArthur Longitudinal Twin Study. *Child Development, 63*, 1437–1455.

Eysenck, H. J. (1956). The questionnaire measurement of neuroticism and extraversion. *Revista Psicologia, 50*, 113–140.

Fenigstein, A., Scheier, M. F., & Buss, A. H. (1975). Public and private self-consciousness: Assessment and theory. *Journal of Consulting and Clinical Psychology, 43,* 522–527.

Fox, N. A., Henderson, H. A., Rubin, K. H., Calkins, S. D., & Schmidt, L. A. (2001). Continuity and discontinuity of behavioral inhibition and exuberance: Psychophysiological and behavioral influences across the first four years of life. *Child Development, 72,* 1–21.

Fox, N. A., Nichols, K. E., Henderson, H. A., Rubin, K. H., Schmidt, L. A., Hamer, D., et al. (2005). Evidence for a gene–environment interaction in predicting behavioral inhibition in middle childhood. *Psychological Science, 16,* 921–926.

Fox, N. A., Rubin, K. H., Calkins, S. D., Marshall, T. R., Coplan, R. J., Porges, S. W., et al. (1995). Frontal activation asymmetry and social competence at four years of age. *Child Development, 66,* 1770–1784.

Garcia-Coll, C., Kagan, J., & Reznick, J. S. (1984). Behavioral inhibition in young children. *Child Development, 55,* 1005–1019.

Goldberg, J. O., & Schmidt, L. A. (2001). Shyness, sociability, and social dysfunction in schizophrenia. *Schizophrenia Research, 48,* 343–349.

Hampton, F. A. (1927). Shyness. *Journal of Neurology and Psychopathology, 8,* 124–131.

Heiser, N. A., Turner, S. M., & Beidel, D. C. (2003). Shyness: Relationship to social phobia and other psychiatric disorders. *Behaviour Research and Therapy, 41,* 209–221.

Jetha, M. K., Schmidt, L. A., & Goldberg, J. O. (2007). Stability of shyness, sociability, and social dysfunction in schizophrenia: A preliminary investigation of the influence of social skills training in a community-based outpatient sample. *European Journal of Psychiatry, 21,* 189–198.

Jones, W. H., Briggs, S. R., & Smith, T. G. (1986). Shyness: Conceptualization and measurement. *Journal of Personality and Social Psychology, 51,* 629–639.

Jones, W. H., Cheek, J. M., & Briggs, S. R. (1986). *Shyness: Perspectives on research and treatment.* New York: Plenum Press.

Kagan, J. (1994). *Galen's prophecy: Temperament in human nature.* New York: Basic Books.

Kagan, J. (1999). The concept of behavioral inhibition. In L. A. Schmidt & J. Schulkin (Eds.), *Extreme fear, shyness, and social phobia: Origins, biological mechanisms, and clinical outcomes* (pp. 3–13). New York: Oxford University Press.

Kagan, J., & Reznick, J. S. (1986). Shyness and temperament. In W. H. Jones, J. M. Cheek, & S. R. Briggs (Eds.), *Shyness: Perspectives on research and treatment* (pp. 81–90). New York: Plenum Press.

Kagan, J., Reznick, J. S., Clarke, C., Snidman, N., & Garcia-Coll, C. (1984). Behavioral inhibition to the unfamiliar. *Child Development, 55,* 2212–2225.

Kagan, J., Reznick, J. S., & Snidman, N. (1987). The physiology and psychology of behavioral inhibition in children. *Child Development, 58,* 1459–1473.

Kagan, J., Reznick, J. S., & Snidman, N. (1988). Biological bases of childhood shyness. *Science, 240,* 167–171.

Kochanska, G. (1991). Patterns of inhibition to the unfamilair in children of normal and affectively ill mothers. *Child Development, 62,* 250–263.

Kochanska, G., & Radke-Yarrow, M. (1992). Inhibition in toddlerhood and the dynamics of the child's interaction with an unfamiliar peer at age five. *Child Development, 63,* 325–335.

Lewinsky, H. H. (1941). The nature of shyness. *British Journal of Psychology, 32,* 105–113.

Miller, J. L., Schmidt, L. A., & Vaillancourt, T. (2008). Shyness, sociability, and eating problems in a non-clinical sample of female undergraduates. *Eating Behaviors, 9,* 352–359.

Neal, J. A., & Edelmann, R. J. (2003). The etiology of social phobia: Toward a developmental profile. *Clinical Psychology Review, 23,* 761–786.

Neto, F. (1996). Correlates of Portuguese college students' shyness and sociability. *Psychological Reports, 78,* 79–82.

Oh, W., Rubin, K. H., Bowker, J. C., Booth-LaForce, C., Rose-Krasnor, L., & Lauresent, B. (2008). Trajectories of social withdrawal from middle childhood to early adolescence. *Journal of Abnormal Child Psychology, 36,* 553–566.

Page, R. M. (1990). Shyness and sociability: A dangerous combination for illicit substance use in adolescent males? *Adolescence, 25,* 803–806.

Perry, M., & Buss, A. H. (1990). *Trait and situational aspects of shyness.* Unpublished manuscript, University of Texas, Austin.

Piaget, J. (1932). *Six psychological studies.* New York: Random House.

Pilkonis, P. A. (1977a). Shyness, private and public, and its relation to other measures of social behavior. *Journal of Personality, 45,* 585–595.

Pilkonis, P. A. (1977b). The behavioral consequences of shyness. *Journal of Personality, 45,* 596–611.

Rapee, R. M., & Spence, S. H. (2004). The etiology of social phobia: Empirical evidence and an initial model. [Special Issue: Social Phobia and Social Anxiety]. *Clinical Psychology Review, 24,* 737–767.

Rowe, D. C., & Plomin, R. (1977). Temperament in early childhood. *Journal of Personality Assessment, 41,* 150–156.

Robinson, T. N., Jr. (1989). *Individual differences in shyness: Psychometric, behavioral and cardiovascular differences for different forms of shyness.* Paper presented at the Fourth Meeting of the International Society for the Study of Individual Differences, Heidelberg, West Germany.

Rubin, K. H. (1993). The Waterloo Longitudinal Project: Correlates and consequences of social withdrawal from childhood to adolescence. In K. H. Rubin & J. B. Asendorpf (Eds.), *Social withdrawal, inhibition, and shyness in childhood* (pp. 291–314). Hillsdale, NJ: Erlbaum.

Rubin, K. H., & Asendorpf, J. (1993a). *Social withdrawal, inhibition, and shyness in childhood.* Hillsdale, NJ: Erlbaum.

Rubin, K. H., & Asendorpf, J. B. (1993b). Social withdrawal, inhibition and shyness: Conceptual and definitional issues. In *Social withdrawal, inhibition, and shyness in childhood* (pp. 3–17). Hillsdale, NJ: Erlbaum.

Rubin, K. H., Burgess, K. B., & Hastings, P. D. (2002). Stability and social-behavioral consequences of toddlers' inhibited temperament and parenting. *Child Development, 73,* 483–495.

Rubin, K. H., Burgess, K., Kennedy, A. E., & Stewart, S. (2003). Social withdrawal and inhibition in childhood. In E. Mash & R. Barkley (Eds.), *Child psychopathology* (2nd ed., pp. 372–406). New York: Guilford Press.

Rubin, K. H., Coplan, R. J., & Bowker, J. C. (2009). Social withdrawal and shyness in childhood and adolescence. *Annual Review of Psychology, 60,* 141–171.

Rubin, K. H., Hastings, P. D., Stewart, S., Henderson, H. A., & Chen, X. (1997). The consistency and concomitants of inhibition: Some of the children, all of the time. *Child Development, 68,* 467–483.

Rubin, K. H., Hymel, S., Mills, R. S. L., & Rose-Krasnor, L. (1991). Conceptualizing different pathways to and from social isolation in childhood. In D. Cicchetti & S. Toth (Eds.), *Internalizing and externalizing expressions of dysfunction: Rochester Symposium on Developmental Psychopathology* (Vol. 2, pp. 91–122). Hillsdale, NJ: Erlbaum.

Rubin, K. H., & Mills, R. S. L. (1988). The many faces of social isolation in childhood. *Journal of Clinical and Consulting Psychology, 56,* 916–924.

Rubin, K. H., Nelson, L. J., Hastings, P. D., & Asendorpf, J. (1999). The transaction between parents' perceptions of their children's shyness and their parenting styles. *International Journal of Behavioral Development, 23,* 937–958.

Santesso, D. L., Lewandowski, M. N., Davis, J. M., & Schmidt, L. A. (2006). Resting and affective frontal brain electrical activity (EEG) in distinguishing fearful and self-conscious shyness: Preliminary findings. In A.V. Clark (Ed.), *Psychology of moods* (pp. 103–116). New York: Nova Science.

Santesso, D. L., Schmidt, L. A., & Fox, N. A. (2004). Are shyness *and* sociability still a dangerous combination for substance use?: Evidence from a U.S. and Canadian sample. *Personality and Individual Differences, 37,* 5–17.

Schmidt, L. A. (1999). Frontal brain electrical activity in shyness and sociability. *Psychological Science, 10,* 316–320.

Schmidt, L. A. (2003). Shyness *and* sociability: A dangerous combination for preschoolers. In S. J. Segalowitz (Guest Ed.), The brain factor in understanding psychological development [Special section]. *International Society for the Study of Behavioural Development Newsletter, 27*(3), 6–8.

Schmidt, L. A., & Fox, N. A. (1994). Patterns of cortical electrophysiology and autonomic activity in adults' shyness and sociability. *Biological Psychology, 38,* 183–198.

Schmidt, L. A., & Fox, N. A. (1995). Individual differences in young adults' shyness and sociability: Personality and health correlates. *Personality and Individual Differences, 19,* 455–462.

Schmidt, L. A., & Fox, N. A. (1999). Conceptual, biological, and behavioral distinctions among different categories of shy children. In L. A. Schmidt & J. Schulkin (Eds.), *Extreme fear, shyness, and social phobia: Origins, biological mechanisms, and clinical outcomes* (pp. 47–66). New York: Oxford University Press.

Schmidt, L. A., Fox, N. A., Rubin, K. H., Sternberg, E. M., Gold, P. W., Smith, C., et al. (1997). Behavioral and neuroendocrine responses in shy children. *Developmental Psychobiology, 30,* 127–140.

Schmidt, L. A., Fox, N. A., Schulkin, J., & Gold, P. W. (1999). Behavioral and psychophysiological correlates of self-presentation in temperamentally shy children. *Developmental Psychobiology, 35,* 119–135.

Schmidt, L. A., Miskovic, V., Boyle, M., & Saigal, S. (2008). Shyness and timidity in young adults who were born at extremely low birth weight. *Pediatrics, 122,* e181–e187.

Schmidt, L. A., Polak, C. P., & Spooner, A. L. (2005). Biological and environmental contributions to childhood shyness: A diathesis–stress model. In W. R. Crozier & L. E. Alden (Eds.), *The essential handbook of social anxiety for clinicians* (pp. 33–55). Chichester, UK: Wiley.

Schmidt, L. A., & Robinson, T. R., Jr. (1992). Low self-esteem in differentiating fearful and self-conscious forms of shyness. *Psychological Reports, 70,* 255–257.

Schmidt, L. A., Santesso, D. L., Schulkin, J., & Segalowitz, S. J. (2007). Shyness is necessary but not sufficient for high salivary cortisol in 10 year-olds. *Personality and Individual Differences, 43,* 1541–1551.

Schmidt, L. A., & Schulkin, J. (Eds.). (1999). *Extreme fear, shyness, and social phobia: Origins, biological mechanisms, and clinical outcomes* (Series in Affective Science). New York: Oxford University Press.

Skinner, B. F. (1938). *The behavior of organisms.* New York: Appleton–Century–Crofts.

Sternberger, R. T., Turner, S. M., Beidel, D. C., & Calhoun, K. S. (1995). Social phobia: An analysis of possible developmental factors. *Journal of Abnormal Psychology, 104,* 526–531.

Theall-Honey, L. A., & Schmidt, L. A. (2006). Do temperamentally shy children process emotion differently than non-shy children?: Behavioral, psychophysiological, and gender differences in reticent preschoolers. *Developmental Psychobiology, 48,* 187–196.

Zimbardo, P. G. (1977). *Shyness: What is it and what to do about it.* New York: Symphony Press.

3

Shyness and the Development of Embarrassment and the Self-Conscious Emotions

W. RAY CROZIER

"Self-consciousness," believing oneself to be the object of others' attention, does not seem to be necessary for early-appearing shyness, but it becomes prominent in the childhood years. A key task that has scarcely begun is to show how and when it becomes an important component of shyness. There exist well-developed theory and research on the development of the "self-conscious emotions," and this would seem to offer a valuable source of insight into the development of self-conscious shyness. However, and puzzlingly, this research has consistently neglected shyness. In this chapter I consider research on the development of shyness and the self-conscious emotions, and ask whether research on these emotions can shed light on the involvement of the self in shyness during the childhood years. Before doing so, I analyze the concept of self-consciousness and discuss the status of shyness as a self-conscious emotion.

It is assumed here that shyness is a multifaceted phenomenon involving cognitive, somatic, and behavioral components. Research distinguishes between state and trait shyness (Crozier, 1990); in this chapter, I focus on the experience of shyness as a state, an emotional experience, rather than on individual differences in a predisposition to state shyness. I consider the implications of the distinction that has been made in trait shyness between fearful and self-conscious forms of shyness given the potential relevance of this to the experience of self-consciousness.

I propose, too, that it is useful to distinguish between shy behaviors and the subjective experience of shyness. Quiet, inhibited behavior in the presence of others may be due to many factors. A child might be reticent or reserved because he or she does not know how to behave in particular circumstances, such as attending a new school for the first time; alternatively, he or she may be comfortable playing by him- or herself (Coplan, Prakash, O'Neil, & Armer, 2004). Children with autism often appear to be shy even though they have not achieved the cognitive capacities that seem to be a prerequisite for self-conscious shyness (Sodian, Hülsken, & Thoermer, 2003). On the other hand, someone might feel shy or regard him- or herself as shy, without other people being aware of it. The distinction is important when interpreting findings from studies undertaken with different age groups. Research on shyness in the early years tends to draw upon observations of children's behavior (e.g., Kagan, 2001), whereas studies in later childhood also draw upon self-report questionnaire and interview methods (e.g., Crozier & Burnham, 1990; Crozier, 1995). This can make it difficult to identify stages in emotional development. For example, children may experience shyness without necessarily being able to represent their experience in language or to answer questions about hypothetical events as described in researcher-generated vignettes. This problem of interpretation is perhaps particularly prominent for the development of self-conscious emotions, since the individual's appraisal of the self is fundamental to these emotions.

I also assume that questions of whether shyness is a discrete emotion or a member of a family of self-conscious emotions are not just a quibble about terminology that can be addressed by means of analysis of how words are used. The position I adopt here is influenced by Sabini and Silver's (2005) work on self-conscious emotion. They argue that emotion words do not correspond on a one-to-one basis to emotion states. The mental and physiological state of the person experiencing, in their example, embarrassment and shame may be the same in each emotion (a hypothetical state X) but is described differently depending on the context. In the case of shame and embarrassment, according to Sabini and Silver, the relevant context concerns the person's character, specifically, whether or not a real character flaw has been revealed. Following this line of argument, questions about whether shyness is a self-conscious emotion or how it relates to, say, embarrassment or anxiety can be framed in terms of whether the internal state in shyness is state X or another state and, if it is state X, the circumstances that result in it being labeled shyness and not embarrassment.

THE SELF IN SHYNESS
AND SELF-CONSCIOUS EMOTIONS

References to the self appear frequently in laypersons' descriptions of the experience of shyness. For example, 85% of respondents to the Stanford

Shyness Survey identified self-consciousness as a symptom of their shyness, and this was the most frequently cited symptom (Zimbardo, 1986). The self is also prominent in psychological theorizing on trait shyness. Shy individuals lack confidence in themselves and have low self-efficacy about social interactions (Hill, 1989). They have lower self-esteem (Crozier, 1995). They are motivated to make an effective presentation of self but doubt their ability to do so (Leary, 2001); consequently, they may adopt self-protective strategies to cope with these doubts (Arkin, 1981). They make stable, internal attributions for their social difficulties—they blame themselves for their predicaments. They report negative, self-deprecatory thoughts during social interaction (Bruch, 2001). They develop self-schemas for shyness that produce cognitive biases in processing information (Baldwin & Fergusson, 2001). The impact of shyness on social behavior is moderated by implicit self-theories of shyness (Beer, 2002).

Despite this prominence, research on trait shyness has paid little attention to developments in selfhood within the child. However, these have been the focus of theorizing and research on the self-conscious emotions (Lagattuta & Thompson, 2007; Tracy & Robins, 2004). These emotions are said to require the child's sense of self-awareness and self-representation; recognition of external standards against which the child can be evaluated; adoption by the child of these standards; the capacity to assess congruence or incongruence between behavior or personal characteristics and these standards; and the capacity to make attributions about the reasons for congruence or incongruence. The experiences of embarrassment, shame, guilt, or pride are said to entail an appraisal process, combined with focus of attention on a representation of the self (Tracy & Robins, 2004). Unsurprisingly, there is consensus that the self-conscious emotions develop later than the "primary" emotions of anger, fear, joy, and sadness. There is no reason why self-conscious shyness should not also entail a complex process of appraisals and self-representations. Before addressing this issue through comparison of accounts of the development of shyness and self-conscious emotion (particularly embarrassment) it is essential to consider what is meant by "self-consciousness." I outline alternative interpretations of this state and consider the implications of variation in their emphasis on the capacity to form sophisticated self- and other representations.

THE NATURE OF SELF-CONSCIOUSNESS

Self-consciousness has been conceptualized in several ways. One approach draws upon research on self-attention processes. Carver (1979) proposed conditions in which self-directed attention produces negative evaluation of behavior, withdrawal from the situation, and the state of being "frozen in self-assessment" (p. 1266) that provide a useful characterization of the experience of shyness. Buss (1980) defined "public self-awareness" as awareness of oneself as a social object, and hypothesized that acute public self-awareness is fundamental to four forms of social anxiety, namely, shyness, embarrassment, shame, and audience anxiety. Self-awareness is most likely to be triggered when we are observed by other people, including being photographed or filmed. A second position characterizes self-consciousness as the intrusion of self-related thoughts into consciousness and as self-focused rumination that interferes with the "flow" of appropriate social involvement (Crozier, 1982). A third approach conceptualizes it as a state of heightened awareness of the self—"our consciousness is filled with self" (Izard, 1977, p. 389). Thus, Harris (1990) defined it as a distinctive state that he labeled "acute negative public self-attention." He considered this to be an inherently aversive state that people try to avoid, the anticipation of which evokes anxiety. Self-consciousness is therefore affective, as well as cognitive. Harris and I have also proposed that it has a distinctive psychophysiological signature, namely, the blush (Harris, 1990, p. 69; Crozier, 2006); as Darwin (1872/1965, p. 325) wrote, "It is the thinking of what others think of us which elicits a blush." This position contrasts the state of self-consciousness with the routine flow of conscious involvement in activities.

A fourth approach emphasizes the perspective taking that is implied by self-consciousness: The individual views the self as if through the eyes of others, whether other people who are actually present or an imagined view of the "other." Taylor (1985) has called this an "objective detached observer view of the self"; Semin and Manstead (1981), the "subjective public image"; and Rochat (2003), "meta-cognitive self-awareness." This position can be traced to Adam Smith's *The Theory of Moral Sentiments* (2002), first published in 1759, wherein Smith described the duality of the self:

> When I endeavour to examine my own conduct. ... I divide myself into two characters, as it were into two persons. ... The first is spectator, whose sentiments with regard to my own conduct I endeavour to enter into, by placing myself in his situation, and by considering how it would appear to me, when seen from that particular point of view. (p. 131)

According to this position, too, self-consciousness is a distinctive state. To illustrate this, consider the example of a child who is talking aloud to himself while playing alone, who blushes when he suddenly realizes that he is being observed by an adult. Nothing in the situation has changed except for a shift in his consciousness. Self-consciousness contrasts with an "unselfconscious" state, where the boy's attention would be focused on his play. It also differs from self-directed, negative rumination, in that it entails second-order processes. It requires a capacity for perspective taking, not only appreciation that others take perspectives but also the ability to imagine how one's conduct looks, or might reasonably look, to the other. Finally, it differs from public self-awareness, since it involves more than the realization that one is the object of attention: It assigns a view to the observer. Zinck (2008, p. 497) wrote, "There is at least one further individual involved (or represented) in the evaluative process taking place for self-referential emotion (this individual does not need to be present in person, it suffices, if she is represented in the subject's mind)."

This position is emphasized in accounts of self-conscious emotions such as shame and embarrassment. Is viewing the self as if through the eyes of the other necessary for the experience of shyness? Is self-focused attention or awareness that one is the object of attention sufficient or does one also have to represent how one's conduct might look to someone else? A recurrent theme in descriptions of shyness takes the form "If I say X, I might appear foolish or stupid, or other people will think less of me in some way." This theme can be identified in cross-cultural studies of emotion language. Many of the languages analyzed have concepts equivalent to the English language concepts of "feeling shy" and "being shy." For example, one specification of shyness in terms of semantic primitives (Harkins, 1990) is "I don't know what things are good to do/say here; I don't want to do/say something bad; I don't want people to think something bad about me." The shy person monitors his or her behavior in terms of how that behavior would influence the view of him or her taken by another; specifically, it is a defensive stance, intended to ward off negative outcomes rather than bring about positive ones. Consider, for example, this scenario: A party of schoolchildren is visiting a museum, and a teacher joins a girl and her classmates in the picnic area. Hitherto the girl had been animated in conversation, but her teacher's arrival induces silence and self-consciousness. Before the teacher's arrival, she was making remarks spontaneously, almost without thinking; now she rehearses possible contributions rather than utter them. She fears that if she were to make a contribution it might not come out right because of her confusion.

Is this experience perhaps characteristic of self-conscious shyness but not of the fearful form? The most robust evidence for this distinction comes from analysis of children's conceptions of shyness (Yuill & Banerjee, 2001), and the finding that the self-conscious form is not apparent in children's descriptions before the age of 4–5 years suggests that it requires development in the capacity for perspective taking that is essential for self-conscious emotion as outlined in this section. I return to this distinction later.

SHYNESS AS A SELF-CONSCIOUS EMOTION

Self-consciousness is not peculiar to self-descriptions of shyness, and it characterizes descriptions of embarrassment and shame as well. These have been variously termed emotions of "self-attention," or "social," "self-referential," or "self-conscious" emotions. They imply a reflective self, an individual who is aware how his or her behavior might appear to others and, specifically, is aware that others can take an adverse view of that behavior, whether or not this view is deserved. As Miller (2001, pp. 293–294) writes, "Neither self-conscious shyness nor embarrassment would occur if people were genuinely heedless of the judgements of others, and it is this core characteristic that links the two states." Nevertheless, the relations among shyness, shame, and embarrassment are little understood, and there is disagreement as to whether they are versions of the same underlying affect or emotion (Izard, 1977; Tomkins, 1963), or whether they constitute distinct emotional states (Keltner & Buswell, 1997).

Recently there has been a revival of interest in the self-conscious emotions, which are taken to include shame, embarrassment, guilt, and pride (Tracy & Robins, 2004). Shyness is not included in the set of emotions analyzed by Tracy and Robins, or by Zinck (2008), and does not figure in the recent edited collection on the self-conscious emotions (Tracy, Robins, & Tangney, 2007). Why does shyness not belong with these emotions? There are several answers to this question.

First, shyness may not be an emotion at all. Miller (2001, p. 285) proposes that shyness is "a mood that comprises a discernibly different mix of affects." Leary (1986, p. 30) defined it as "an affective–behavioral syndrome characterized by social anxiety and interpersonal inhibition that results from the prospect or presence of interpersonal evaluation." Yet, historically, influential writers on emotion have regarded shyness as a member of a family of emotions that includes shame and embarrassment, and that has characteristic cognitions, behaviors, facial expression, and physiological components (Izard, 1977; Tomkins, 1963). Respondents to the Stanford Shyness Survey describe a coherent emotional experience—with cognitive, somatic, and behavioral components—that is consistent with the theorizing of Tomkins and Izard.

A second possible answer is that shyness is an emotion but not a distinct one. It might be a mix of affects, as Miller (2001) suggests. Or it might be the expression in particular kinds of circumstances of another emotion, for example, anxiety during or in anticipation of certain kinds of social encounters. Much research on shyness relates it to the fear system (Schmidt & Fox, 1999); the self-presentation perspective characterizes it as a form of anxiety (Leary, 1986). These perspectives provide valuable insights into shyness. They draw attention to the connections between shyness and states of chronic anxiety, such as social phobia/social anxiety disorder, that are supported by evidence of the association between shyness and anxiety problems (reviewed by Rubin, Coplan, & Bowker, 2009). Nevertheless, the relations among shyness, embarrassment, and anxiety warrant further examination. For example, blushing frequently accompanies shyness and embarrassment, without being a typical sign of fear or anxiety. Recent research (reviewed by Crozier, 2006) shows that heightened sympathetic innervation of beta-adrenergic receptors in the facial veins produces increases in blood flow in the facial area, a form of sympathetic arousal that does not typically accompany other fear reactions; indeed, blushing and embarrassment can be associated with heart rate deceleration rather than acceleration (Miller, 2001).

Another candidate emotion is embarrassment. Because shy behaviors are often awkward or inappropriate, or the shy person believes that his or her behavior is inadequate in some way, he or she may experience embarrassment at behaving in a shy manner and being observed to do so. The blushing that is commonly reported as a reaction to shyness-eliciting situations may express the embarrassment about shyness or social predicaments to which, shy people believe, their shyness has contributed. The relations between shyness and embarrassment have been little studied. A review of the literature by Miller (2001) set out several differences between embarrassment and state shyness in antecedents, phenomenology, behaviors, physiological reactions, consequences for social interaction, and development. Miller argued that although the actor in both states is concerned about how his or her conduct appears to others and about others' view of the actor, the differences between the states warrant their separate consideration in psychological research. He concluded that "shyness is an anticipatory mood state, whereas embarrassment is an emotion elicited by events that have already occurred" (p. 296). Shyness here resembles anxiety, which also is an emotional state that occurs in anticipation of events that have yet to happen.

Nevertheless, the differences between the two states can be overemphasized. It can be difficult to determine whether a state is shyness or embarrassment. For example, an adult asks a young boy in the presence of others if he has a girl friend. The boy colors visibly, looks downward and away from the adult, and remains silent. "Ah, he's gone all shy," the adult says. We might think instead that he is embarrassed. Many would label the schoolgirl's reticence when her teacher joined her in the museum as shyness; the Stanford Shyness Survey identifies the presence of authority figures as a common elicitor of shyness. This pattern could also be described as embarrassment, where the girl is flustered by the teacher's presence. Some argue that the blush distinguishes the emotions, claiming that it is specific to embarrassment (Buss, 1985; Miller, 2001). Yet empirical research shows that blushing is frequently reported as a symptom of shyness (Ishiyama, 1984; Zimbardo,

1986), with rates of reports similar to those found in surveys of embarrassment (Parrott & Smith, 1991).

Self-conscious emotion and anxiety often co-occur. Fear of embarrassment exerts a powerful influence on behavior; for example, it prevents many children from sharing their worries with others. Malicious teasing, name-calling, coining cruel nicknames, making derogatory remarks about a child or his or her family, playing practical jokes and tricks, and circulating messages and photographs by cell phone or on the Internet are all forms of bullying in school that create anxiety because of their capacity to induce embarrassment, shame, and humiliation.

In this section, I have argued that shyness is a plausible candidate for a self-conscious emotion, that it shares characteristics with embarrassment, and that these emotions are distinguishable from anxiety. However, this still leaves the question of whether self-consciousness is necessary for shyness. In the next section, I consider whether shyness and embarrassment are experienced prior to the development of self-consciousness.

SELF-CONSCIOUSNESS IN THE DEVELOPMENT OF SHYNESS

Two approaches to the emergence of the self in shyness can be identified, one that implies an essential continuity in the development of shyness, another that argues for distinct stages. Rubin and his associates (Rubin, Burgess, Kennedy, & Stewart, 2003; Rubin et al., 2009) propose that the negative social experiences of shy children, contingent on their reticent and withdrawn behavior, result in low self-esteem. At the age when the child's peers judge this pattern of behavior to deviate from norms, the shy child is likely to be rejected and unpopular. The avoidance of novel situations that characterizes shyness reduces opportunities for the acquisition of confident, skilled social behavior, which in turn leads to unsuccessful interactions with peers. The shy child suffers negative experiences, such as victimization and rejection, and also finds it difficult to bring about successful outcomes, for example, influencing others. These experiences provide the basis for negative self-perceptions of social skills and peer relationships. These self-perceptions may be reinforced when parents, teachers, or peers label the child as "shy."

Kagan (2001) suggests an alternative explanation. Inhibited children have a physiology that produces more intense negative emotional reactions. Their characteristic dysphoric body tone may predispose them toward negative interpretations of social events. These predispositions result in more intense fear of criticism and rejection, and a greater tendency to perceive social situations as threatening to the self. There is substantial evidence that relates inhibition to reticence, and social withdrawal to rejection by peers, and also evidence that shy, withdrawn children have negative self-perceptions and low social self-esteem from about 7 years of age (Rubin et al., 2009).

Although there is no inexorable route from early temperament to a shy, withdrawn "personality"—parent–child attachment relationships, parenting beliefs and styles, and children's friendships can act as moderating factors—the model proposes an essential continuity in development. Temperament produces patterns of behavior that acquire meanings in the social world and have implications for the child's social standing. In contrast with the position outlined below, no new form of shyness is proposed. The child's behavior, the effects it produces in others, and the child's awareness and evaluation of others' reactions provide the basis for the involvement of the self in shyness: low social self-esteem or self-efficacy. Clearly, this must be contingent upon developments within the child, including the acquisition and elaboration of a self-concept, increased understanding of the social environment, appreciation that others may view the child's behavior in a negative light, and attribution of negative social experiences to the self.

An alternative approach to conceptualizing the emergence of the self is to propose two different kinds of shyness, one that does not require a developed self-concept and another that does. Buss (1985, 1986) distinguished between early-appearing fearful shyness and later-appearing self-conscious shyness. The former is elicited by social novelty, intrusion into personal space, and social evaluation; the latter, by conspicuousness, being the focus of attention, being noticeably different from others, and breaches of privacy. Buss (1986, p. 43) wrote, "Fearful shyness requires no special, advanced sense of self. . . . Self-conscious shyness involves public self-awareness, which requires an advanced, cognitive self, and is therefore present only in older human children and adults." The self-conscious kind appears at age 4–5 years and requires the development of a sense of oneself as a social object and a focus on those aspects of the self that are observable and noticeable.

There is little direct evidence related to the theory. Research has relied on studies of children's conceptions of shyness, whether through content analysis of descriptions of shyness or children's responses to vignettes. Analysis shows that younger children's conceptions are dominated by references to fearful shyness, whereas from about 4 years of age on, references to the self-conscious kind predominate (Yuill & Banerjee, 2001). These references do not displace the fearful kind, and both kinds can be identified in the responses of older children and adults (Crozier, 1999). The two forms can be distinguished in terms of eliciting circumstances and reactions: Four-year-old children report that meeting a stranger is more likely to elicit shyness than singing alone in front of the class, whereas the latter situation is more frequently nominated by 5- and 6-year-olds (Yuill & Banerjee, 2001).

Younger children refer to being frightened or hiding, whereas older children also refer to blushing, feeling nervous, feeling embarrassed, and smiling (Crozier, 1999). Parallel evidence comes from research involving children's descriptions of their own shyness (Crozier & Burnham, 1990), hypothetical children's shyness (Yuill & Banerjee, 2001), and peer nomination techniques (Younger, Schneider, Wadeson, Guirguis, & Bergeron, 2000). Nevertheless, the differences between the two forms of shyness may be exaggerated, as indications of both forms are evident in the responses of younger children (Crozier, 1999). Research into different forms of shyness has been hampered by the dearth of measures: Apart from the peer nomination technique reported by Younger et al. (2000), there exist no established measures of individual differences in fearful and self-conscious shyness. Proposals for indirect approaches, for example, by categorizing research participants on the basis of their patterns of scores on measures of shyness, fearfulness, and public self-consciousness (Bruch, Giordano, & Pearl, 1986), have not been developed into reliable psychometric instruments, nor have they been applied to the study of children.

The distinction between fearful and self-conscious forms is not the only distinction that has been made in accounts of shyness. Asendorpf (1989) identified two classes of situations—novel and evaluative—that elicit shyness. Coplan et al. (2004) distinguished between conflicted shyness, where the child would like to interact with others but is constrained by anxiety, and social disinterest, where the child plays alone because he or she does not have strong motivation for social interaction. Schmidt and Fox (1999) mapped fearful and self-conscious shyness onto a distinction between avoidant and conflicted subtypes of childhood shyness, proposing "avoidant shyness" that comprises fearful shyness and avoidant behavior, and "conflicted shyness" that comprises self-conscious shyness and approach–avoidance conflict. However, whereas the link between fear and avoidance is consistent with findings about shyness and inhibition (Rubin et al., 2003), there is no evidence that conflict necessarily entails self-consciousness.

It is important to construct robust measures of self-conscious shyness to test the validity of these proposed types and to investigate implications of age-related developments in self-consciousness for individual differences in shyness. Self-report measures might be appropriate for older children; nevertheless, it would be useful to explore the relevance of observational and psychophysiological measures developed in the field of embarrassment and self-conscious emotion. For example, significant progress has been made in the detailed analysis of facial expression and in the physiological recording of blushing that uses measures of cheek temperature and blood flow (Shearn, Bergman, Hill, Abel, & Hinds, 1990). To date, this research has focused on adults and on exposure embarrassment, where participants have to perform "embarrassing" activities in front of an audience or watch a video recording of their performance in the presence of others. Unfortunately, research into blushing in childhood has scarcely begun (Crozier, 2006).

In the next section, I outline a distinction in the study of self-conscious emotion that resembles that between early- and late-appearing shyness.

SELF-CONSCIOUSNESS IN THE DEVELOPMENT OF EMBARRASSMENT

The self has attracted substantially more theorizing and empirical research in the development of embarrassment (and other self-conscious emotions, including shame, guilt, and pride) than in shyness. For example, Lewis (1992) distinguished between exposed emotions and self-conscious evaluative emotions. "Exposed emotions" are contingent upon the acquisition of objective self-awareness or "metarepresentation," or "idea of me," which normally emerges between 15 and 24 months of age and is indexed by a child's capacity for visual self-recognition, the emergence of self-referential language, and the capacity for pretense. Exposed emotions precede evaluative emotions, which require cognitive developments over and above the acquisition of a sense of self: The child must be able to absorb and "own" (p. 92) a set of standards, rules, and goals, and to evaluate his or her actions, thoughts, and feelings in terms of these. The child must be able to determine success or failure outcomes in attaining these standards and to attribute these outcomes to the self. Lewis's account does not specify the timing of the emergence of evaluative emotions, other than to suggest that they emerge at around 3 years of age.

This account of the onset of exposure embarrassment is supported by findings from visual self-recognition tasks. Lewis, Sullivan, Stanger, and Weiss (1989) found that 22-month-old children show overt signs of embarrassment when viewing themselves in a mirror while other people look on, when profusely complimented, or when asked to perform (e.g., dance) for adults. Specifically, signs of embarrassment during these tasks were observed only among those children who had previously shown self-recognition to the mirror (touched their nose after rouge had been applied surreptitiously).

Lewis distinguishes exposure embarrassment from shyness: Although visual self-recognition was correlated with signs of embarrassment, it was not associated with observed wariness expressed in response to the approach of a stranger. However, individual differences in embarrassment and the onset of visual self-recognition were influenced by the child's temperament (DiBiase & Lewis, 1997; Lewis, 2001). Children who were fearful, withdrawn, and with predominantly negative mood showed earlier self-recognition and were more likely to show embarrassment. Once visual self-recognition was acquired they were also more likely than children with a less difficult temperament to show signs of embarrassment, whereas temperament was unrelated to embarrassment among children who did not show self-recognition (DiBiase & Lewis, 1997).

Comparison of Buss and Lewis

Both Buss (1985) and Lewis (2001) distinguish two forms of self-conscious emotions and regard them as appearing in sequence, with the emergence of each contingent upon cognitive developments. Table 3.1 compares the two theories on prerequisites for their emergence, approximate age of onset, and eliciting circumstances. It is evident that the two accounts do not map onto one another. They differ in their view of self-consciousness, in the significance of conspicuousness, and in their treatment of self-evaluation. Buss (1985) identifies social evaluation with fearful shyness, although he admits that evaluation concerns are found only among older children and adults who have sufficient socialization experience to be aware of a discrepancy between their behavior and standards of evaluation. He acknowledges the apparent paradox in assigning a cause of early-appearing shyness to a factor that is evident in behavior only later, arguing that later events "maintain or intensify" this form of shyness (p. 70). In contrast, Lewis (2001) maintains that the evaluative embarrassment comes later in development, when the child has internalized standards of evaluation. He also makes a sharper distinction between shyness and evaluative embarrassment, arguing that evaluation is not necessary for shyness. Buss's construct of self-conscious shyness resembles embarrassment. Its description in terms of fluster and disorganization of behavior, blushing, and acute awareness of self as a social object could equally well serve as a description of embarrassment.

STAGES IN THE DEVELOPMENT OF SELF-CONSCIOUS EMOTIONS

Lewis's work is consistent with trends in research into development of the self and self-conscious emotions that propose two important developmental milestones. One takes place in the second year and the other at around the third to fourth year, when children show emerging awareness of their own and others' mental states as indexed, for example, by performance on second-order false belief tasks. As stated earlier, self-conscious emotion requires not only a capacity for self-awareness but also the capacities to adopt and internalize standards, and to construct attributions for (in)congruence with these standards.

TABLE 3.1. Comparison of Buss and Lewis Theories of Development

	Buss	Lewis
	Fearful shyness	Exposure embarrassment
Prerequisite	Not specified—discriminate unfamiliar others	Self-awareness (idea of "me"/ metarepresentation)
Age of onset	7–9 months	15–18 months
Elicitors	Strangers, unfamiliar people Intrusion Social evaluation	Being observed Performing in front of audience View self in mirror Being complimented
	Self-conscious shyness	Self-conscious evaluative embarrassment
Prerequisite	Advanced cognitive self as basis for public self-awareness	Self-attribution of internalized standards, rules
Age of onset	4–5 years	3 years
Elicitors	Conspicuousness Distinctiveness Attention of others	Social evaluation Task failure in front of audience Faux pas

Note. Based on descriptions provided by Buss (1985) and Lewis (2001).

The second year is significant not only for evidence of the capacity for visual self-recognition but also for developments on many fronts, for example, in vocabulary, the use of self-referential language, symbolic representation, pretend play, empathic behavior, and ideas of causality (Courage & Howe, 2002). There is evidence that children begin to appreciate adult standards for behavior and evaluate themselves relative to standards, for example, showing distress when they commit acts that fall short (Kagan, 1981), showing signs of apologies and self-blame (Kochanska, Casey, & Fukumoto, 1995), anticipating adult reactions to their success or failure, and looking to adults for recognition of their achievements (Barrett, 2005).

However, the thesis that "an idea of me" is a prerequisite for embarrassment is disputed. Reddy (2000) reported evidence of "coyness"—an ambivalent pattern of smiling and gaze or head aversion—in children as young as 2 months of age, which was elicited not just by strangers but also when the infant was greeted by a familiar adult after a brief separation or when viewing his or her reflection in a mirror. Barrett (2005) found that success at visual self-recognition tasks (VSRTs) did not predict embarrassment, shame, or guilt among a sample of children age 17 months. Indeed, VSRT performance was negatively related to embarrassment, qualified by an interaction with gender: Boys who had passed the VSRT showed less embarrassment than boys who had not passed, whereas there was no relation between VSRT and embarrassment among girls. At first sight, these results appear inconsistent with Lewis's theory. However, Lewis (2001) claims that success at the VSRT is a prerequisite for exposure embarrassment, and there is no evidence reported in Barrett's study that relates to exposure embarrassment. According to Lewis, the children would be too young to show evaluative embarrassment, and this may explain the nonsignificant relations with shame and guilt (the findings on embarrassment surely need replicating). One important finding from this study is that factor analysis applied to the measures of overt behavior identified three factors that could be labeled embarrassment, shame and guilt. Even at 17 months, children are showing distinctive reactions to predicaments.

The next milestone that has been emphasized is children's acquisition of a theory of mind. Lagattuta and Thompson (2007, p. 106) suggest that children's knowledge about mental states is significant for the emergence of self-conscious emotions. Yuill and Banerjee (2001, p. 123) propose that the child's acquisition of a theory of mind is prerequisite for "self-conscious shyness": understanding how one is represented by others is necessary in order to feel concern about being evaluated by others. Age of theory of mind acquisition is associated with awareness of being evaluated by others; for example, Dunn (1995) found that success at the false belief test predicted children's sensitivity to teachers' criticism of their work. Zinck (2008, p. 500) takes a different view, arguing that self-conscious emotions (she labels them "self-referential emotions") do not require an elaborate "proposition-based" theory of mind or language-based self-representations. Zinck refers to Reddy's work on coy smiles, as well as evidence of infant's apparent pride in producing changes in the environment, and argues that these are forms of self-conscious emotion that do not require a theory of mind (nor do they need a representational self, in Lewis's terms). Furthermore, the child can participate effectively in social interaction prior to success on theory of mind tasks. Banerjee and Henderson (2001) found that performance on a second-order false belief task did not discriminate between children (between age 6 and 11 years) who scored high and low in shyness, whereas shy children performed less well on measures of their understanding of vignettes describing faux pas and self-presentation goals.

Whether the role of the acquisition of theory of mind as indexed by the false belief task is necessary or sufficient for self-conscious emotion or shyness, it seems essential for the experience of self-consciousness that children attain "awareness of *how* they are in the mind of others" (Rochat, 2003, p. 722, emphasis in original). It is likely that this is acquired when the child who has acquired an "idea of me" coordinates cognitions, affect, and behavior in interactions with others, and reflects on these and on how his or her behavior impacts others. What is crucial is that self-conscious emotion is inherently social. It is clear that when children do become aware of how they are, or might be, in the mind of others, this self-consciousness becomes salient in shyness.

This is apparent by age 7 years. La Greca, Dandes, Wick, Shaw, and Stone (1988) identified a fear of negative evaluation factor in factor analysis of a social anxiety scale administered to 7-year-olds. The analysis replicated the factor structure found in the adult version of the scale. Gesell and Ilg's (1946) detailed descriptions of "typical" children illustrate changes in concerns between ages 7 and 9 years. Seven-year-olds worry that their peers might not like them; they are "very much aware of what others might think, and are careful not to expose themselves to criticism. They cringe when they are laughed at or made fun of" (pp. 147–148). An 8-year-old is "increasingly aware of himself as a person ... is more conscious of himself in the ways he differs from other people" (p. 176). At 9 years, "a good relationship with others is important. ... He is anxious to please, he wants to be liked and he loves to be chosen ... but he is still sensitive to correction and may be embarrassed by it" (p. 202). Data on children's fears and worries also show increasing reference to social concerns in the middle-childhood years. Silverman, La Greca, and Wasserstein (1995) found that children ages 7 to 12 years reported worries about being called on in class, being picked on, ignored or being rejected by friends or classmates, and saying something to hurt someone's feelings. The children expressed concerns about their appearance and about what others thought of their performance, although events and situations of a social nature did not elicit their most intense or frequent worries. Spence and McCathie (1993) found that fears of "giving a spoken report" in class increased significantly from ages 8 to 10 years.

Research with children from about age 7 onward indicates the prominence of self-conscious concerns in shyness: how one is viewed by others; fear of looking foolish or being criticized; and sensitivity to embarrassment. Studies of children's understanding of shyness show that these concerns augment, and do not displace, anxieties about meeting new people or encountering novel social situations. Children can be shy in the presence of familiar others.

This research provides insight into self-consciousness and the nature of children's self-presentation concerns, and it can provide a basis for devising age-appropriate self-report questionnaire items and parent–teacher checklist items to construct reliable measures of individual differences in self-conscious shyness. In combination with observational measures and the microanalysis of facial expressions and blushing, this could help overcome limitations in current understanding of self-conscious shyness and its development.

CONCLUSIONS

Shyness involves the state of self-consciousness and in this respect belongs with self-conscious emotions such as embarrassment and shame. The study of this state within research into self-conscious emotion emphasizes an "other perspective" that is taken on the self, together with an appraisal process that involves standards, rules, and goals.

The capacity to adopt another perspective on the self represents a cognitively complex achievement that has been addressed by researchers on the development of perspective taking (Selman, 1980; Harter, 1998), the self (Rochat, 2003), self-conscious emotion (Lagattuta & Thompson, 2007), shyness (Yuill & Banerjee, 2001), and the influence of social withdrawal on the development of perspective-taking skills (LeMare & Rubin, 1987). In self-conscious emotion, the "other perspective" that is imagined is evaluative and regards the self as falling short of standards; the individual understands that he or she can be regarded as doing so, whether or not he or she believes this is deserved. This is not merely a cognitive assessment process; it is an emotional experience. A substantial body of research identifies key developments in these capacities in the second year, for example, the child's capacity for visual self-recognition, which Lewis (2001) argues is a prerequisite for the emergence of embarrassment. It is not, he argues, sufficient for evaluative embarrassment, shame, guilt or pride, since these also require the capacity for learning and adopting standards and rules, evaluating success and failure, and attributing these to the self. Less research has investigated the development of metacognitive self-awareness or "thinking of what others think of us" as a prerequisite for either evaluative emotion or shyness. Philosophers such as Taylor (1985) regard this form of self-awareness as fundamental to the self-conscious emotions; Miller (2001) argues that it is central to both shyness and embarrassment. However, there is a dearth of empirical research on its development.

Although children in the second year demonstrate awareness of standards and discrepancies from standards in task performance, and look to adults for approval or disapproval, this does not necessarily constitute evidence of awareness of standards for social behavior. Signs of social success and failure may be subtle and more difficult to discern than, say, standards for well-defined problems. Also, success and failure are defined in terms of identity goals and standards. There is little systematic evidence on children's acquisition of identity goals and standards, or evaluation of their own behavior according to these. The notion of standards is important in Goffman's (1972) account of shyness. Goffman related shyness and embarrassment to the attributes and capacities that participants in social encounters are expected to have in order to present "a self that is at once coherently unified and appropriate for the occasion" (p. 10). He explained shyness in terms of the person's belief that he or she lacks social poise, and that this "disqualifies" him or her from claiming an appropriate identity; the inability to project an appropriate self into encounters increases the likelihood of embarrassment. Here shyness is close to evaluative embarrassment. Cognitive and emotional developments of the kind studied by theorists of social emotions are necessary for beliefs about qualifications for social participation. So, too, are the kinds of social experiences identified by Rubin et al. (2003), as are labels, such as "being shy" and "feeling shy," that are available in society to be appropriated by individuals to describe their own and others' behavior and experience.

Research on the development of embarrassment proposes three stages: (1) early coyness or bashfulness, which can be detected in the first months; (2) embarrassment that requires the emergence of self-awareness, which is evidenced in the second year; (3) embarrassment at failing to meet standards and attributing failure to the self, which appears, as far as we know, from about the third year on. The first stage is neither self-referential nor evaluative. However, it is difficult to believe that these experiences would not soon become self-referential and evaluative as children develop identity goals and the capacity to attribute outcomes to the self, and enter the social world of school where identities have to be constructed, social interactions managed, and friendships and social groups formed.

Are there parallel developments in shyness? Individual differences in behavioral inhibition are apparent in the second year, when children are also acquiring self-awareness (in one sense of this) and awareness of standards and rules. How temperament is related to these developments and the contribution of the emerging self to shyness in both novel and familiar settings are important questions for research. Although the details of Buss's account of self-awareness have been challenged, and are inconsistent with the account offered by Lewis (2001) and research more generally into the development of self-conscious emotion, Buss's account (1985) does outline a progression toward increasing involvement of the self in shyness. When and how this takes place warrants further research, and it would be productive to relate this research to developments in embarrassment. Children are sensitive to parental approval and disapproval from an early age. Standards for social behavior involving peers become fluid, fluctuate, and indeed salient as children enter the social world of childhood, for example, standards for appearance, whether the right label or logo is worn, and whether interests in particular computer games or music are "cool." Skills have to be acquired: how to engage in banter, to tease or be teased, to initiate and sustain conversation. All are subject to the judgments of peers, and all require, in Goffman's terms, the projection of an appropriate and "qualified" self. All have potential for eliciting self-conscious emotion, for feeling embarrassed and ashamed, and, I argue here, for feeling shy. Temperament can make these tasks more difficult and the acquisition of "qualifications" harder; just how is a matter of further research.

Approaches to the emergence of the self in shyness and embarrassment advocate different forms: fearful and self-conscious shyness; exposure and evaluative embarrassment. Do these forms represent different kinds of experience, or do the differences lie in the eliciting circumstances? It is not yet established whether the distinction between fearful and self-conscious shyness maps onto the distinction between avoidant and conflicted subtypes of childhood shyness, as proposed by Schmidt and Fox (1999). Do different types of shyness imply different states or a common state that is elicited by different types of circumstances, for example, by novel and evaluative situations (Asendorpf, 1989)? Nor is it clear whether the emergence of the self-conscious kind implies that children who hitherto have not been shy become shy at this stage, yielding different types of shy child. Asendorpf (1989) has argued for the former position, while the findings reported by Younger et al. (2000) imply the latter, if peer-nomination measures can be said to differentiate types of withdrawn children. It would be parsimonious to adopt the first position until convincing evidence provides support for separate forms. Research to date has been hampered by the lack of measures of the two forms of shyness, an absence that may be telling in itself.

Studying subjective states in children is a challenging task, and reliance on verbal descriptions and responses to vignettes has its limitations. Yet even self-conscious emotions have their overt expressions, and research into embarrassment has identified distinctive displays in young children (Barrett, 2005; Lewis, 2001). Recent research has produced techniques for measuring the blush, a transient and elusive expression that is reported to accompany both shyness and embarrassment (Crozier, 2006). Technological advances, extension of the research to children, and exploration of eliciting circumstances other than embarrassment could yield insight into the development of self-conscious shyness.

In conclusion, research into social emotions has begun to map the development of self-awareness, although work remains to be done on children's acquisition of an "other perspective" and their awareness of social standards and rules. Developments in embarrassment seem to parallel the emergence of self-conscious shyness, but there is a dearth of research on its emergence. Bringing together these strands of research and, in particular, investigating the role of self-consciousness in shyness would advance our understanding of the development of shyness during childhood and adolescence.

REFERENCES

Arkin, R. M. (1981). Self-presentation styles. In J. T. Tedeschi (Ed.), *Impression management theory and social psychological research* (pp. 311–333). New York: Academic Press.

Asendorpf, J. B. (1989). Shyness as a final common pathway for two different kinds of inhibition. *Journal of Personality and Social Psychology, 57,* 481–492.

Baldwin, M., & Fergusson, P. (2001). Relational schemas: The activation of interpersonal knowledge structures in social anxiety. In W. R. Crozier & L. E. Alden (Eds.), *International handbook of social anxiety* (pp. 235–257). Chichester, UK: Wiley.

Banerjee, R., & Henderson, L. (2001). Social-cognitive factors in childhood social anxiety: A preliminary analysis. *Social Development, 10,* 558–572.

Barrett, K. C. (2005). The origins of social emotions and self-regulation in toddlerhood: New evidence. *Cognition and Emotion, 19,* 953–979.

Beer, J. S. (2002). Implicit self-theories of shyness. *Journal of Personality and Social Psychology, 83,* 1009–1024.

Bruch, M. A. (2001). Shyness and social interaction. In W. R. Crozier & L. E. Alden (Eds.), *International handbook of social anxiety* (pp. 195–215). Chichester, UK: Wiley.

Bruch, M. A., Giordano, S., & Pearl, L. (1986). Differences between fearful and self-conscious shy subtypes in background and current adjustment. *Journal of Research in Personality, 20,* 172–186.

Buss, A. H. (1980). *Self-consciousness and social anxiety.* San Francisco: Freeman.

Buss, A. H. (1985). Two kinds of shyness. In R. Schwarzer (Ed.), *Self-related cognition in anxiety and motivation* (pp. 65–75). Hillsdale, NJ: Erlbaum.

Buss, A. H. (1986). A theory of shyness. In W. H. Jones, J. M. Cheek, & S. R. Briggs (Eds.), *Shyness: Perspectives on research and treatment* (pp. 39–46). New York: Plenum Press.

Carver, C. S. (1979). A cybernetic model of self-attention processes. *Journal of Personality and Social Psychology, 37,* 1251–1281.

Coplan, R. J., Prakash, K., O'Neil, K., & Armer, M. (2004). Do you "want" to play?: Distinguishing between conflicted shyness and social disinterest in early childhood. *Developmental Psychology, 40,* 244–258.

Courage, M. L., & Howe, M. L. (2002). From infant to child: The dynamics of cognitive change in the second year of life. *Psychological Bulletin, 128,* 250–277.

Crozier, W. R. (1982). Explanations of social shyness. *Current Psychological Reviews, 2,* 47–59.

Crozier, W. R. (1990). Social psychological perspectives on shyness, embarrassment and shame. In *Shyness and embarrassment: Perspectives from social psychology* (pp. 19–58). New York: Cambridge University Press.

Crozier, W. R. (1995). Shyness and self-esteem in middle childhood. *British Journal of Educational Psychology, 65,* 85–95.

Crozier, W. R. (1999). Individual differences in childhood shyness. In L. Schmidt & J. Chaulkin (Eds.), *Extreme fear and shyness: Origins, neuroendocrine mechanisms, and clinical outcomes* (pp. 14–29). New York: Oxford University Press.

Crozier, W. R. (2006). *Blushing and the social emotions: The self unmasked.* London: Palgrave/Macmillan.

Crozier, W. R., & Burnham, M. (1990). Age-related differences in children's understanding of shyness. *British Journal of Developmental Psychology, 8,* 179–185.

Darwin, C. (1965). *The expression of emotions in man and animals.* Chicago: University of Chicago Press. (Original work published 1872)

DiBiase, R., & Lewis, M. (1997). The relation between temperament and embarrassment. *Cognition and Emotion, 11,* 259–271.

Dunn, J. (1995). Children as psychologists: The later correlates of individual differences in understanding of emotions and other minds. *Cognition and Emotion, 9,* 187–201.

Gesell, A. L., & Ilg, F. L. (1946). *The child from five to ten.* New York: Harper.

Goffman, E. (1972). *Interaction ritual.* Harmondsworth, UK: Penguin.

Harkins, J. (1990). Shame and shyness in the Aboriginal classroom: A case for "practical semantics." *Australian Journal of Linguistics, 10,* 293–306.

Harris, P. R. (1990). Shyness and embarrassment in psychological theory and ordinary language. In W. R. Crozier (Ed.), *Shyness and embarrassment: Perspectives from social psychology* (pp. 59–86). New York: Cambridge University Press.

Harter, S. (1998). Developmental perspectives on the self-system. In N. Eisenberg & W. Damon (Eds.), *Handbook of child psychology: Vol. 3. Social, emotional, and personality development* (5th ed., pp. 102–132). New York: Wiley.

Hill, G. J. (1989). An unwillingness to act: Behavioral appropriateness, situational constraint, and self-efficacy in shyness. *Journal of Personality, 57,* 871–890.

Ishiyama, F. I. (1984). Shyness: Anxious social sensitivity and self-isolating tendency. *Adolescence, 19,* 903–911.

Izard, C. E. (1977). *Human emotions.* New York: Plenum Press.

Kagan, J. (1981). *The second year.* Cambridge, MA: Harvard University Press.

Kagan, J. (2001). Temperamental contributions to affective and behavioral profiles in childhood. In S. G. Hofmann & P. M. DiBartolo (Eds.), *From social anxiety to social phobia: Multiple perspectives* (pp. 216–234). Boston: Allyn & Bacon.

Keltner, D., & Buswell, B. N. (1997). Embarrassment: Its distinct form and appeasement functions. *Psychological Bulletin, 122,* 250–270.

Kochanska, G., Casey, R. J., & Fukumoto, A. (1995). Toddlers' sensitivity to standard violations. *Child Development, 66,* 643–656.

Lagattuta, K. H., & Thompson, R. A. (2007). The development of self-conscious emotions: Cognitive processes and social influences. In J. L. Tracy, R. W. Robins, & J. P. Tangney (Eds.), *The self-conscious emotions: Theory and research* (pp. 91–113). New York: Guilford Press.

La Greca, A. M., Dandes, S. K., Wick, P., Shaw, K., & Stone, W. L. (1988). Development of the Social Anxiety Scale for Children: Reliability and concurrent validity. *Journal of Clinical Child Psychology, 17,* 84–91.

Leary, M. R. (1986). Affective and behavioral components of shyness: Implications for theory, measurement, and research. In W. H. Jones, J. M. Cheek, & S. R. Briggs (Eds.), *Shyness: Perspectives on research and treatment* (pp. 27–38). New York: Plenum Press.

Leary, M. R. (2001). Social anxiety as an early warning system: A refinement and extension of the self-presentation theory of social anxiety. In S. G. Hofmann & P. M. DiBartolo (Eds.), *From social anxiety to social phobia: Multiple perspectives* (pp. 321–334). Boston: Allyn & Bacon.

LeMare, L. J., & Rubin, K. H. (1987). Perspective-taking and peer interaction: Structural and developmental analyses. *Child Development, 58,* 306–315.

Lewis, M. (1992). *Shame: The exposed self.* New York: Free Press.

Lewis, M. (2001). The origins of the self-conscious child. In W. R. Crozier & L. E. Alden (Eds.), *International handbook of social anxiety* (pp. 101–118). Chichester, UK: Wiley.

Lewis, M., Sullivan, M. W., Stanger, C., & Weiss, M. (1989). Self-development and self-conscious emotions. *Child Development, 60,* 146–156.

Miller, R. S. (2001). Shyness and embarrassment compared: Siblings in the service of social evaluation. In W. R. Crozier & L. E. Alden (Eds.), *International handbook of social anxiety* (pp. 281–300). Chichester, UK: Wiley.

Parrott, W. G., & Smith, S. F. (1991). Embarrassment: Actual vs. typical cases, classical vs. prototypical representations. *Cognition and Emotion, 5,* 467–488.

Reddy, V. (2000). Coyness in early infancy. *Developmental Science, 3,* 186–192.

Rochat, P. (2003). Five levels of self-awareness as they unfold early in life. *Consciousness and Cognition, 12,* 717–731.

Rubin, K. H., Burgess, K. B., Kennedy, A. E., & Stewart, S. L. (2003). Social withdrawal in childhood. In E. J. Mash & R. A. Barkley (Eds.), *Child psychopathology* (2nd ed., pp. 372–406). New York: Guilford Press.

Rubin, K. H., Coplan, R. J., & Bowker, J. C. (2009). Social withdrawal in childhood. *Annual Review of Psychology, 60,* 141–171.

Sabini, J., & Silver, M. (2005). Why emotion names and experiences don't neatly pair. *Psychological Inquiry, 16,* 1–10.

Schmidt, L. A., & Fox, N. A. (1999). Conceptual, biological, and behavioral distinctions among different categories of shy children. In L. A. Schmidt & J. Schulkin (Eds.), *Extreme fear, shyness, and social phobia: Origins, biological mechanisms, and clinical outcomes* (pp. 47–66). New York: Oxford University Press.

Selman, R. (1980). *The growth of interpersonal understanding.* New York: Academic Press.

Semin, G. R., & Manstead, A. S. R. (1981). The beholder beheld: A study of social emotionality. *European Journal of Social Psychology, 11,* 253–265.

Shearn, D., Bergman, E., Hill, K., Abel, A., & Hinds, L. (1990). Facial coloration and temperature responses in blushing. *Psychophysiology, 27,* 687–693.

Silverman, W. K., La Greca, A. M., & Wasserstein, S. (1995). What do children worry about?: Worries and their relation to anxiety. *Child Development, 66,* 671–686.

Smith, A. (2002). *The theory of moral sentiments.* Cambridge, UK: Cambridge University Press. (Original work published 1759)

Sodian, B., Hülsken, C., & Thoermer, C. (2003). The self and action in theory of mind research. *Consciousness and Cognition, 12,* 777–782.

Spence, S. H., & McCathie, H. M. (1993). The stability of fears in children: A two-year prospective study: A research note. *Journal of Child Psychology and Psychiatry, 34,* 579–585.

Taylor, G. (1985). *Pride, shame and guilt: Emotions of self-assessment.* Oxford, UK: Clarendon.

Tomkins, S. S. (1963). *Affect, imagery, consciousness: Vol. 2. The negative affects.* New York: Springer.

Tracy, J. L., & Robins, R. W. (2004). Putting the self into self-conscious emotions: A theoretical model. *Psychological Inquiry, 15,* 103–125.

Tracy, J. L., Robins, R. W., & Tangney, J. P. (Eds.). (2007). *The self-conscious emotions: Theory and research.* New York: Guilford Press.

Younger, A. J., Schneider, B. H., Wadeson, R., Guirguis, M., & Bergeron, N. (2000). A behaviour-based peer-nomination measure of social withdrawal in children. *Social Development, 9,* 544–564.

Yuill, N., & Banerjee, R. (2001). Children's conceptions of shyness. In W. R. Crozier & L. E. Alden (Eds.), *International handbook of social anxiety* (pp. 119–136). Chichester, UK: Wiley.

Zimbardo, P. G. (1986). The Stanford Shyness Project. In W. H. Jones, J. M. Cheek, & S. R. Briggs (Eds.), *Shyness: Perspectives on research and treatment* (pp. 17–25). New York: Plenum Press.

Zinck, A. (2008). Self-referential emotions. *Consciousness and Cognition, 17,* 496–505.

4

Unsociability and the Preference for Solitude in Childhood

ROBERT J. COPLAN
MURRAY WEEKS

The happiest of all lives is a busy solitude.
—VOLTAIRE

I have never found a companion so companionable
as solitude.
—HENRY DAVID THOREAU

In previous conceptual writings, researchers have placed the construct of "unsociability" (also sometimes called "social disinterest") within a taxonomy and theoretical framework that "carves up" the experience of behavioral solitude by virtue of different social and motivational processes (e.g., Asendorpf, 1990, 1993; Coplan & Armer, 2007; Rubin & Asendorpf, 1993; Rubin & Coplan, 2004; Rubin, Coplan, & Bowker, 2009). Simply put, it is argued that in the presence of potential playmates and opportunities for peer interaction, children may end up spending time alone for a number of different reasons.

Within this framework, "social withdrawal" refers to the process whereby a child removes him- or herself (for whatever reason) from opportunities to engage in social interaction with peers. This is contrasted with "active isolation," whereby the child is excluded by peers (i.e., spends frequent time alone because other children do not want to play with him or her). "Unsociability" is conceptualized within this typology as a subtype of social withdrawal arising from a child's preference for playing alone. This is contrasted with another subtype of withdrawal, "shyness," which refers to social fear and anxiety in the presence of peers that inhibit the child's desire to engage in social interaction (e.g., Coplan, Prakash, O'Neil, & Armer, 2004).

We define "unsociability" in childhood as the expression of individual differences in the preference for solitude and solitary activities. This definition is consistent with the previous conceptualizations described earlier. However, we offer three additional points of clarification (on which we expand in this chapter): (1) Unsociability represents an affinity for being alone, in contrast to simply a tolerance or acceptance of being placed in or having to endure periods of solitude; (2) unsociability is indicative of a motivation to be alone that reflects the positive appeal that solitude and solitary activities hold for the child; and (3) unsociability does *not* refer to a desire for solitude derived from social fear or self-consciousness, sadness or lethargy, a need for privacy, or as a means of avoiding or seeking solace from unpleasant social circumstances.

As compared to shyness, and even the more general construct of social withdrawal, unsociability in childhood has received only scant research attention. Indeed, despite some recent methodological advances, there are still only a handful of empirical studies that have specifically assessed unsociability in childhood. In this chapter we explore the historical and theoretical roots of the study of unsociability (with both adults and children), review the relevant empirical research (with careful attention to conceptualization and assessment issues), and offer suggestions for future research.

CONCEPTUAL AND HISTORICAL OVERVIEW

The study of the *preference for solitude* has a long history in the adult personality literature. For example, affiliation motivation was an important part of the adult personality dimension of *extraversion–introversion* described by Eysenck (1947). Despite a focus on individuals' sensitivity to cortical arousal, "introverts," by definition, were also described as being inclined to prefer solitude. In subsequent writings, Eysenck (1956; Eysenck & Eysenck, 1969) specifically differentiated between the adult personality traits of "neurotic" shyness, involving self-consciousness, insecurity, and anxiety in the face of social interactions, and "introverted" shyness, where the individual would rather be alone but could also effectively participate in social interaction. This conceptual distinction was reinforced by Cheek and Buss (1981), who provided evidence of the empirical distinctiveness between "shyness" (tension and inhibition with others), and "low sociability" (preference for being alone rather than being with others).

Building from these early roots, later studies of unsociability in adulthood continued to examine individual differences in the preference for solitude (e.g., Burger, 1995) and also explored people's different potential motivations for wanting to spend time alone (e.g., Hill, 1987). More recently, Leary, Herbst, and McCrary (2003) suggested that unsociability is most strongly influenced by a strong desire to be alone. In their study, Leary et al. described a "sociotropic" orientation as reflecting the strength of one's desire to affiliate with others. It should be noted that although *low* sociotropy might suggest a lesser desire for social interaction, it does not necessarily reflect a strong motivation to avoid others. A "solitropic" orientation, on the other hand, reflects the strength of one's desire to be alone, which can be conceptualized as the *need* for solitude. Leary et al. (2003) found that the reasons people tend to spend time alone have more to do with high solitropy than with low sociotropy. This suggests that being an unsociable adult appears to have more to do with a strong desire for being alone (i.e., high solitropy) than a lack of desire to be around others (i.e., low sociotropy). Thus, unsociable people may not necessarily be averse to social interaction when opportunities present themselves; rather, they are more highly motivated to spend time by themselves.

It is this conceptual approach that we draw upon and adapt to understand and explain the construct of unsociability in childhood. However, it should be noted that other researchers have highlighted additional "reasons" why individuals may seek out solitude, including a desire for privacy (Pedersen, 1979) or to limit how much other people know about them (Berscheid, 1977). As well, individuals may seek solace in solitude when they are upset or trying to avoid something undesirable (Larson, 1990). To us, these descriptions may be more akin to another subtype of social withdrawal, "social avoidance," which Asendorpf (1990, 1993) characterized as the combination of low social approach and high social avoidance motivations.

Finally, researchers have also emphasized several "positive" reasons why people may seek solitude (e.g., Bates, 1964; Burke, 1991). For example, solitude has been described as an important context for religious experiences (Hay & Morisey, 1978), creativity and insights (Storr, 1988), and the simple enjoyment of leisure activities (Purcell & Keller, 1989). Long, Seburn, Averill, and More (2003) suggested that the more positive aspects of solitude can be divided into two dimensions—inner directed (e.g., inner peace) and outer directed (e.g., spirituality)—that reflect potentially beneficial uses for solitude.

Early Studies in Childhood

The earliest studies of constructs related to a preference for solitude in childhood focused on the differential hereditability of sociability and shyness (e.g., Plomin & Rowe, 1977; Scarr, 1969). However, we would argue that two early observational studies (Jennings, 1975; Rubin, 1982) and the theoretical writings of Asendorpf (1990, 1993) established the foundations for the empirical study of unsociability in childhood.

Jennings (1975) observed 30 young children during free play at preschool. Aspects of children's "focus" during play (i.e., people-centered vs. object-centered attention) and the social "context" of their play (i.e., solitary vs. cooperative) were coded. From these data, Jennings created an index of object–person orientation. Children higher in object orientation displayed more social difficulties and were more adult-oriented, but they also tended to perform better on tests of ability to organize and classify physical materials. Jennings concluded that "preferences for activities with objects provide opportunities for more learning about the physical environment" (p. 516). This study was among the first to suggest that some children have a preference for toys over peers—a premise that went on to become closely linked to the construct of unsociability (Coplan et al., 2004).

Rubin (1982) also observed young children (N = 144) during free play at school. Rubin's observational taxonomy focused on the display of specific types of nonsocial play, including solitary–constructive activities (e.g., building with blocks, drawing a picture). Children who were frequently observed to display solitary–constructive play received fewer social initiations from peers and spent less time engaged in peer conversation. However, this form of nonsocial play was unrelated to teacher ratings of social competence or assessments of role-taking and social problem-solving ability. Rubin concluded that this form of solitary activity was "somewhat benign" (p. 654). This study is noteworthy for not only establishing the premise that not all forms of social withdrawal are necessarily problematic but also suggesting that unsociable children might be identified by the behavioral display of solitary–constructive activities (later referred to as "solitary–passive" play, Coplan, Rubin, Fox, Calkins, & Stewart, 1994) during free play with peers.

In a series of conceptual writings, Asendorpf (1990, 1993) described a detailed and theoretically derived taxonomy for distinguishing between different forms of social withdrawal (including unsociability) in childhood. This conceptual framework has been extremely influential in our own work (e.g., Coplan, Wilson, Frohlick, & Zelenski, 2006; Coplan & Armer, 2007; Coplan et al., 2004) and adopted by other social withdrawal researchers in the study of both children (e.g., Bowker, Bukowski, Zargarpour, & Hoza, 1998; Eisenberg, Shepard, Fabes, Murphy, & Guthrie, 1998; Gazelle & Rudolph, 2004; Harrist, Zaia, Bates, Dodge, & Pettit, 1997; Thijs, Koomen, de Jong, van der Leij, & van Leeuwen, 2004; Xu, Farver, Chang, Zhang, & Yu, 2007) and adults (e.g., Nikitin & Freund, 2008). However, operationalizing the constructs described in this model remains an ongoing challenge.

Drawing upon the early work of Gray (1972), Asendorpf (1990, 1993) described different psychosocial outcomes for children as a function of the combination of social approach and social avoidance motivations. In this model, unsociable children were characterized by low social approach and low social avoidance motivations. Thus, unsociable children might be content to play alone without initiating social contacts but also be willing to engage in more socially oriented activities if provided an attractive social invitation (Asendorpf, 1993). This was contrasted with shyness, which was characterized by the presence of both high social approach and high social avoidance motivations (i.e., an approach–avoidance conflict). In this regard, the shy child's desire to interact with peers is thought to be inhibited by social fear and anxiety simultaneously.

It has also been argued that although unsociability might be a relatively benign form of social withdrawal in early childhood, it might become increasingly maladaptive in later years, and may in fact merge with other forms of social withdrawal in middle or late childhood (Rubin & Asendorpf, 1993). The rationale for these hypotheses was that regardless of the *type* of social withdrawal, a continued lack of social interaction over time (for whatever reason) may interfere with the acquisition of age-appropriate social and social-cognitive skills, become viewed as increasingly deviant by peers, and ultimately lead to rejection (Rubin & Mills, 1988; Younger & Piccinin, 1989).

Taken together, these studies provided the core set of *conceptual assertions* in a developmental model of unsociability in childhood. These can be broadly summarized as follows: (1) Unsociability is a distinct form of social withdrawal in childhood; (2) unsociable children have a preference for solitary activities but are not otherwise averse to engaging in social interactions; and (3) unsociability is a comparatively benign form of social withdrawal in early childhood, but unsociable children will experience greater socioemotional difficulties later on. In the following pages, we focus on how subsequent empirical studies of unsociability in childhood have provided support (or, in some cases, called into question) these original theoretical assumptions.

Unsociability: A Distinct Form of Childhood Social Withdrawal?

In their earlier writings, Asendorpf (1990, 1993) and Rubin (1982; Rubin & Mills, 1988) established the conceptual grounds for establishing unsociability as a distinct form of social withdrawal. More recent empirical support for this assertion can be found in a series of studies indicating that parents, teachers, and even young children distinguish between unsociability and shyness in early childhood.

Coplan et al. (2004) developed a parental rating scale specifically to distinguish between shyness and unsociability (which they labeled "social disinterest") in young children. The conceptualization of unsociability (and shyness) for this measure was derived from Asendorpf's (1990, 1993) motivational model. Thus, unsociable items denote a preference for solitary activities (e.g., "My child often seems content to play alone"), whereas shyness items reference an approach–avoidance conflict (e.g., "My child seems to want to play with other children, but is sometimes nervous to"). Results from factor analysis (with a sample of 274 preschool-aged children) indicated a two-factor solution, with high factor loadings and strong internal consistency for both subscales, and a modest correlation ($r = .29$) between factors. From these findings, it can be inferred that mothers can provide psychometrically sound assessments of unsociability in their young children (distinct from an assessment of shyness).

Some teacher rating scales have also been developed that assess constructs conceptually related to unsociability (e.g., Child Behavior Scale, Ladd & Profilet, 1996). Thijs et al. (2004) modified previous questionnaires to create a measure of subtypes of social withdrawal in kindergarten children. Their results indicated orthogonal factors conceptually similar to unsociability (labeled "solitary behavior"; e.g., "often plays alone") and shyness (labeled "social inhibition"; e.g., "rather quiet, does not say anything spontaneously").

Harrist et al. (1997) used cluster analyses of various teacher ratings to identify subtypes of kindergarten children who previously had been observed to engage frequently in solitary behaviors. One group was labeled "unsociable," because although these children interacted with peers less frequently, they were otherwise undifferentiated from their nonwithdrawn counterparts in terms of social and social-cognitive variables. Arbeau and Coplan (2007) asked a sample of 202 kindergarten teachers about their attitudes and beliefs in response to a series of hypothetical vignettes describing the behaviors of shy, unsociable, aggressive, and prosocial children. The hypothetical *unsociable* child was described as playing quietly away from the other children, not appearing anxious or upset, and, if left undisturbed, would happily continue playing on his or her own. Teachers reported that the behaviors of the unsociable child were more intentional and less problematic (both socially and academically) compared to the hypothetical *shy* child, and that they would be less likely to intervene to alter the unsociable child's behavior. These findings provide more direct empirical support for the contention that teachers distinguish between unsociability and other forms of social withdrawal.

In terms of the abilities of children to make these types of distinctions, results have been more mixed. To begin with, it has been previously argued that socially withdrawn behaviors are less salient (e.g., as compared to aggression) for younger children, who do not have a well-developed social schema for social withdrawal (e.g., Bukowski, 1990; Younger & Boyko, 1987; Younger & Piccinin, 1989). Indeed, consistent with this notion, factor analyses of the peer nomination measures (i.e., Revised Class Play; Masten, Morison, & Pellegrini, 1985) typically indicate a single factor containing items related to shyness (e.g., "someone who is very shy"), unsociability (e.g., "someone who would rather play alone than with others"), and isolation by the peer group (e.g., "can't get others to listen"; Masten et al., 1985; Rubin & Mills, 1988; Wichmann, Coplan, & Daniels, 2004).

However, results from other studies suggest that under the right "circumstances," children (even young children) do make distinctions between different types of socially withdrawn peers (Galanaki, 2004). For example, using open-ended questions, Gavinski-Molina, Coplan, and Younger (2003) asked children in grades 1 (6 years old) and 5 (10 years old) to describe peers they knew who frequently "played alone at school." Content analyses of their responses indicated that even the youngest children in the sample provided descriptions of "solitary" children that included unsociable, shy, and actively isolated exemplars.

Coplan, Girardi, Findlay, and Frohlick (2007) asked 5- to 6-year-old children ($N = 137$) about their perceptions, attitudes, and responses to hypothetical vignettes of peers displaying shy, unsociable, aggressive, and prosocial behaviors. Results suggested that even young children made surprisingly "fine-grained" distinctions between shy and unsociable peers. For example, the behaviors of the hypothetical unsociable child were characterized as being more intentional than those of the shy child. As well, unsociable children were also explicitly described as having a lesser desire to play with others than did shy children.

Taken together, these findings provide converging evidence that unsociability in childhood is a distinct form of social withdrawal that is distinguished as such by parents, teachers, and peers. However, results from a recent study by Spangler and Gazelle (2009) raise serious questions about the assessment of unsociability. These researchers conducted a multimethod analysis of social withdrawal with a sample of children ages 8 to 9 years ($N = 163$). Measures of unsociability and "anxious solitude" (a construct similar to shyness), as well as peer exclusion, were obtained from peer nominations, teacher and parent ratings, self-reports, and behavioral observations. An analysis of the multitrait–multimethod matrix indicated that unsociability had poorer convergent and divergent validity than both anxious solitude and peer rejection. As well, there were strong associations between latent estimates of these three constructs. It should be noted that most of the assessments of unsociability were created by the authors for this particular study. Notwithstanding, as we discuss in a later section, these findings reinforce the need for continued development of measures designed specifically to assess unsociability.

CHARACTERISTICS AND BEHAVIORS
OF UNSOCIABLE CHILDREN

The core characteristic underlying unsociability is the expressed preference for solitary activities (e.g., Asendorpf, 1990). Results from empirical studies have largely supported this conceptualization. For example, Coplan et al. (2004) reported that unsociability was positively related to a greater expressed preference for playing alone. Affinity for solitary versus group activities was assessed by having preschool-age children indicate (by pointing to appropriate pictures) whether they would prefer to play with a series of pictured toys (i.e., blocks, slide, dress-up clothes) alone, with a friend, or with an grown-up. Similarly, Coplan et al. (2007) found that, compared to shy and comparison children, young unsociable children indicated that they were less interested in playing and being friends with described hypothetical peers. Most recently, Coplan and Weeks (in press) reported that although unsociable 6- to 8-year-old children were rated by teachers as more socially withdrawn at school, they did not report feeling more lonely than their more sociable counterparts. These findings suggest that unsociable children (at least, as identified by the parental rating scale used in these three studies) do in fact have an expressed preference for solitary activities.

It has also been speculated that although unsociable children may not seek out social activities, they are capable of engaging in competent social interactions when called upon to do so (Asendorpf, 1993). There also appears to be empirical support for this claim. For example, Asendorpf and Meier (1993) monitored the conversations of forty-one 7- to 8-year-old children over a 7-day period. They found that unsociable children (as identified by parent ratings) spent less time engaged in conversation with their peers than did their more sociable agemates. This is consistent with results by Coplan et al. (2004), who reported a negative relation between child unsociability and observed social initiations to peers during free play in preschool.

Notwithstanding, Asendopf and Meier (1993) also reported that despite talking less, unsociable children did not differ from peers in terms of their verbal participation *within* the conversations. Similarly, Harrist et al. (1997) reported that although unsociable young children spent more time alone, they did not differ from their peers in terms of social-cognitive abilities. Thus, despite a lower observed frequency of social initiations and social participation, unsociable children (at least in early childhood) do not appear to have deficits in social-cognitive and social-communicative competence that would interfere with age-appropriate peer interaction.

Finally, we thought it was important to consider specifically the purported link between unsociability and "solitary–passive play," which includes engaging in quiet exploratory and constructive activities while playing alone in the presence of peers (Coplan et al., 1994; Rubin, 1982).

As described earlier, Rubin first suggested that this form of nonsocial play might be comparatively benign in early childhood. Results from several subsequent studies have supported this assertion, largely by failing to find significant associations between observed solitary–passive play and indices of socioemotional maladjustment (Coplan, 2000; Coplan et al., 1994; Coplan & Rubin, 1998; Rubin, 1982; Rubin, Coplan, Fox, & Calkins, 1995). Not surprisingly, this pattern of results led to speculation that solitary–passive play was in fact a "behavioral marker" of unsociability (e.g., Rubin & Asendorpf, 1993).

We have come to believe that this is not the case. Asendorpf (1991) actually postulated that some temperamentally shy children may retreat to solitary–passive play as a means of resolving their approach–avoidance conflicts. In support of this notion, the later findings of Henderson, Marshall, Fox, and Rubin (2004) suggest that engaging in solitary–passive play among peers may also serve as a strategy for shy children to cope with feelings of social unease. There is also evidence linking solitary–passive play in early childhood to externalizing problems and peer rejection (Spinrad et al., 2004), suggesting that some children may retreat into solitary–passive play in response to being excluded by peers. Along these lines, other researchers have suggested that this form of nonsocial play may not be so benign in early childhood, particularly for boys (Coplan, Gavinski-Molina, Lagacé-Séguin, & Wichmann, 2001; Nelson, Rubin, & Fox, 2005).

As well, Coplan et al. (2004) reported that parent-rated unsociability (although related to teacher-rated social withdrawal and fewer observed social initiations made to peers) was not significantly associated with any observed form of social withdrawal during free play (including solitary–passive play). It was speculated that the proximity of other children in the preschool playroom may have resulted in unsociable children spending less time in solitary activities (despite their relatively low rates of social initiations). Similarly, Spangler and Gazelle (2009) failed to find significant associations between observed solitary–passive play and assessments of unsociability from other sources (i.e., parents, teachers, peers, and self-reports).

To us, these findings suggest that an important distinction needs to be made. It may indeed be the case that when playing alone among peers, some unsociable children tend to engage in solitary–passive activities. However, it also appears that other children may engage in frequent solitary–passive play for reasons *other* than preference for solitude. For example, shy children may attempt to regulate their social wariness by engaging in constructive solitary activities, or rejected children may play quietly alone because others do not want to play with them. Consequently, we argue that there is not a "one-to-one" correspondence between solitary–passive behavior and unsociability. As such, an observed high frequency of solitary–passive play should not be the sole criterion for identifying unsociable children.

DEVELOPMENTAL CONSEQUENCES
AND IMPLICATIONS OF UNSOCIABILITY
IN CHILDHOOD

Winnicott (1965) suggested that "many people become able to enjoy solitude before they are out of childhood, and they may even value solitude as a most precious possession" (p. 30). Consistent with these ideas, unsociability has generally been considered a comparatively benign form of social withdrawal, particularly in early childhood (Asendorpf, 1990; Rubin, 1993). However, empirical support for this contention has been somewhat mixed, and the implications of unsociable behavior in the peer group at large are still not well understood.

On the one hand, results from several studies employing direct assessments of unsociability in early childhood indicate an overall lack of associations between this form of social withdrawal and indices of socioemotional difficulties (e.g., Asendorpf & Meier, 1993; Coplan et al., 2004, 2006; Harrist et al., 1997). Moreover, Coplan and Weeks (in press) recently reported that unsociable 6- to 8-year-old children did not differ from their nonwithdrawn counterparts in terms of parent and teacher ratings of internalizing problems, self-reported loneliness, or self-reported school avoidance. Indeed, unsociable children reported liking school even more than did comparison children.

In contrast, it has also been suggested that socially withdrawn children may be perceived to be less approachable than more outgoing children (Richmond, Beatty, & Dyba, 1985). In support of this notion, Coplan and colleagues (2004) reported a positive association between parent-rated unsociability and teacher-rated peer exclusion in their study of preschool-age children. This finding was recently replicated with 6- to 8-year-old children (Coplan & Weeks, in press). These authors speculated that peers may come to feel "put off" by children who rarely invite others to play. Indeed, Coplan et al. (2007) found that unsociable children (as described with hypothetical vignettes) were seen as less attractive playmates and were liked less than both comparison and shy children.

Taken together these findings suggest that despite experiencing some degree of difficulties with their peer relationships, young unsociable children do not appear to feel particularly lonely, poorly about themselves, or anxious. This represents an interesting "disconnect" between the peer group experiences of unsociable children and their socioemotional well-being. A possible explanation for this finding could be the lack of importance that unsociable children may place on their peer relationships. For example, Coplan et al. (2007) recently reported that, compared to their more sociable peers, unsociable children rated hypothetical children displaying peer problem behaviors (e.g., aggression, shyness) as having less of a "negative impact" in class.

The authors speculated that because unsociable children are more socially disconnected from the peer group, they would less likely be influenced by the social behaviors of others. This may be similar to the construct of "rejection sensitivity," which refers to the tendency toward anxious expectation and perception of rejection by peers (Purdie & Downey, 2000). Rejection sensitivity is associated with social anxiety and other internalizing problems (e.g., London, Downey, Bonica, & Paltin, 2007; Sandstrom, Cillessen, & Eisenhower, 2003). It may be the case that unsociable children, who are not thought to be anxious, may also be particularly "insensitive" to being rejected by peers.

To date, we are unaware of any published research specifically assessing the correlates and outcomes of unsociability in later childhood or adolescence. It has been argued that with increasing age, unsociability becomes increasingly associated with negative outcomes (Rubin & Asendorpf, 1993). From this perspective, it can be postulated that even if unsociable young children are not "bothered" at this stage by peer relationship difficulties, poor peer relations have long-term negative effects that have been well documented (Rubin, Bukowski, & Parker, 2006). Thus, if unsociable children continue to be the target of peer exclusion, they may come to experience the pervasive socioemotional difficulties that typically accompany problems with peers. As well, as described earlier, with increasing age, any form of social withdrawal may become viewed as increasingly deviant by peers and lead to rejection (Nelson et al., 2005; Rubin, Hymel, & Mills, 1989; Younger & Piccinin, 1989).

It may be the case that the compounded effects of peer exclusion and increasing perceptions of deviance from age-normal social expectations contribute to greater socioemotional difficulties for unsociable children in middle- and later childhood. This is consistent with the "cumulative deficit" hypothesis forwarded by peer relationship researchers (Rubin et al., 2006). Indeed, this further suggests that unsociable children would continue to experience increasing difficulties through adolescence and into adulthood.

However, it is also possible that the relation between unsociability and outcomes does not follow a linear developmental trend. The amount of time people spend alone during waking hours appears to increase with age, with adults reporting that they spend more time alone than adolescents, and retired adults spending more time alone than adults (Larson, 1990). From a developmental perspective, it has been argued that adolescence may be the developmental period during which we begin to appreciate the benefits of solitude (Larson, 1990; Marcoen, Goossens, & Caes, 1987). For example, Larson (1990) found that adolescents reported more positive affect following periods of solitude versus periods of time with others, although this was not the case for preadolescents. Similarly, adolescence is also marked by an increase in the uses of privacy (e.g., Wolfe & Laufer, 1974), and a greater ability and need to be alone (e.g., Freeman, Csikszentmihalyi, & Larson, 1986; Marcoen & Goossens, 1993).

Moreover, as described earlier, many researchers have stressed the potential positive benefits of solitude in adulthood (e.g., Burke, 1991; Long & Averill, 2003; Long et al., 2003; Maslow, 1970). Indeed, there is some empirical support linking constructs related to unsociability with positive outcomes in adulthood. For example, Eisenberg, Fabes, and Murphy (1995) found that adults who scored low in sociability did not display negative emotionality or maladaptive coping styles, although these *were* attributes of shy adults. Similarly, Hills and Argyle (2001) reported that although extraversion is generally associated with feelings of happiness, a number of introverts also reported being happy. These researchers also found no relation between preference for solitude and happiness, suggesting that both sociable and unsociable people are able to be happy but may find happiness in different ways.

UNANSWERED QUESTIONS AND FUTURE RESEARCH

The study of unsociability in childhood is still very much in its infancy. The recent increased involvement of new researchers bodes well for the future of this research area, but there are still many important issues to be resolved and questions to be answered.

To begin with, we know almost nothing about the etiology of unsociability in childhood. There is some indirect evidence from twins research to suggest that unsociability is influenced both by genetics and a shared environment (e.g., Plomin & Rowe, 1977; Scarr, 1969; Silberg et al., 2005). However, it remains unclear whether unsociability should be classified as a temperamental trait. There is also a clear need for further research examining the role of parents. Coplan et al. (2004) reported that parents of unsociable children placed a lower importance on social goals (i.e., "It is important for my child to make friends") than did parents of more sociable children. These authors suggested that unsociable children might be modeling parental unsociable attitudes and behaviors. Longitudinal studies are required to explore the role of various parental characteristics (e.g., personality, parenting beliefs, parenting styles; cf. Rubin, Mills, & Krasnor, 1989) in the development of unsociability in childhood. Moreover, research from the personality literature suggests that other family factors (e.g., birth order, number of siblings) may also be related to unsociability (e.g., Beck, Burnet, & Vosper, 2006; Nakao et al., 2000). The goal of this research should be to establish a developmental model of unsociability that describes the role of biological, familial, sociodemographic, and extrafamilial factors. Such models have proven to be extremely beneficial in guiding research in the development of shyness and social withdrawal (e.g., Rubin & Mills, 1988).

With continued advancements in the conceptualization of unsociability, current measures need to be revised to reflect changing ideas. Indeed, as noted by Spangler and Gazelle (2009), assessments of unsociability appear to "lag behind" measures of other forms of social withdrawal in terms of their psychometric properties and construct validity. As well, in a research area that historically has been plagued by a lack of conceptual clarity (Rubin & Coplan, 2004), we need to be vigilant about the definition and use of related terms. For example, some researchers are still using the label "unsociability" when measuring constructs such as behavior problems and peer rejection (e.g., Giannopulu, Escolano, Cusin, Citeau, & Dellatolas, 2008).

The creation of new measures will also likely require new methodological approaches. For example, some researchers have attempted to use Gray's (1972) concept of the behavioral inhibition and activation systems (i.e., BIS–BAS) to identify unsociable children thought to exhibit low behavioral activation and low behavioral inhibition (e.g., Coplan et al., 2006). The development and validation of new self-report measures for use with older children is also required. In older children and adolescents, self-reports appear to have the highest face validity in terms of the assessment of internal motivational states that are presumed to underlie unsociability.

Further exploration of potential sex differences in unsociability would also seem warranted. Results from a growing number of studies suggest that shyness and social withdrawal (in general) may be a greater risk factor for boys than for girls (e.g., Coplan et al., 2004; Eisenberg et al., 1998; Gazelle & Ladd, 2003; Morison & Masten, 1991). Rubin and Coplan (2004) argued that these findings reflect a greater social acceptance of shyness for girls than for boys in Western cultures. There is some preliminary evidence that these same attitudes may apply to unsociability. Results from a few recent studies suggest that unsociability is also more strongly associated with peer exclusion and social difficulties for boys than for girls (Coplan et al., 2004; Coplan & Weeks, in press; Spangler & Gazelle, 2009).

Larson (1997) noted that although research on solitude in children typically occurs in the school setting, much of children's time alone actually occurs outside of school. This highlights the importance of examining the behavior of unsociable children across different contexts (i.e., home, school, neighborhood). It remains to be seen whether unsociability is stable across contexts. Indeed, different social contexts impart a different level of "control" to children with regard to their social interactions. For example, at school, where activities are more structured, unsociable children may end up spending more time interacting with peers. However, if unsociable children do indeed prefer to play alone, we might expect them to spend considerably more time by themselves while at home.

We also need to explore the "quality" of the activities in which children engage when alone. Long et al. (2003) reported that while at home alone, adults tend to engage in distracting activities, possibly because more productive activities require more inner resources when other people are absent (Long & Averill, 2003). Unsociable children, who are presumably more content spending time alone, might feel less of a need to distract themselves and thus use their time in more productive ways. Moreover, we need to carefully define exactly what it means to be "alone." Is an adolescent in her room by herself, working on homework while simultaneously exchanging e-mails, texts, or instant messages with friends, considered to be "alone"?

As well, the meaning and implication of unsociability needs to be explored in different cultures. Growing evidence suggests that shyness is more positively evaluated in China because of its more collectivistic nature (Chen, Cen, Li, & Hi, 2005; Chen, Rubin, & Li, 1995). The consequences of unsociability may also vary across cultural contexts. Indeed, Chen (2008) speculated that unsociable children would face more problems than shy children in China, because they are intentionally removing themselves from the collective. However, it remains to be seen whether reliable and valid distinctions between the subtypes of social withdrawal are even made in other cultures.

Finally, from a conceptual and methodological perspective, we also need to bridge the existing gap between unsociability in childhood and similar constructs in the adult personality literature. Indeed, without longitudinal studies, we cannot be sure of the continuity of these constructs across the lifespan (see Asendorpf, Chapter 8, this volume). In this regard, it remains unknown what types of long-term consequences might be associated with unsociability over time. As described earlier, there exist competing hypotheses. If all forms of social withdrawal become increasingly maladaptive with age (e.g., Nelson et al., 2005; Rubin & Asendorpf, 1993), then unsociable children would be predicted to experience more socioemotional problems in adolescence and into adulthood. In contrast, if unsociability leads to a greater appreciation of solitude in adulthood, unsociable children might grow up to become content, contemplative, and self-actualized (Maslow, 1970).

Thus, we must continue to explore both the negative and potentially positive implications of solitude across the lifespan. Although extremely shy children may benefit from targeted early intervention and prevention, it remains unclear as to when, or even whether, ameliorative intervention programs should be administered in the case of extreme unsociability. We remain hopeful that future research will help to clarify when it might be acceptable to "leave a child alone."

ACKNOWLEDGMENTS

This research was supported by a Social Science and Humanities Research Council of Canada Research Grant to Robert J. Coplan and a Social Science and Humanities Research Council of Canada Doctoral Fellowship to Murray Weeks.

REFERENCES

Arbeau, K. A., & Coplan, R. J. (2007). Kindergarten teachers' beliefs and responses to hypothetical prosocial, asocial, and antisocial children. *Merrill–Palmer Quarterly, 53*, 291–318.

Asendorpf, J. B. (1990). Beyond social withdrawal: Shyness, unsociability, and peer avoidance.*Human Development, 33*, 250–259.

Asendorpf, J. B. (1991). Development of inhibited children's coping with unfamiliarity. *Child Development, 62*, 1460–1474.

Asendorpf, J. B. (1993). Abnormal shyness in children. *Journal of Child Psychology and Psychiatry, 34*, 1069–1081.

Asendorpf, J. B., & Meier, G. H. (1993). Personality effects on children's speech in everyday life: Sociability-mediated exposure and shyness-mediated reactivity to social situations. *Journal of Personality and Social Psychology, 64*, 1072–1083.

Bates, A. P. (1964). Privacy—a useful concept? *Social Forces, 42*, 429–434.

Beck, E., Burnet, K. L., & Vosper, J. (2006). Birth-order effects on facets of extraversion. *Personality and Individual Differences, 40*(5), 953–959.

Berscheid, E. (1977). Privacy: A hidden variable in experimental social psychology. *Journal of Social Issues, 33*, 85–101.

Bowker, A., Bukowski, W., Zargarpour, S., & Hoza, B. (1998). A structural and functional analysis of a two-dimensional model of withdrawal. *Merrill–Palmer Quarterly, 44*, 447–463

Bukowski, W. M. (1990). Age differences in children's memory of information about aggressive, socially withdrawn, and prosociable boys. *Child Development, 61*(5), 1326–1334.

Burger, J. M. (1995). Individual differences in preference for solitude. *Journal of Research in Personality, 29*, 85–108.

Burke, N. (1991). College psychotherapy and the development of a capacity for solitude. *Journal of College Student Psychotherapy, 6*, 59–86.

Cheek, J. M., & Buss, A. H. (1981). Shyness and sociability. *Journal of Personality and Social Psychology, 41*, 330–339.

Chen, X. (2008). Shyness and unsociability in cultural context. In A. S. LoCoco, K. H. Rubin, & C. Zappulla (Eds.), *L'isolamento sociale durante l'infanzia [Social withdrawal in childhood]* (pp. 143–160). Milan: Unicopli.

Chen, X., Cen, G., Li, D., & He, Y. (2005). Social functioning and adjustment in Chinese children: The imprint of historical time. *Child Development, 76*, 182–195.

Chen, X., Rubin, K. H., & Li, Z. (1995). Social functioning and adjustment in Chinese children: A longitudinal study. *Developmental Psychology, 31*, 531–539.

Coplan, R. J. (2000). Assessing nonsocial play in early childhood: Conceptual and methodological approaches. In K. Gitlin-Weiner, A. Sangdrund, & C. Schaefer (Eds.), *Play diagnosis and assessment* (2nd ed., pp. 563–598). New York: Wiley.

Coplan, R. J., & Armer, M. (2007). A "multitude" of solitude: A closer look at social withdrawal and nonsocial play in early childhood. *Child Development Perspectives, 1,* 26–32.

Coplan, R. J., Gavinski-Molina, M. H., Lagacé-Séguin, D. G., & Wichmann, C. (2001). When girls versus boys play alone: Nonsocial play and adjustment in kindergarten. *Developmental Psychology, 37,* 464–474.

Coplan, R. J., Girardi, A., Findlay, L. C., & Frohlick, S. L. (2007). Understanding solitude: Young children's attitudes and responses towards hypothetical socially withdrawn peers. *Social Development, 16,* 390–409.

Coplan, R. J., Prakash, K., O'Neil, K., & Armer, M. (2004). Do you "want" to play?: Distinguishing between conflicted shyness and social disinterest in early childhood. *Developmental Psychology, 40,* 244–258.

Coplan, R. J., & Rubin, K. H. (1998). Exploring and assessing non-social play in the preschool: The development and validation of the Preschool Play Behavior Scale. *Social Development, 7,* 72–91.

Coplan, R. J., Rubin, K. H., Fox, N. A., Calkins, S. D., & Stewart, S. L. (1994). Being alone, playing alone, and acting alone: Distinguishing among reticence and passive and active solitude in young children. *Child Development, 65,* 129–137.

Coplan, R. J., & Weeks, M. (in press). Unsociability in middle childhood: Conceptualization, assessment, and associations with socio-emotional functioning. *Merrill–Palmer Quarterly.*

Coplan, R. J ., Wilson, J., Frohlick, S. L., & Zelenski, J. (2006). A person-oriented analysis of behavioral inhibition and behavioral activation in childhood. *Personality and Individual Differences, 41,* 917–927.

Eisenberg, N., Fabes, R. A., & Murphy, B. C. (1995). Relations of shyness and low sociability to regulation and emotionality. *Journal of Personality and Social Psychology, 68,* 505–517.

Eisenberg, N., Shepard, S. A., Fabes, R. A., Murphy, B. C., & Guthrie, I. K. (1998). Shyness and children's emotionality, regulation, and coping: Contemporaneous, longitudinal, and across-context relations. *Child Development, 69,* 767–790.

Eysenck, H. J. (1947). *Dimensions of personality.* Oxford, UK: Kegan Paul.

Eysenck, H. J. (1956). The questionnaire measurement of neuroticism and extraversion. *Revista de Psicologia, 50,* 113–140.

Eysenck, H. J., & Eysenck, S. B. G. (1969). *Personality structure and measurement.* London: Routledge & Kegan Paul.

Freeman, M., Csikszentmihalyi, M., & Larson, R. (1986). Adolescence and its recollection: Towards an interpretive model of development. *Merrill–Palmer Quarterly, 32,* 167–185.

Galanaki, E. (2004). Are children able to distinguish among the concepts of aloneness, loneliness, and solitude? *International Journal of Behavioral Development, 28,* 435–443.

Gavinski-Molina, M. H., Coplan, R. J., & Younger, A. (2003). A closer look at children's knowledge about social isolation. *Journal of Research in Childhood Education, 18,* 93–104.

Gazelle, H., & Ladd, G. W. (2003). Anxious solitude and peer exclusion: A diathesis–stress model of internalizing trajectories in childhood. *Child Development, 74,* 257–278.

Gazelle, H., & Rudolph, K. D. (2004). Moving toward and away from the world: Social approach and avoidance trajectories in anxious solitary youth. *Child Development, 75,* 1–21.

Giannopulu, I., Escolano, S., Cusin, F., Citeau, H., & Dellatolas, G. (2008). Teachers' reporting of behavioural problems and cognitive–academic performances in children aged 5–7 years. *British Journal of Educational Psychology, 78,* 127–147.

Gray, J. A. (1972). The psychophysiological nature of introversion–extraversion: A modification of Eysenck's Theory. In V. D. Nebylitsyn & J. A. Gray (Eds.), *Biological bases of individual behaviour* (pp. 182–205). New York and London: Academic Press.

Harrist, A. W., Zaia, A. F., Bates, J. E., Dodge, K. A., & Pettit, G. S. (1997). Subtypes of social withdrawal in early childhood: Sociometric status and social-cognitive differences across four years. *Child Development, 68,* 278–294.

Hay, D., & Morisey, A. (1978). Reports of ecstatic, paranormal, or religious experience in Great Britain and the United States—a comparison of trends. *Journal for the Scientific Study of Religion, 17,* 255–268.

Henderson, H. A., Marshall, P. J., Fox, N. A., & Rubin, K. H. (2004). Psychophysiological and behavioral evidence for varying forms and functions of nonsocial behavior in preschoolers. *Child Development, 75,* 251–263.

Hill, C. A. (1987). Affiliation motivation: people who need people ... but in different ways. *Journal of Personality and Social Psychology, 52,* 1008–1018.

Hills, P., & Argyle, M. (2001). Happiness, introversion–extraversion and happy introverts. *Personality and Individual Differences, 30,* 595–608.

Jennings, K. D. (1975). People versus object orientation, social behavior, and intellectual abilities in children. *Developmental Psychology, 11,* 511–519.

Ladd, G. W., & Profilet, S. M. (1996). The Child Behavior Scale: A teacher-report measure of young children's aggressive, withdrawn, and prosocial behaviors. *Developmental Psychology, 32*(6), 1008–1024.

Larson, R. W. (1990). The solitary side of life: An examination of the time people spend alone from childhood to old age. *Developmental Review, 10,* 155–183.

Leary, M. R., Herbst, K. C., & McCrary, F. (2003). Finding pleasure in solitary activities: Desire for aloneness or disinterest in social contact? *Personality and Individual Differences, 35,* 59–68.

London, B., Downey, G., Bonica, C., & Paltin, I. (2007). Social causes and consequences of rejection sensitivity. *Journal of Research on Adolescence, 17*(3), 481–506.

Long, C. R., & Averill, J. R. (2003). Solitude: An exploration of benefits of being alone. *Journal for the Theory of Social Behavior, 33,* 21–44.

Long, C. R., Seburn, M., Averill, J. R., & More, T. A. (2003). Solitude experiences:

Varieties, settings, and individual differences. *Personality and Social Psychology Bulletin, 29*(5), 578–583.

Marcoen, A., & Goossens, L. (1993). Loneliness, attitude towards aloneness, and solitude: Age differences and development significance during adolescence. In S. Jackson & H. Rodriguez-Tome (Eds.), *Adolescence and its social worlds* (pp. 197–227). Hillsdale, NJ: Erlbaum.

Marcoen, A., Goossens, L., & Caes, P. (1987). Loneliness in pre- through late adolescence: Exploring the contributions of a multidimentional approach. *Journal of Youth and Adolescence, 16*(6), 561–577.

Maslow, A. H. (1970). *Motivation and personality* (2nd ed.). New York: Harper & Row.

Masten, A. S., Morison, P., & Pellegrini, D. S. (1985). A Revised Class Play method of peer assessment. *Developmental Psychology, 21*, 523–533.

Morison, P., & Masten, A. S. (1991). Peer reputation in middle childhood as a predictor of adaptation in adolescence: A seven-year follow-up. *Child Development, 62*, 991–1007.

Nakao, K., Takaishi, J., Tatsuta, K., Katayama, H., Iwase, M., Yorifuji, K., et al. (2000). The influences of family environment on personality traits. *Psychiatry and Clinical Neurosciences, 54*(1), 91–95.

Nelson, L. J., Rubin, K. H., & Fox, N. A. (2005). Social withdrawal, observed peer acceptance, and the development of self-perceptions in children ages 4 to 7 years. *Early Childhood Research Quarterly, 20*, 185–200.

Nikitin, J., & Freund, A. M. (2008). The role of social approach and avoidance motives for subjective well-being and the successful transition to adulthood. *Applied Psychology, 57*, 90–111.

Pedersen, D. M. (1979). Dimensions of privacy. *Perceptual and Motor Skills, 48*, 1291–1297.

Plomin, R., & Rowe, D. C. (1977). A twin study of temperament in young children. *Journal of Psychology, 97*, 107–113.

Purcell, R. Z., & Keller, M. J. (1989). Characteristics of leisure activities which may lead to leisure satisfaction among older adults. *Activities, Adaptation and Aging, 13*(4), 17–29.

Purdie, V., & Downey, G. (2000). Rejection sensitivity and adolescent girls' vulnerability to relationship-centered difficulties. *Child Maltreatment, 5*(4), 339–349.

Richmond, V. P., Beatty, M. J., & Dyba, P. (1985). Shyness and popularity: Children's views. *Western Journal of Speech Communication, 49*, 116–125.

Rubin, K. H. (1982). Nonsocial play in preschoolers: Necessarily evil? *Child Development, 53*, 651–657.

Rubin, K. H. (1993). The Waterloo Longitudinal Project: Correlates and consequences of social withdrawal from childhood to adolescence. In K. H. Rubin & J. B. Asendorpf (Eds.), *Social withdrawal, inhibition, and shyness in childhood* (pp. 291–314). Hillsdale, NJ: Erlbaum.

Rubin, K. H., & Asendorpf, J. B. (1993). Social withdrawal, inhibition, and shyness in childhood: Conceptual and definitional issues. In K. H. Rubin & J. B. Asendorpf (Eds.), *Social withdrawal, inhibition, and shyness in childhood* (pp. 3–17). Hillsdale, NJ: Erlbaum.

Rubin, K. H., Bukowski, W., & Parker, J. (2006). Peer interactions, relationships, and groups. In N. Eisenberg, W. Damon, & R.M. Lerner (Eds.), *Handbook of child psychology: Social, emotional, and personality development* (6th ed., pp. 571–645). New York: Wiley.

Rubin, K. H., & Coplan, R. J. (2004). Paying attention to and not neglecting social withdrawal and social isolation. *Merrill–Palmer Quarterly, 50,* 506–534.

Rubin, K. H., Coplan, R. J., & Bowker, J. (2009). Social withdrawal in childhood. *Annual Review of Psychology, 60,* 141–171.

Rubin, K. H., Coplan, R. J., Fox, N. A., & Calkins, S. D. (1995). Emotionality, emotion regulation, and preschoolers' social adaptation. *Development and Psychopathology, 7,* 49–62.

Rubin, K. H., Hymel, S., & Mills, R. S. (1989). Sociability and social withdrawal in childhood: Stability and outcomes. *Journal of Personality* [Special issue: Long-term stability and change in personality], *57*(2), 237–255.

Rubin, K. H., & Mills, R. S L. (1988). The many faces of social isolation in childhood. *Journal of Consulting and Clinical Psychology, 56,* 916–924.

Rubin, K. H., Mills, R. S. L., & Krasnor, L. R. (1989). Parental beliefs and children's social competence. In B. Schneider, G. Atilli, J. Nadel, & R. Weissberg (Eds.), *Social competence in developmental perspective* (pp. 313–331). Dordrecht, Netherlands: Kluwer International.

Sandstrom, M. J., Cillessen, A. H. N., & Eisenhower, A. (2003). Children's appraisal of peer rejection experiences: Impact on social and emotional adjustment. *Social Development, 12,* 530–550.

Scarr, S. (1969). Social introversion–extroversion as a heritable response. *Child Development, 40,* 823–832.

Silberg, J. L., San Miguel, V. F., Murrelle, E. L., Prom, E., Bates, J. E., Canino, G., et al. (2005). Genetic and environmental influences on temperament in the first year of life: The Puerto Rico Infant Twin Study (PRINTS). *Twin Research and Human Genetics, 8*(4), 328–336.

Spangler, T., & Gazelle, H. (2009). Anxious solitude, unsociability, and peer exclusion in middle childhood: A multitrait–multimethod matrix. *Social Development, 18,* 833–856.

Spinrad, T. L., Eisenberg, N., Harris, E., Hanish, L., Fabes, R. A., Kupanoff, K., et al. (2004). The relation of children's everyday nonsocial peer play behavior to their emotionality, regulation, and social functioning. *Child Development, 40,* 67–80.

Storr, A. (1988). *Solitude: A return to the self.* New York: Free Press.

Thijs, J. T., Koomen, H. M. Y., de Jong, P. F., van der Leij, A., & van Leeuwen, M. G. P. (2004). Internalizing behaviors among kindergarten children: Measuring dimensions of social withdrawal with a checklist. *Journal of Clinical Child and Adolescent Psychology, 33,* 802–812.

Wichmann, C., Coplan, R. J., & Daniels, T. (2004). The social cognitions of socially withdrawn children. *Social Development, 13*(3), 377–392.

Winnicott, D. W. (1965). *The maturational processes and the facilitating environment: Studies in the theory of emotional development.* New York: International Universities Press.

Wolfe, M., & Laufer, R. (1974). The concept of privacy in childhood and adolescence. In D. Carson (Ed.), *Man–environment interactions, Part II*. Stroudsburg, PA: Dowden, Hutchinson & Ross.

Xu, Y., Farver, J., Chang, L., Zhang, Z., & Yu, L. (2007). Moving away or fitting in?: Understanding shyness in Chinese children. *Merrill–Palmer Quarterly, 53*, 527–556.

Younger, A. J., & Boyko, K. A. (1987). Aggression and withdrawal as social schemas underlying children's peer perceptions. *Child Development, 58*, 1094–1100.

Younger, A. J., & Piccinin, A. M. (1989). Children's recall of aggressive and withdrawn behaviors: Recognition memory and likability judgments. *Child Development, 60*, 580–590.

5

Biological Moderators of Infant Temperament and Its Relation to Social Withdrawal

NATHAN A. FOX
BETHANY C. REEB-SUTHERLAND

It has been 25 years since Jerome Kagan and his colleagues published their first of several articles describing the behavior of children they called "behaviorally inhibited." In that original article, Garcia-Coll, Kagan, and Reznick (1984) presented data on children (21–24 months of age) who had been identified via a two-stage process: Parents were recruited by letter or phone call, then interviewed with a version of the Toddler Temperament Scale (Fullard, McDevitt, & Carey, 1984), which asked about their child's approach–withdrawal behavior. These questions pertained to the child's behavior in novel or unfamiliar situations. Based upon their answers, a subset of children was classified as "inhibited" (those who were reported as being fearful or withdrawn in novel or unfamiliar situations) or "noninhibited" (those who were reported as being fearless or approach-oriented in these novel or unfamiliar situations) and invited to the laboratory to participate in two behavioral sessions (3–5 weeks apart). In the laboratory, children's behavioral responses to novel social and nonsocial challenges were observed and coded. In addition, heart rate was recorded while the child was presented with visual and auditory stimuli. The authors reported that the tendency to remain behaviorally inhibited, to display vigilance to novel events and withdraw from social interaction, was stable over the two laboratory sessions, and that behaviorally inhibited children had rapid and

84

stable heart rates. As well, a follow-up of these children 10 months later found moderate stability across time.

Since their initial observations, Kagan and colleagues have gone on to identify physiological differences in reactivity between inhibited and non-inhibited children (Kagan, Reznick, & Snidman, 1987, 1988a; McManis, Kagan, Snidman, & Woodward, 2002; Woodward et al., 2001) and patterns of behavioral reactivity observed during early infancy that identify those children who display behavioral inhibition later in childhood (Kagan & Snidman, 1991). In addition, Kagan observed and described the continuity of behavioral inhibition from early toddlerhood to middle childhood (Kagan, 1994; Kagan, Reznick, Snidman, Gibbons, & Johnson, 1988b).

Kagan's approach to the study of temperament was groundbreaking in a crucial aspect. Reading widely the then-current neuroscience literature on the circuitry involved in fear conditioning, particularly the role of the amygdala, he linked the behaviors and physiological responses of behaviorally inhibited children to that structure and circuit (Kagan, 1994; Kagan et al., 1988a). He reasoned that the responses to novelty he observed (i.e., freezing behavior, increased latency to approach) were similar to behaviors observed in animal models of fear conditioning and, as in animals, these behaviors were the result of a hyperactive amygdala (Davis, 1986; LeDoux, 2000; LeDoux, Iwata, Cicchetti, & Reis, 1988). Indeed, Kagan, along with others, found support for this hypothesis examining physiological responses in behaviorally inhibited children that reflected outputs of a hyperactive amygdala (Gunnar, Tout, de Haan, Pierce, & Stansbury, 1997; Kagan et al., 1987, 1988a; Pérez-Edgar, Schmidt, Henderson, Schulkin, & Fox, 2008; Schmidt et al., 1997). Specifically, behaviorally inhibited children tended to have increased baseline measures of the stress hormone cortisol compared to uninhibited children (Kagan et al., 1987; Pérez-Edgar et al., 2008; Schmidt et al., 1997), as well as increased cortisol reactivity during interaction with unfamiliar peers (Gunnar et al., 1997), although these results have not been entirely consistent (de Haan, Gunnar, Tout, Hart, & Stansbury, 1998; Nachmias, Gunnar, Mangelsdorf, Parritz, & Buss, 1996; Schmidt, Fox, Schulkin, & Gold, 1999). In addition, behaviorally inhibited children displayed increased heart rate compared to uninhibited children in response to novelty (Kagan et al., 1987, 1988a). Elevated stable heart rate, as well, has been found to predict stability in behavioral inhibition (Marshall & Stevenson-Hinde, 1998). In linking his work to that of LeDoux et al. (1988) and Davis (1986), as well as other neuroscientists working in the area of fear conditioning, Kagan placed the study of behavioral inhibition squarely within the context of biological psychiatry and the development of anxiety disorders. Much of the research by neuroscientists studying fear conditioning had already been framed to address issues of mechanisms underlying anxiety. Understanding the neural mechanisms involved in fear learning was thought to provide insight into the etiology of anxiety and possible treatment interventions. Linking this animal work to the study of temperamental behavioral inhibition was a key element toward understanding the importance of this temperament for later psychopathology.

There have been a number of longitudinal studies in which children observed to display behavioral inhibition are followed up in adolescence and screened for psychiatric disorders. The findings from these studies have been mixed. The presence of behavioral inhibition in early childhood has been shown to be a risk factor for anxiety in childhood (Hirshfeld et al., 1992; Rosenbaum et al., 1991, 1992) and adolescence (Schwartz, Snidman, & Kagan, 1996a, 1999), particularly with regard to social phobia (Biederman et al., 2001; Schwartz et al., 1999). The link is strongest among adolescents who display consistent signs of inhibition across multiple testing points in childhood (Biederman et al., 1993). For example, Biederman et al. (2001) found that 15% of young adults identified previously as behaviorally inhibited toddlers were diagnosed with generalized social phobia. In addition, Schwartz and colleagues (1999) found that adolescents who were inhibited at the age of 2 years were more likely than their uninhibited peers to show symptoms of social anxiety, as assessed by a semistructured diagnostic interview (i.e., Diagnostic Interview Schedule for Children [DISC]). Indeed, 61% of the adolescents had current symptoms, and 80% had shown symptoms of anxiety at one point in their lifetime. Although these studies suggest that many behaviorally inhibited individuals go on to develop anxiety disorders, many—in fact, the majority—do not. This discontinuity from childhood to adolescence is similar to the discontinuity between adolescence and adulthood in the incidence of anxiety disorders. For example, Pine (2001, 2002) found that most adolescents diagnosed with an anxiety disorder do not continue to display this disorder as adults. In both instances, the relation between temperamental behavioral inhibition and anxiety disorders, and between adolescent anxiety and incidence of anxiety in adulthood, certain factors must moderate these relations. In our research over the past number of years, we have attempted to identify just what these factors may be. Possible candidates include neural or psychological processes that are involved in the regulation of emotion, including approach–withdrawal motivational bias, threat perception, and attention control. In addition, there may be underlying genetic differences between those behaviorally inhibited children who maintain this profile and those who change over time. In this chapter, we review our work examining these factors as they pertain to a longitudinal cohort we have been studying over the past 18 years.

CONTEXT FOR THE RESEARCH

Kagan and colleagues hypothesized that one can identify infants who will exhibit behavioral inhibition later in childhood based upon initial levels of reactivity to novelty. Kagan and Snidman (1991) presented novel auditory and visual stimuli to a sample of 4-month-old infants and selected those infants who displayed heightened motor reactivity and negative affect. They reported that a significant percentage of these infants exhibited signs of behavioral inhibition in early childhood. Based upon these findings, N. Fox, Henderson, Rubin, Calkins, and Schmidt (2001) screened over 400 typically developing 4-month-old infants, using stimuli similar to those described by Kagan, and coded their motor and emotional reactivity in a similar manner. Roughly 15% of the sample displayed high motor and negative reactivity, 15% displayed high motor and positive reactivity, and 15% displayed low motor and low-positive or negative reactivity. These children ($N = 155$) were subsequently followed up at the University of Maryland's Child Development Laboratory when they were 9, 14, 24, 48, and 84 months of age. At 9 months of age, brain electrical activity was recorded by electroencephalogram (EEG), while infants attended to an attractive event. At 14 months of age, EEG data were collected and infants were observed in the Ainsworth Strange Situation and in a set of protocols thought to elicit behaviors reflecting behavioral inhibition. These included interaction with an unfamiliar adult and a clown, and presentation of a mechanical robot and a tunnel with an attractive toy placed inside. At 24 months, children were again observed in a similar set of protocols in the lab. At both ages, latency to approach, proximity to mother, and affect were coded for each episode, and these variables were aggregated at each age to create a composite score of behavioral inhibition. At ages 4 and 7 years, in collaboration with Kenneth Rubin, play quartets were formed (same-age, same-sex children), with an attempt to place one behaviorally inhibited child and three noninhibited children in the same playgroup. The children were observed in a set of structured and semistructured interactions, and their behaviors were coded by Rubin and colleagues using his Play Observation Scale (POS; Rubin, 1989; Rubin, Maioni, & Hornung, 1976). A measure of social reticence (unoccupied, onlooking behavior plus anxious behaviors during free play) was computed (Coplan, Rubin, Fox, & Calkins, 1994).

These assessments led to a series of manuscripts (Calkins, Fox, & Marshall, 1996; N. Fox et al., 2001; Henderson, Fox, & Rubin, 2001; Henderson, Marshall, Fox, & Rubin, 2004; Rubin, Hastings, Stewart, Henderson, & Chen, 1997) that catalogued the trajectories of infants selected as high motor/high cry at 4 months of age, and the continuity of behavioral inhibition from age 14 months through age 7 years. In general, there was modest continuity in the sample, with behaviorally inhibited boys more likely to remain so over time. For a full review of this work, readers are referred to N. Fox, Henderson, et al. (2005).

Further follow-up of this sample took place when children were between the ages of 13 and 16 years. At that time, participants again returned to the Child Development Laboratory, where they underwent intensive assessments of their physiological reactivity, attention, and social behavior. A number of articles detailing the data from these assessments are recently published or "in press" (McDermott, Pérez-Edgar, Henderson, Pine, & Fox, 2009; Pérez-Edgar, Fox, Bar-Haim, Martin McDermott, & Pine, in press; Pérez-Edgar et al., 2007; Reeb-Sutherland et al., 2009; Reeb-Sutherland et al., 2009). The data presented in this chapter represent work from this longitudinal effort and as such are informed by the patterns of continuity and discontinuity found within this sample.

FRONTAL ACTIVATION ASYMMETRY

Previous studies have examined asymmetry in EEG activity, particularly in the frontal regions of the cortex, as a trait measure reflecting dispositions related to motivationally biased behavior (N. Fox et al., 2001; Schmidt & Fox, 1994; Tomarken, Davidson, Wheeler, & Doss, 1992; Wheeler, Davidson, & Tomarken, 1993). Davidson was first to hypothesize that increased activation of the left-frontal cortex, as measured by alpha EEG suppression in left-frontal EEG electrode sites, reflects a disposition related to approach motivation, whereas increased right-frontal activation, as measured by right-frontal EEG alpha suppression, reflected a disposition related to withdrawal motivation (Davidson, 1995; Fox, 1991; Fox, Calkins, & Bell, 1994). Several studies examining EEG frontal activation differences between behaviorally inhibited and noninhibited children from our own and Kagan's laboratory provide evidence to support this hypothesis. Specifically, we found that behaviorally inhibited individuals display greater right-frontal EEG activation compared to noninhibited individuals during infancy (Calkins et al., 1996), early childhood (Fox, Schmidt, Calkins, Rubin, & Coplan, 1996; Henderson et al., 2004), and late childhood (McManis et al., 2002). In addition, children who displayed continuity in their behavioral inhibition from infancy to childhood also showed greater right-frontal activation during infancy compared to those who did not show continuity (N. Fox et al., 2001). In a study examining the moderating role of EEG asymmetry on the relation between infant reactivity and childhood social reticence, Henderson et al. (2001) found that infants displaying negative reactivity to novelty at 9 months of age demonstrated socially reticent behavior at age 4 years if they also displayed relative increases in right-frontal activation at 9 months of age. No relation was found between negative reactivity and social wariness in infants who displayed greater left-frontal activation during infancy. To summarize, these results suggested that frontal EEG asymmetry might be a reliable biological marker to distinguish between inhibited and noninhibited individuals. As well, the data suggest that frontal EEG asymmetry may also be a predictor of children who are more likely to remain behaviorally inhibited throughout childhood and who, therefore, are more likely to develop an anxiety disorder.

NOVELTY DETECTION

One of the primary descriptors of behavioral inhibition in the first reports by Kagan and colleagues was that behaviorally inhibited children manifest signs of heightened vigilance to novelty (Garcia-Coll, Kagan, & Reznick, 1984; Kagan, Reznick, Clarke, Snidman, & Garcia-Coll, 1984; Kagan, Reznick, & Gibbons, 1989). The propensity to display increased vigilance among behaviorally inhibited children may prevent effective regulation of emotional responses to novel situations, and may both sustain and exacerbate social and affective maladjustment (E. Fox, Russo, Bowles, & Dutton, 2001; E. Fox, Russo, & Georgiou, 2005). Kagan suggested that the heightened vigilance toward novelty displayed by behaviorally inhibited children is the result of a hyperactive amygdala (Kagan, 1994; Kagan et al., 1987, 1988a). The amygdala, a region of the brain that is part of the limbic system, has long been associated with emotion processing, particularly the processing of fear stimuli (Davis, 1998; LeDoux, 2000, 2008). Initial studies examining amygdala hyperactivity in behaviorally inhibited children used indirect measures of amygdala output, such as the stress hormone cortisol (Kagan et al., 1987, 1988a; Schmidt et al., 1997) and heart rate (Kagan et al., 1987, 1988a; Marshall & Stevenson-Hinde, 1998). However, recent studies have examined direct measures of amygdala activation during the presentation of novel stimuli in behaviorally inhibited and noninhibited individuals using functional magnetic resonance imaging (fMRI). Schwartz, Wright, Shin, Kagan, and Rauch (2003) compared amygdala activation during the viewing of familiar and novel emotionally neutral faces of adults identified as either behaviorally inhibited or noninhibited at 2 years of age. Compared to noninhibited adults, behaviorally inhibited adults displayed increased amygdala activation in response to viewing novel versus familiar faces. Consistent with these results, adults rated as being high on measures of shyness showed greater amygdala activation than bold adults when viewing emotionally neutral faces of unfamiliar strangers compared to neutral faces of personally familiar individuals (Beaton et al., 2008).

Expanding upon these studies, Pérez-Edgar et al. (2007) examined neural activation using functional neuroimaging in adolescents characterized as behaviorally inhibited in our longitudinal study, using an emotion face-rating task. Participants were presented with multiple exemplars of faces displaying a range of emotions (happy, fearful, angry, neutral) and were asked to view the face passively, rate the width of the nose, and report on how afraid they were or how hostile the face appeared to them. Two interesting results were found. First, as predicted, behaviorally inhibited adolescents displayed heightened amygdala activation when shown a fearful face and asked to rate how afraid they were of the face (compared to their passive viewing of that face). Second, when shown a happy face and asked to rate how afraid they were of that face, these same behaviorally inhibited participants displayed increased amygdala activation as well. The authors interpreted this latter result as reflecting a condition of increased uncertainty and novelty that elicited the heightened amygdala activity.

Studies in our lab have also used event-related potentials (ERPs) to examine differences in the neural activation associated with novelty detection between behaviorally inhibited and noninhibited children. Bar-Haim, Marshall, Fox, Schorr, and Gordon-Salant (2003), for example, examined individual differences in novelty detection by presenting to these children (7 to 12 years old) an auditory oddball paradigm with two tones, a frequent (standard) tone and an infrequent (deviant) tone. The mismatch negativity (MMN), an electrophysiological marker of auditory preperceptual novelty detection (Naatanen & Alho, 1995; Naatanen, Paavilainen, Tiitinen, Jiang, & Alho, 1993), was then computed and examined. Unexpectedly, inhibited children displayed decreased MMN amplitude compared to noninhibited children (Bar-Haim et al., 2003). The authors speculated that these differences might be the consequence of individual differences in either top-down or bottom-up processes. Therefore, the observed difference in MMN between inhibited and noninhibited children may be driven by either higher-order affective areas of the brain, such as the amygdala, or by lower-order processes that feed forward and influence the later processing and evaluation of change in sensory information. Using a somewhat different paradigm in which complex, novel sounds (e.g., cork popping, dog barking) were presented in addition to standard and deviant tones, Marshall, Reeb, and Fox (2009) examined novelty detection in 9-month-old infants selected for high-motor/high-distress reactivity at 4 months of age. They found that these negatively reactive infants displayed an increased response to deviant versus standard tones compared to positively reactive infants. Surprisingly, the positively reactive infants showed an increased response to the novel sounds compared to that of the negatively reactive infants. The authors suggest that these differences in novelty processing may reflect individual differences in novelty preference (Berlyne, 1960). These results, along with the previously discussed findings on amygdala activation, suggest that behaviorally inhibited and noninhibited individuals differ in their processing of novel information, and that these underlying neural differences may influence the expression of behavioral withdrawal in the presence of novel stimuli.

To further investigate the possibility that measures of novelty detection serve as a potential moderator of the relation between behavioral inhibition and anxiety disorders, Reeb-Sutherland, Vanderwert, et al. (2009) studied the longitudinal cohort during adolescence using a novel auditory oddball task to examine P3 amplitude. In contrast to the MMN, which is an early ERP difference wave reflecting automatic novelty detection, the P3 component is associated with later attention processes, particularly the orienting response (Cycowicz & Friedman, 1998; Friedman, Cycowicz, & Gaeta, 2001). Reeb-Sutherland, Vanderwert, et al. (2009) reported that increased P3 amplitude in response to novel, complex sounds moderated the relation between behavioral inhibition and anxiety during adolescence. Specifically, behaviorally inhibited adolescents with large P3 responses to novelty were at greater risk for an anxiety diagnosis compared to those with small P3 responses. Together, these results suggest that behaviorally inhibited children display perturbations in early processing of auditory novelty detection, and that increased neural responses to novelty may modulate the development of anxiety disorders. It should be noted that an anxiety diagnosis was assessed at the same time psychophysiological measures were collected; therefore, this study was unable to determine whether increased response to novelty can predict anxiety or is the result of a child being both behaviorally inhibited and anxious.

ATTENTION

Recent literature has linked perturbations in attention processes, particularly attention bias to threat, to the development of social withdrawal and anxiety disorders (Pine, 2007; Rothbart & Posner, 2006). It is likely that behaviorally inhibited children who can harness attention may mitigate underlying reactive tendencies and avoid deleterious effects of negative affect. In contrast, behaviorally inhibited children with poor attention control skills may be more beholden to initial affective reactions and attention biases to external stimuli. Over time, this may lead them to display signs of enhanced social reticence. Thus, behavioral inhibition may modify the mechanisms of attention involved in the detection of threat in the environment (Derryberry & Reed, 1994). Indeed, studies have demonstrated that behaviorally inhibited children display perturbations in attention processing when emotionally threatening stimuli are used (Pérez-Edgar & Fox, 2005, 2007; Schwartz, Snidman, & Kagan, 1996b). It has been suggested that these perturbations in attention moderate the association between behavioral inhibition and later anxiety disorders (Fox, Hane, & Pine, 2007).

A number of researchers have found increased attention bias toward threat in adult and pediatric populations (Bar-Haim, Lamy, Pergamin, Bakermans-Kranenburg, & van IJzendoorn, 2007; Pine, 2007; Roy et al., 2008). One task used to assess attention bias toward threat is the dot-probe task (MacLeod, Mathews, & Tata, 1986; Mogg, Philippot, & Bradley, 2004), during which the participant typically is presented with two faces side-by-side; one face is neutral and the other is threatening. The faces are then followed by a neutral target probe (an arrow pointing up or down) that appears at the location of one of the faces. The participant has to indicate the direction of the probe by pressing one of two buttons as quickly and accurately as possible. Individuals who show an attention bias toward threat have faster reaction times to the probes that appear on the same side as threatening stimuli compared to neutral stimuli. Pérez-Edgar, Fox, Bar-Haim, Martin McDermott, and Pine (in press) used this paradigm to assess attention bias toward threat in our sample when participants were adolescents. Pérez-Edgar et al. asked two questions: First, do adolescents in our sample, previously characterized as behaviorally inhibited, display heightened attention bias toward threat using the dot-probe task? Second, do perturbations in attention to threat (heightened orienting to threat) moderate the relation between behavioral inhibition in childhood, and anxiety disorders and social withdrawal in adolescents? Data from this study revealed that, similar to children with anxiety disorders (Roy et al., 2008), behaviorally inhibited adolescents display increased attention bias toward threat compared to noninhibited adolescents. In addition, magnitude of attention bias toward threat moderated the relation between childhood behavioral inhibition and maternal report of adolescent social withdrawal (as assessed by the Child Behavior Checklist (CBCL, Achenbach, 2001).

Heightened vigilance toward novelty or threat may affect learning which cues in the environment are "safe" and which are "threatening." In a recent meta-analysis of conditioning studies in the clinical anxiety literature, Lissek et al. (2005) reported that anxious adults could not discriminate between a cue predicting the presentation of an aversive stimulus and a cue predicting the absence of an aversive stimulus. This lack of differentiation may be a result of failure to learn the discrimination or, more likely, overgeneralization of threat to nonthreatening stimuli. In an attempt to examine this issue using a fear-potentiated startle paradigm, Reeb-Sutherland and colleagues (2009) studied adolescents from our cohort during their lab visit. In this study, the electromyographic (EMG) blink reflex response was recorded in behaviorally inhibited and noninhibited adolescents as they listened to bursts of white noise (startle probe) while viewing different colored squares (blue and green). Participants were told that one of the colors (e.g., green) signaled a possibility of receiving an air blast to the larynx (threat cue), and the other colored square (e.g., blue) signaled no possibility of receiving an air blast (safety cue). The startle probe was presented after the onset of the colored squares during the safe and threat conditions. Individual differences in startle amplitude to the probe during safety and threat cues were examined. The authors reported that startle amplitude to the safety cue rather than to the threat cue modulated the relation between behavioral inhibition and anxiety. Specifically, only behaviorally inhibited adolescents with increased startle response to safety were at risk for having a lifetime anxiety diagnosis. The results are consistent with findings reported in children at risk for anxiety disorders (Grillon, Dierker, & Merikangas, 1997, 1998) as well as adult populations with anxiety disorders (Lissek et al., 2005). These studies suggested that an increased startle response to safety cues reflects generalization from threat to safety in behaviorally inhibited adolescents who develop anxiety. This generalization may be due to an inability to inhibit their startle response or to disengage attention from threat even when the environment is safe.

Differences in attention processes between behaviorally inhibited and noninhibited children are not exclusive to threat processing. As reviewed earlier, the P3 component, which is associated with orientation to novelty, was shown to moderate the relation between early behavioral inhibition and anxiety (Reeb-Sutherland et al., 2009). A recent study has investigated error-related negativity (ERN) as an additional moderator of the relation between behavioral inhibition and anxiety (McDermott et al., 2009). To elicit the ERN, adolescents participated in a flanker task that required them to respond quickly and accurately over the course of multiple trials. During this specific task, they were asked to identify the middle letter in each row during both congruent (HHHHH or SSSSS) and incongruent (HHSHH or SSHSS) trials. Errors during these tasks are relatively rare and are thought to be due to impulsive responding prior to complete processing of the stimulus (Rabbitt & Vyas, 1981). McDermott et al. (2009) found that behaviorally inhibited adolescents showed increased ERN amplitude compared to noninhibited adolescents. Furthermore, ERN amplitude moderated the relation between behavioral inhibition and anxiety such that behaviorally inhibited adolescents with increased ERN amplitude were at significant risk for anxiety diagnosis, particularly among boys. These results are consistent with other studies showing that anxiety disorders are related to increased ERN amplitude (Olvet & Hajcak, 2008). It has been suggested that ERN amplitude is related to individual differences in punishment sensitivity (Boksem, Tops, Wester, Meijman, & Lorist, 2006). Therefore, this increased ERN response among anxious behaviorally inhibited adolescents suggests that these individuals may view commission of errors as more aversive than do other behaviorally inhibited children who do not develop anxiety.

ENVIRONMENTAL FACTORS

A number of studies have suggested that environmental factors, such as maternal behavior and child care context, may influence the continuity of behavioral inhibition across childhood (for extensive review, see Degnan & Fox, 2007; Hane & Fox, 2007). Parenting styles can moderate the continuity of behavioral inhibition across development by continuously molding attention processes used to regulate emotions. Briefly, several studies from our laboratory and from Kenneth Rubin's lab report that oversolicitous maternal behavior that is intrusive and overcontrolling is typically related to behavioral inhibition (Rubin, Cheah, & Fox, 2001; Rubin et al., 1997), while others have reported that maternal sensitivity and warmth are related to less inhibition (Park, Belsky, Putnam, & Crnic, 1997; Wood, McLeod, Sigman, Hwang, & Chu, 2003). However, some research has reported that overly warm maternal care, paired with oversolicitousness (Degnan, Henderson, Fox, & Rubin, 2008; Rubin, Burgess, & Coplan, 2002), as well as low intrusiveness, have been related to behavioral inhibition (Park et al., 1997; Rubin et al., 1997; van Brakel, Muris, Bogels, & Thomassen, 2006). These findings are interpreted to reflect the possibility that the mother "caters" to the child's fears, therefore reinforcing patterns of withdrawal behavior, as well as decreasing the child's ability to learn self-regulatory processes (see Hastings, Nuselovici, Rubin, & Cheah, Chpater 6, this volume, for a relevant review).

Nonparental child care has also been investigated as a potential moderator for behavioral inhibition continuity. Through external child care, behaviorally inhibited children may gain additional social experience through interactions with several peers within a variety of situations and contexts. Because behaviorally inhibited children show increased fear and withdrawal in social situations, increased exposure to such social situations may increase inhibited children's chance to learn how to self-regulate during these seemingly stressful situations. In fact, a study by N. Fox and colleagues (2001) provides evidence for such an hypothesis. They found that 4-month-old negatively reactive infants were less likely to be characterized as behaviorally inhibited during toddlerhood if placed in nonparental child care environments with one or more nonsibling peers for at least 10 hours per week. Other researchers have reported similar findings (Arcus & McCartney, 1989; Furman, Rahe, & Hartup, 1979). Although it is not necessarily known what specific qualities of nonparental child care (i.e., amount of time spent, number of peer interactions, quality of care) influence behavioral inhibition, it is clear that this type of care is a potential moderator of behavioral inhibition continuity.

GENE–ENVIRONMENT INTERACTION

Although there are many possible genes that separately and together may influence the expression of behavioral inhibition, studies have primarily focused on polymorphisms in the promoter region of the gene for the serotonin transporter (*5-HTT*). The *5-HTT* gene comprises a long (*l*) and short (*s*) allele. The *s* allele results in lower *5-HTT* levels and reduced serotonin uptake, thus having effects on neural circuits regulated by serotonin (Hariri et al., 2002), and has been associated with anxiety and negative emotionality (Munafo et al., 2003). Studies examining group differences between behaviorally inhibited and noninhibited children have found inconsistent results. Battaglia et al. (2005) reported that an increased level of shyness was associated with being homozygous for the short *5-HTT* allele (*s-s*). In contrast, Schmidt, Fox, Rubin, Hu, and Hamer (2002) found no relation between the *5-HTT* gene and behavioral inhibition.

Environmental factors, such as stress, have been shown to interact with 5-HTT status to predict psychopathology in humans (Caspi et al., 2003; Kaufman et al., 2004) and fearfulness in animals (Suomi, 2004), suggesting that environmental stress may interact with *5-HTT* gene status to predict behavioral inhibition. Indeed, a study by N. Fox, Nichols, et al. (2005) found that 7-year-old children with both a short *5-HTT* allele and maternal report of low social support displayed increased measures of behavioral inhibition, as well as increased levels of maternally reported shyness. These results are the first to describe a gene–environment interaction for the temperamental trait of behavioral inhibition in children.

SUMMARY AND CONCLUSION

Over the past 18 years, our studies of behavioral inhibition have attempted to identify a number of mechanisms that account for both the continuity and discontinuity of this temperament over development. As well, this work has attempted to determine what factors may be involved in moderating the relations between childhood behavioral inhibition and the emergence of anxiety disorders in adolescence. A number of processes have been identified. First, it appears that, from an early age, behaviorally inhibited infants are "primed" to detect novelty in their environments. This heightened detection may lead to an overgeneralization of threat by young children and, in response to this, increased social withdrawal. Second, attention mechanisms appear to moderate relations between childhood behavioral inhibition and adolescent anxiety disorders. Those behaviorally inhibited individuals who display heightened orienting to threat, enhanced novelty detection, and greater error monitoring are more likely to develop anxiety disorders. It appears that perturbations in attention that persist into early adolescence exacerbate the tendency of behaviorally inhibited individuals to withdraw from social situations in a persistent and maladaptive manner, resulting in the development of anxiety disorders. Finally, the maintenance of these attention styles over time is most probably a result of the context of caregiving and the manner in which parents and peers respond to the child's initial reactivity and hypervigilance. We have suggested (Fox et al., 2007) that maternal behaviors may in fact turn children's dispositional tendencies toward novelty detection into bias toward viewing novelty as threat in the environment. Evidence of maternal behavior in the case of children with anxiety disorders supports this supposition (Barrett, Rapee, & Dadds, 1996).

Our recent studies described in this chapter point to potential neurobiological moderators of anxiety. However, because diagnosis and electrophysiological measures were assessed concurrently, it is impossible to tease apart whether the increased novelty detection, attention bias to threat, and error monitoring observed in anxious behaviorally inhibited adolescents are predictors of anxiety risk or the result of being both behaviorally inhibited and diagnosed with an anxiety disorder. To determine whether these measures are potential predictors for anxiety risk, they must be examined during childhood, prior to the manifestation of anxiety disorders. To address this issue, we are currently conducting studies in 7-year-old children who were selected on measures of negative reactivity at 4 months of age and have been assessed on measures of behavioral inhibition throughout toddlerhood and childhood. Included in this study are measures assessing novelty detection, attention bias to threat, and error monitoring. In addition, because the majority of our studies thus far have employed measures of EEG or ERP, we are unable to draw any conclusions about the underlying brain structures involved in the moderation of behavioral inhibition and anxiety. Therefore, future studies should use fMRI to examine activation, as well as the interaction of different brain regions known to be involved in individuals with anxiety disorders, including the amygdala and prefrontal cortex in behaviorally inhibited individuals. Follow-up studies using fMRI are currently underway in our sample of behaviorally inhibited adolescents now entering young adulthood. Additionally, we are planning future studies to investigate individual differences in brain activation among behaviorally inhibited children.

REFERENCES

Achenbach, T. M. (2001). *Child Behavior Checklist for ages 6 to 18*. Burlington: University of Vermont, Research Center for Children, Youth, and Families.

Arcus, D., & McCartney, K. (1989). When baby makes four: Family influences in the stability of behavioral inhibition. In J. S. Reznick (Ed.), *Perspectives on behavioral inhibition* (pp. 197–218). Chicago: University of Chicago Press.

Bar-Haim, Y., Lamy, D., Pergamin, L., Bakermans-Kranenburg, M. J., & van IJzendoorn, M. H. (2007). Threat-related attentional bias in anxious and nonanxious individuals: A meta-analytic study. *Psychological Bulletin, 133*, 1–24.

Bar-Haim, Y., Marshall, P. J., Fox, N. A., Schorr, E. A., & Gordon-Salant, S. (2003). Mismatch negativity in socially withdrawn children. *Biological Psychiatry, 54*, 17–24.

Barrett, P. M., Rapee, R. M., & Dadds, M. M. (1996). Family enhancement of cognitive style in anxious and aggressive children. *Journal of Abnormal Child Psychology, 24*, 187–203.

Battaglia, M., Ogliari, A., Zanoni, A., Citterio, A., Pozzoli, U., Giora, R., et al. (2005). Influence of the serotonin transporter promoter gene and shyness on children's cerebral responses to facial expressions. *Archives of General Psychiatry, 62*, 85–94.

Beaton, E. A., Schmidt, L. A., Schulkin, J., Antony, M. M., Swinson, R. P., & Hall, G. B. (2008). Different neural responses to stranger and personally familiar faces in shy and bold adults. *Behavioral Neuroscience, 122*, 704–709.

Berlyne, D. E. (1960). *Conflict, arousal, and curiosity*. New York: McGraw-Hill.

Biederman, J., Hirshfeld-Becker, D. R., Rosenbaum, J. F., Herot, C., Friedman, D., Snidman, N., et al. (2001). Further evidence of association between behavioral inhibition and social anxiety in children. *American Journal of Psychiatry, 158*, 1673–1679.

Biederman, J., Jerrold, M. A., Rosenbaum, J. F., Bolduc-Murphy, E. A., Faraone, S. V., Chaloff, J., et al. (1993). A 3-year follow-up of children with and without behavioral inhibition. *Journal of the American Academy of Child and Adolescent Psychiatry, 32*, 814–821.

Boksem, M. A., Tops, M., Wester, A. E., Meijman, T. F., & Lorist, M. M. (2006). Error-related ERP components and individual differences in punishment and reward sensitivity. *Brain Research, 1101*, 92–101.

Calkins, S. D., Fox, N. A., & Marshall, T. R. (1996). Behavioral and physiological antecedents of inhibited and uninhibited behavior. *Child Development, 67*, 523–540.

Caspi, A., Snugden, K., Moffitt, T. E., Taylor, A., Craig, I. W., Harrington, H., et al. (2003). Influence of life stress on depression: Moderation by a polymorphism in the 5-HTT gene. *Science, 301*, 386–389.

Coplan, R. J., Rubin, K. H., Fox, N. A., & Calkins, S. D. (1994). Being alone, playing alone, and acting alone: Distinguishing among reticence and passive and active solitude in young children. *Child Development, 65*, 129–138.

Cycowicz, Y. M., & Friedman, D. (1998). Effect of sound familiarity on the event-related potentials elicited by novel environmental sounds. *Brain and Cognition, 36,* 30–51.

Davidson, R. J. (1995). Cerebral asymmetry, emotion, and affective style. In R. J. Davidson & K. Hugdahl (Eds.), *Brain asymmetry* (pp. 361–387). Cambridge, MA: MIT Press.

Davis, M. (1986). Pharmacological and anatomical analysis of fear conditioning using the fear-potentiated startle paradigm. *Behavioral Neuroscience, 100,* 814–824.

Davis, M. (1998). Are different parts of the extended amygdala involved in fear versus anxiety? *Biological Psychiatry, 44,* 407–422.

de Haan, M., Gunnar, M. R., Tout, K., Hart, J., & Stansbury, K. (1998). Familiar and novel contexts yield different associations between cortisol and behavior among 2-year-old children. *Developmental Psychobiology, 33,* 93–101.

Degnan, K. A., & Fox, N. A. (2007). Behavioral inhibition and anxiety disorders: Multiple levels of a resilience process. *Development and Psychopathology, 19,* 729–746.

Degnan, K. A., Henderson, H. A., Fox, N. A., & Rubin, K. H. (2008). Predicting social wariness in middle childhood: The moderating roles of child history, maternal personality and maternal behavior. *Social Development, 17,* 471–487.

Derryberry, D., & Reed, M. A. (1994). Temperament and attention: Orienting toward and away from positive and negative signals. *Journal of Personality and Social Psychology, 66,* 1128–1139.

Fox, E., Russo, R., Bowles, R., & Dutton, K. (2001). Do threatening stimuli draw or hold visual attention in subclinical anxiety? *Journal of Experimental Psychology: General, 130,* 681–700.

Fox, E., Russo, R., & Georgiou, G. A. (2005). Anxiety modulates the degree of attentive resources required to process emotional faces. *Cognitive Affective and Behavioral Neuroscience, 5*(4), 396–404.

Fox, N. A. (1991). If it's not left, it's right: Electroencephalograph asymmetry and the development of emotion. *American Psychologist, 46,* 863–872.

Fox, N. A., Calkins, S. D., & Bell, M. A. (1994). Neural plasticity and development in the first two years of life: Evidence from cognitive and socioemotional domains of research. *Development and Psychopathology, 6,* 677–696.

Fox, N. A., Hane, A. A., & Pine, D. S. (2007). Plasticity for affective neurocircuitry. *Current Directions in Psychological Science, 16,* 1–5.

Fox, N. A., Henderson, H. A., Marshall, P. J., Nichols, K. E., & Ghera, M. M. (2005). Behavioral inhibition: Linking biology and behavior within a developmental framework. *Annual Review of Psychology, 56,* 235–262.

Fox, N. A., Henderson, H. A., Rubin, K. H., Calkins, S. D., & Schmidt, L. A. (2001). Continuity and discontinuity of behavioral inhibition and exuberance: Psychophysiological and behavioral influences across the first four years of life. *Child Development, 72,* 1–21.

Fox, N. A., Nichols, K. E., Henderson, H. A., Rubin, K. H., Schmidt, L. A., Hamer, D., et al. (2005). Evidence for a gene–environment interaction in predicting behavioral inhibition in middle childhood. *Psychological Science, 16,* 921–926.

Fox, N. A., Schmidt, L. A., Calkins, S. D., Rubin, K. H., & Coplan, R. J. (1996). The role of frontal activation in the regulation and dysregulation of social behavior during the preschool years. *Development and Psychopathology, 8,* 89–102.

Friedman, D., Cycowicz, Y. M., & Gaeta, H. (2001). The novelty P3: An event-related brain potential (ERP) sign of the brain's evaluation of novelty. *Neuroscience and Biobehavioral Reviews, 25,* 355–373.

Fullard, W., McDevitt, S. C., & Carey, W. B. (1984). Assessing temperament in one-to three-year-old children. *Journal of Pediatric Psychology, 9,* 205–217.

Furman, W., Rahe, D. F., & Hartup, W. W. (1979). Rehabilitation of socially withdrawn preschool children through mix-age and same-age socialization. *Child Development, 50,* 915–922.

Garcia-Coll, C., Kagan, J., & Reznick, J. S. (1984). Behavioral inhibition in young children. *Child Development, 55,* 1005–1019.

Grillon, C., Dierker, L., & Merikangas, K. R. (1997). Startle modulation in children at risk for anxiety disorders and/or alcoholism. *Journal of the American Academy of Child and Adolescent Psychiatry, 36,* 925–936.

Grillon, C., Dierker, L., & Merikangas, K. R. (1998). Fear-potentiated startle in adolescent offspring of parents with anxiety disorders. *Biological Psychiatry, 44,* 990–997.

Gunnar, M. R., Tout, K., de Haan, M., Pierce, S., & Stansbury, K. (1997). Temperament, social competence, and adrenocortical activity in preschoolers. *Developmental Psychobiology, 31,* 65–85.

Hane, A. A., & Fox, N. A. (2007). A closer look at the transactional nature of early social development: The relations among early caregiving environments, temperament, and early social development. In F. Santoianni & C. Sabatano (Eds.), *Brain development in learning environments: Embodied and perceptual advancements* (pp. 1–15). Newcastle upon Tyne: Cambridge Scholars Press.

Hariri, A. R., Mattay, V. S., Tessitore, A., Kolachana, B., Fera, F., Goldman, D., et al. (2002). Serotonin transporter genetic variation and the response of the human amygdala. *Science, 297,* 400–403.

Henderson, H. A., Fox, N. A., & Rubin, K. H. (2001). Temperamental contributions to social behavior: the moderating roles of frontal EEG asymmetry and gender. *Journal of the American Academy of Child and Adolescent Psychiatry, 40,* 68–74.

Henderson, H. A., Marshall, P. J., Fox, N. A., & Rubin, K. H. (2004). Psychophysiological and behavioral evidence for varying forms and functions of nonsocial behavior in preschoolers. *Child Development, 75,* 251–263.

Hirshfeld, D. R., Jerrold, M. A., Rosenbaum, J. F., Biederman, J., Bolduc, E. A., Faraone, S. V., et al. (1992). Stable behavioral inhibition and its association with anxiety disorder. *Journal of the American Academy of Child and Adolescent Psychiatry, 31,* 103–111.

Kagan, J. (1994). *Galen's prophecy.* New York: Basic Books.

Kagan, J., Reznick, J. S., Clarke, C., Snidman, N., & Garcia-Coll, C. (1984). Behavioral inhibition to the unfamiliar. *Child Development, 55,* 2212–2225.

Kagan, J., Reznick, J. S., & Gibbons, J. (1989). Inhibited and uninhibited types of children. *Child Development, 60,* 838–845.

Kagan, J., Reznick, J. S., & Snidman, N. (1987). The physiology and psychology of behavioral inhibition in children. *Child Development, 58,* 1459–1473.

Kagan, J., Reznick, J. S., & Snidman, N. (1988a). Biological bases of childhood shyness. *Science, 240,* 167–171.

Kagan, J., Reznick, J. S., Snidman, N., Gibbons, J., & Johnson, M. O. (1988b). Childhood derivatives of inhibition and lack of inhibition to the unfamiliar. *Child Development, 59,* 1580–1589.

Kagan, J., & Snidman, N. (1991). Infant predictors of inhibited and uninhibited profiles. *Psychological Science, 2,* 40–44.

Kaufman, J., Yang, B. Z., Douglas-Palumberi, H., Houshyar, S., Lipschitz, D., Krystal, J. H., et al. (2004). Social supports and serotonin transporter gene moderate depression in maltreated children. *Proceedings of the National Academy of Sciences USA, 101,* 17316–17421.

LeDoux, J. E. (2000). Emotion circuits in the brain. *Annual Review of Neuroscience, 23,* 155–184.

LeDoux, J. E. (2008). The amygdala. *Current Biology, 17,* R868–R874.

LeDoux, J. E., Iwata, J., Cicchetti, P., & Reis, D. J. (1988). Different projections of the central amygdoid nucleus mediate autonomic and behavioral correlates of conditioned fear. *Journal of Neuroscience, 8,* 2517–2529.

Lissek, S., Powers, A. S., McClure, E. B., Phelps, E. A., Woldehawariat, G., Grillon, C., et al. (2005). Classical fear conditioning in the anxiety disorders: A meta-analysis. *Behaviour Research and Therapy, 43,* 1391–1424.

MacLeod, C., Mathews, A., & Tata, P. (1986). Attentional bias in emotional disorders. *Journal of Abnormal Psychology, 95,* 15–20.

Marshall, P. J., Reeb, B. C., & Fox, N. A. (2009). Electrophysiological responses to auditory novelty in temperamentally different 9-month-old infants. *Developmental Science, 12,* 568–582.

Marshall, P. J., & Stevenson-Hinde, J. (1998). Behavioral inhibition, heart period, and respiratory sinus arrhythmia in young children. *Developmental Psychobiology, 33,* 283–292.

McDermott, J. M., Pérez-Edgar, K., Henderson, H. A., Pine, D. S., & Fox, N. A. (2009). A history of childhood behavioral inhibition and enhanced self-monitoring lead to clinical anxiety in adolescence. *Biological Psychiatry, 65,* 445–448.

McManis, M. H., Kagan, J., Snidman, N., & Woodward, S. A. (2002). EEG asymmetry, power, and temperament in children. *Developmental Psychobiology, 41,* 169–177.

Mogg, K., Philippot, P., & Bradley, B. P. (2004). Selective attention to angry faces in clinical social phobia. *Journal of Abnormal Psychology, 113,* 160–165.

Munafo, M. R., Clark, T. G., Moore, L. R., Payne, E., Walton, R., & Flint, J. (2003). Genetic polymorphisms and personality in healthy adults: A systematic review and meta-analysis. *Molecular Psychiatry, 8,* 471–484.

Naatanen, R., & Alho, K. (1995). Mismatch negativity—a unique measure of sensory processing in audition. *International Journal of Neuroscience, 80,* 317–337.

Naatanen, R., Paavilainen, P., Tiitinen, H., Jiang, D., & Alho, K. (1993). Attention and mismatch negativity. *Psychophysiology, 30,* 436–450.

Nachmias, M., Gunnar, M., Mangelsdorf, S., Parritz, R. H., & Buss, K. (1996). Behavioral inhibition and stress reactivity: The moderating role of attachment security. *Child Development, 67,* 508–522.

Olvet, D. M., & Hajcak, G. (2008). The error-related negativity (ERN) and psychopathology: toward an endophenotype. *Clinical Psychology Review, 28,* 1343–1354.

Park, S., Belsky, J., Putnam, S., & Crnic, K. (1997). Infant emotionality, parenting, and 3-year inhibition: Exploring stability and lawful discontinuity in a male sample. *Developmental Psychology, 33,* 218–227.

Pérez-Edgar, K., & Fox, N. A. (2005). A behavioral and electrophysiological study of children's selective attention under neutral and affective conditions. *Journal of Cognition and Development, 6,* 89–118.

Pérez-Edgar, K., & Fox, N. A. (2007). Temperamental contributions to children's performance in an emotion-word processing task: A behavioral and electrophysiological study. *Brain and Cognition, 65,* 22–35.

Pérez-Edgar, K., Fox, N. A., Bar-Haim, Y., Martin McDermott, J., & Pine, D. S. (in press). Attention bias to threat link behavioral inhibition in early childhood to adolescent social withdrawal. *Emotion.*

Pérez-Edgar, K., Roberson-Nay, R., Hardin, M. G., Poeth, K., Guyer, A. E., Nelson, E. E., et al. (2007). Attention alters neural responses to evocative faces in behaviorally inhibited adolescents. *NeuroImage, 35,* 1538–1546.

Pérez-Edgar, K., Schmidt, L. A., Henderson, H. A., Schulkin, J., & Fox, N. A. (2008). Salivary cortisol levels and infant temperament shape developmental trajectories in boys at risk for behavioral maladjustment. *Psychoneuroendocrinology, 33,* 916–925.

Pine, D. S. (2001). Affective neuroscience and the development of social anxiety. *Psychiatric Clinics of North America, 24,* 689–705.

Pine, D. S. (2002). Brain development and the onset of mood disorders. *Seminars in Clinical Neuropsychiatry, 7,* 223–233.

Pine, D. S. (2007). Research review: A neuroscience framework for pediatric anxiety disorders. *Journal of Child Psychology and Psychiatry, 48,* 631–648.

Rabbitt, P., & Vyas, S. (1981). Processing a display even after you make a response to it: How perceptual errors can be corrected. *Quarterly Journal of Experimental Psychology, 33A,* 223–239.

Reeb-Sutherland, B. C., Helfinstein, S. M., Degnan, K. A., Pérez-Edgar, K., Henderson, H. A., Lissek, S., et al. (2009). Startle response in behaviorally inhibited adolescents with a lifetime occurrence of anxiety disorders. *Journal of the American Academy of Child and Adolescent Psychiatry, 48,* 610–617.

Reeb-Sutherland, B. C., Vanderwert, R. E., Marshall, P. J., Pérez-Edgar, K., Chronis-Tuscano, A., Pine, D. S., et al. (2009). Attention to novelty in behaviorally inhibited adolescents moderates risk for anxiety. *Journal of Child Psychology and Psychiatry, 50,* 1365–1372.

Rosenbaum, J. F., Biederman, J., Bolduc, E. A., Hirshfeld, D. R., Faraone, S. V., & Kagan, J. (1992). Comorbidity of parental anxiety disorders as risk for childhood-onset anxiety in inhibited children. *American Journal of Psychiatry, 149,* 475–481.

Rosenbaum, J. F., Biederman, J., Hirshfeld, D. R., Bolduc, E. A., Faraone, S. V.,

Kagan, J., et al. (1991). Further evidence of an association between behavioral inhibition and anxiety disorders: Results from a family study of children from a non-clinical sample. *Journal of Psychiatry Research, 25,* 49–65.

Rothbart, M. K., & Posner, M. I. (2006). Temperament, attention, and developmental psychopathology. In D. Cicchetti & D. J. Cohen (Eds.), *Handbook of developmental psychopathology* (2nd ed., Vol. 2, pp. 465–501). Hoboken, NJ: Wiley.

Roy, A. K., Vasa, R. A., Bruck, M., Mogg, K., Bradley, B. P., Sweeney, M., et al. (2008). Attention bias toward threat in pediatric anxiety disorders. *Journal of the American Academy of Child and Adolescent Psychiatry, 47,* 1189–1196.

Rubin, K. H. (1989). *The Play Observation Scale (POS).* Waterloo, Ontario, Canada: University of Waterloo.

Rubin, K. H., Burgess, K. B., & Coplan, R. J. (2002). Social withdrawal and shyness. In P. K. Smith & C. H. Hart (Eds.), *Blackwell handbook of childhood social development* (pp. 330–352). Malden, MA: Blackwell.

Rubin, K. H., Cheah, C. S. L., & Fox, N. A. (2001). Emotion regulation, parenting, and display of social reticence in preschoolers. *Early Education and Development, 12,* 97–115.

Rubin, K. H., Hastings, P., Stewart, S., Henderson, H. A., & Chen, X. (1997). The consistency and concomitants of inhibition: some of the children, all of the time. *Child Development, 68,* 467–483.

Rubin, K. H., Maioni, T. L., & Hornung, M. (1976). Free play behaviors in middle- and lower-class preschoolers: Parten and Piaget revisited. *Child Development, 47,* 414–419.

Schmidt, L. A., & Fox, N. A. (1994). Patterns of cortical electrophysiology and autonomic activity in adults' shyness and sociability. *Biological Psychology, 38,* 183–198.

Schmidt, L. A., Fox, N. A., Rubin, K. H., Hu, S., & Hamer, D. H. (2002). Molecular genetics of shyness and aggression in preschoolers. *Personality and Individual Differences, 33,* 227–238.

Schmidt, L. A., Fox, N. A., Rubin, K. H., Sternberg, E., Gold, P. W., Smith, C. C., et al. (1997). Behavioral and neuroendocrine responses in shy children. *Developmental Psychobiology, 30,* 127–140.

Schmidt, L. A., Fox, N. A., Schulkin, J., & Gold, P. W. (1999). Behavioral and psychophysiological correlates of self-presentation in temperamentally shy children. *Developmental Psychobiology, 35,* 119–135.

Schwartz, C. E., Snidman, N., & Kagan, J. (1996a). Early childhood temperament as a determinant of externalizing behavior in adolescence. *Development and Psychopathology, 8,* 527–537.

Schwartz, C. E., Snidman, N., & Kagan, J. (1996b). Early temperamental predictors of Stroop interference to threatening information at adolescence. *Journal of Anxiety Disorders, 10,* 89–96.

Schwartz, C. E., Snidman, N., & Kagan, J. (1999). Adolescent social anxiety as an outcome of inhibited temperament in childhood. *Journal of the American Academy of Child and Adolescent Psychiatry, 38*(8), 1008–1015.

Schwartz, C. E., Wright, C. I., Shin, L. M., Kagan, J., & Rauch, S. L. (2003). Inhibited and uninhibited infants "grown up": Adult amygdalar response to novelty. *Science, 300*(5627), 1952–1953.

Suomi, S. J. (2004). How gene–environment interaction shape biobehavioral development: Lessons from studies with rhesus monkeys. *Research in Human Development, 3,* 205–222.

Tomarken, A. J., Davidson, R. J., Wheeler, R. E., & Doss, R. C. (1992). Individual differences in anterior brain asymmetry and fundamental dimensions of emotion. *Journal of Personality and Social Psychology, 62,* 676–687.

van Brakel, A. M. L., Muris, P., Bogels, S. M., & Thomassen, C. (2006). A multifactorial model for the etiology of anxiety in non-clinical adolescents: Main and interactive effects of behavioral inhibition, attachment, and parental rearing. *Journal of Child and Family Studies, 15,* 569–579.

Wheeler, R. W., Davidson, R. J., & Tomarken, A. J. (1993). Frontal brain asymmetry and emotional reactivity: A biological substrate of affective style. *Psychophysiology, 30,* 82–89.

Wood, J. J., McLeod, B. D., Sigman, M., Hwang, W. C., & Chu, B. C. (2003). Parenting and childhood anxiety: Theory empirical findings, and future directions. *Journal of Child Psychology and Psychiatry, 44,* 134–151.

Woodward, S. A., McManis, M. H., Kagan, J., Deldin, P., Snidman, N., Lewis, M., et al. (2001). Infant temperament and the brainstem auditory evoked response in later childhood. *Developmental Psychology, 37,* 533–538.

PART III

PERSONAL AND INTERPERSONAL PROCESSES

6

Shyness, Parenting, and Parent–Child Relationships

PAUL D. HASTINGS
JACOB N. NUSELOVICI
KENNETH H. RUBIN
CHARISSA S. L. CHEAH

The mother and her daughter were seated on the floor, looking at a set of dolls and toys before them. The experimenter had just set up a situation in which the mother and daughter arrived late at day care to find three other children playing while the teacher looked on. The experimenter looked at them and said, "Now you finish the story. What happens next?"

In response, the 2½-year-old girl happily moved "her doll" toward the other doll "children." She took the ball from the other "children" and showed her mother how she could kick it. Her mother said, "You can kick it to the other kids," and the girl did. As she continued to play with the dolls, her mother said: "OK, it's time for Mommy to go to work." "No!" the girl said, her eyes wide. She took the "mother" doll and moved it further into the room, beside her own doll. "No, you stay," the girl asserted, and then resumed her play with the ball. The mother turned to the experimenter with a surprised expression and said, "Well, I guess I know what to expect in September when she starts day care!"

Three months later, when the girl was visited at day care, she was observed to be calm and happy, sometimes playing with her classmates and at other times coloring on her own. According to her teacher, this was a normal day for this sociable little girl.

This anecdote was taken from one family that participated in one of our studies of young children's early social and emotional development. Most children are socially competent and comfortable with engaging in mutually pleasing interactions with their peers, like this little girl. Some children are not. An expression of distress at the prospect of being separated from their parents can foretell such children's difficulty with social activities, their reluctance to play, and their tendency to withdraw from others—although this was not the case with this girl. There has been a great deal of interest in understanding why some children are shy, whereas others are sociable, even though they might show some early "warning signs" for shyness. In this chapter, we consider the evidence that parents play a substantial role in shaping their children's development of shyness and social withdrawal.

RELEVANT THEORY

In paraphrasing the old African proverb "It takes a village to raise a child," Hillary Clinton (1996) emphasized that children are socialized not only by parents and families, but also by their surrounding community and culture. In doing so, she echoed the tenets of Bronfenbrenner's bioecological model of development (Bronfenbrenner & Morris, 2006). A child's direct interactions with parents and other people in day-to-day life form a social microsystem, which is embedded within ever-broadening social structures, such as neighborhoods and schools (mesosystem), community resources (exosystem), and cultural practices and values (macrosystem). Connections between and across these systems unfold over time (chronosystem), shaping the child's immediate behavior and longer-term development. Until later childhood or adolescence, however, children have less direct contact with the broader, external systems than with the microsystem; therefore, many of these broader systems' influences are filtered through the child's day-to-day social partners. Thus, the stresses and strengths of neighborhoods, communities, and cultures principally have indirect effects on young children via their effects upon parents. Children's parents are their first and most enduring social partners, and for most children, parents have the greatest responsibility and opportunity to contribute to the course of their development.

This is not to disregard the active roles of children themselves in their own development. The individual temperaments of children, their innate behavioral and emotional tendencies, make them more or less prone to shyness, or a consistent and persistent tendency to avoid or withdraw from others in social situations (e.g., Degnan & Fox, 2007; Fox, Henderson, Marshall, Nichols, & Ghera, 2005). Children's characteristics also serve as stimuli that elicit parental responses and create opportunities for socialization (e.g., Rubin, Nelson, Hastings, & Asendorpf, 1999). Thus, as well as being influenced by parents, children influence their parents' child-rearing behaviors, in accord with bidirectional (Bell, 1979) and transactional (Sameroff, 1975) perspectives on socialization. A child and a parent are continuously acting and reacting to each other, creating a dynamic and developing relationship that can be regarded as the context of socialization (Kuczynski & Parkin, 2007). These transactional processes are nested within the history of the parent–child relationship; parents and children perceive, interpret, respond to, and learn from each other's actions based on their past shared experiences and their future expectations.

PARENTING AND THE DEVELOPMENT OF SHYNESS

Socialization researchers have approached the study of parenting from myriad perspectives, each of which has informed our understanding of the links between parenting and children's shyness. More than 40 years ago, Schaeffer (1959) and Becker (1964) identified parental psychological control, reflected in practices such as manipulating the parent–child emotional bond (e.g., love withdrawal) and anxious overintrusiveness, as likely to undermine children's development of autonomy. Psychological control was somewhat neglected by parenting researchers for almost 30 years, however, before renewed interest began to confirm its role in children's risk for shyness (e.g., Barber, Olsen, & Shagle, 1994; Mills & Rubin, 1998). Rather, the majority of socialization research in the latter quarter of the 20th century used the framework of broad parenting styles, and particularly Baumrind's (1971) conceptualization of authoritative, authoritarian, permissive, and neglectful parenting (Maccoby & Martin, 1983). This approach identified "authoritarian parenting," or a pattern of rigid, punitive, or harshly restrictive control, as likely to lead to withdrawal and shyness in children—along with a host of other emotional and behavioral problems. Simultaneously, attachment researchers examined young children's sense of security within the parent–child relationship as the foundation for their confident engagement with the social world (Ainsworth, Blehar, Waters, & Wall, 1978). Failing to establish a secure working relationship with the primary caregiver was expected to set a child on a path toward social difficulties. These three lines of research—attachment, parenting styles, and psychological control— continue to dominate the study of the socialization of shyness.

In addition, researchers have recently begun to consider how a range of more specific parenting behaviors might contribute to children's development of shyness and related problems (e.g., Bayer, Sanson, & Hemphill, 2006; McLeod, Wood, & Weisz, 2007). In accord with risk and protective models that characterize developmental psychopathology (Cummings, Davies, & Campbell, 2000), these studies not only focus on maladaptive parenting but also include consideration of positive parenting practices, such as warmth and induction that might diminish children's shyness and promote social competence. Studying specific parenting practices can complement the other lines of research by identifying which particular components of, for example, authoritarian styles are most closely linked to children's risk of developing shyness rather than other adjustment problems. Knowing what aspects of parenting "matter most" for shyness can in turn help to inform the design of targeted prevention and intervention efforts to address maladaptive parenting.

We now consider the literature on the links between children's shyness and parenting styles, attachment relationships, psychological control, and other parenting behaviors. This review is organized developmentally, from infancy through adolescence. It should be recognized that the vast majority of research on parental socialization of shyness has involved mothers but not fathers; thus, less is known about the possible contributions of paternal socialization to the development of shyness. We consider the limited research on fathers after reviewing the more substantive literature on mothers' parenting.

Infancy and Toddlerhood (0–24 Months)

The earliest roots of shyness and social withdrawal lie in infants' temperamental reactivity, the sensitivity and appropriateness of maternal care, and the formation of the mother–infant attachment relationship. Young infants who show strongly negative emotional reactions are likely to develop inhibited temperaments, showing wariness of novelty and withdrawing from unfamiliar people (Degnan & Fox, 2007). Caring for these infants is demanding for parents, and some mothers of reactive and inhibited infants can have difficulty being sensitive, responsive, and appropriately supportive of their infants' needs (Kiang, Moreno, & Robinson, 2004). This combination of temperamental vulnerability and maternal insensitivity increases the likelihood that infants will fail to establish a secure attachment (Bowlby, 1980). Securely attached infants appear capable of using their mothers as a trustworthy source of support and assurance, such that they can leave the mothers' immediate proximity to explore their surroundings with a sense of safety. Infants who form an insecure attachment relationship do not benefit from these competencies, and it has been suggested that temperamentally inhibited infants with insensitive mothers may be particularly likely to form an ambivalent (C) attachment (Booth-LaForce & Oxford, 2008). Ambivalently attached infants do not seem able to cope with new challenges or social situations; thus, fearing failure or rejection, they withdraw from interactions.

Several studies have provided support for this model. Insecurely attached infants, and particularly infants with ambivalent attachments, are more likely to be fearful and inhibited toddlers (Calkins & Fox, 1992; Kochanska, 1998; Matas, Arend, & Sroufe, 1978; Spangler & Schieche, 1998) and to be withdrawn or lacking confidence in the preschool- and school-age years (Erickson, Sroufe, & Egeland, 1985; Renken, Egeland, Marvinney, Mangelsdorf, & Sroufe, 1989). Recently, Booth-LaForce and Oxford (2008) demonstrated that children with less secure attachment at 24 months were described by teachers as more shy throughout the elementary school-age period. Clearly, children's early attachment relationships are important foundations for their later social development. This does not imply that children's social proclivities have been set in stone by age 24 months, regardless of subsequent parental socialization experiences. In fact, Booth-LaForce and Oxford showed that early attachment did not directly predict later shyness when maternal parenting in the preschool years was taken into account. Thus, children's social tendencies continue to be malleable and subject to influence by maternal socialization.

Psychological control is particularly linked to young children's propensity for shyness and social withdrawal. Rubin, Hastings, Stewart, Henderson, and Chen (1997) identified a pattern of overprotective control, or oversolicitous parenting, that includes intrusive and unnecessary micromanagement of a child's independent activities, and strong affection in the absence of child distress or need for comforting. This pattern of parenting undermines the young child's autonomy by denying opportunities to practice coping with developmentally normative challenges, and by communicating that the child is incapable of handling tasks without parental assistance. More oversolicitous mothers had 24-month-old-children who were more withdrawn from an unfamiliar peer and inhibited with an unfamiliar adult (Rubin et al., 1997). This was particularly true of toddlers who were highly temperamentally fearful, indicating that vulnerable children might be more prone to the adverse effects of inappropriate maternal socialization. Recently, Bayer and colleagues (2006) replicated the association between mothers' overprotective control and toddlers' anxious difficulties, including withdrawal from unfamiliar peers.

Mothers' psychological control also contributes to toddlers' later development of shyness. Rubin, Burgess, and Hastings (2002) found that withdrawn toddlers with highly oversolicitous mothers were still likely to be reticent with unfamiliar peers 2 years hence, but withdrawn toddlers with less solicitous mothers were not. Similarly, Bayer and colleagues (2006) found that mothers who were overprotective of toddlers had children with more anxiety-related problems 2 years later. In addition, Rubin and colleagues

(2002) noted parallel relations for a second feature of psychological control, derisive or overcritical parenting. Parents who are derogatory and rejecting threaten their children's confidence in the parent–child relationship, eroding children's self-worth and trust in others (Barber & Harmon, 2002). Withdrawn toddlers with derisive mothers were likely to become reticent preschoolers, but withdrawn toddlers with mothers who did not express derision were not likely to maintain reticent behaviors (Rubin et al., 2002). Thus, emotionally manipulative overcontrol, whether effusively affectionate or chillingly negative, appears to keep toddlers on stable trajectories toward shyness and withdrawal.

One group of researchers has reported that mothers who were more intrusive during interactions with their 18-month-old boys at home had sons who were less inhibited during laboratory tasks when they were 3 years old, especially if the boys had shown high negative emotionality in infancy (Park, Belsky, Putnam, & Crnic, 1997). On first glance, this might appear to contradict the previously described studies of psychological control. However, Park et al.'s conceptualization of "intrusive parenting" reflected mothers making their infant sons engage in activities that appeared to be counter to the boys' wishes, which is rather the opposite of placing limits on children's activities (characteristic of overprotective control). Emotionally reactive children might show some distress at being made to handle normative events they would rather not confront, but when mothers provide these experiences, they might promote their children's ability to cope with such everyday challenges.

It is fortunate that research has not only identified "poor parenting" that increases children's risk for the development of shyness. Importantly, we know that there are also maternal actions that might protect young children from following trajectories toward shyness. For example, mothers' sensitivity to infants' cues diminishes the likelihood that highly wary infants will be nervous and withdrawn in kindergarten (Early et al., 2002). Similarly, mothers who engage with their toddlers, appropriately structuring activities and showing warmth through praise and positive affect, have children who displayed fewer anxiety-related problems as preschoolers (Bayer et al., 2006). These positive features of mothers' care for infants and toddlers appear to set the stage for young children's progression toward the development of greater social competence.

Preschool (2–5 Years)

The research on the associations between maternal socialization and shyness in the preschool period is largely consistent with the pattern just described in infancy. More shy, withdrawn and inhibited preschoolers have more overprotective mothers (e.g., McShane & Hastings, 2009), less authoritative mothers (e.g., Coplan, Findlay, & Nelson, 2004), or mothers who are less sensitive, supportive, and encouraging of autonomous activities (e.g., Dumas, LaFrenière, & Serketich, 1995), and the children and mothers are less likely to have secure attachment relationships (LaFrenière, Provost, & Dubeau, 1992; Shamir-Essakow et al., 2005). Studies have also indicated the contexts in which inappropriate maternal parenting has greater influence on children's shyness, how various child vulnerabilities make children more susceptible to maternal influence, and how socialization in preschool continues to shape children's social behavior in later years.

One aspect of overprotective or oversolicitous parenting that has confounded some socialization researchers is that it appears to contain elements of "good" parenting. Are parents not *supposed* to be highly involved and affectionate with their young children? Alas, mothers who are *too* contingent (Malatesta, Culver, Tesman, & Shepard, 1989) or *too* comforting (Denham, 1993) can undermine children's socioemotional competence. Thomasgard and Metz (1993) proposed that one of the features distinguishing normative and appropriate parental protection from maladaptive overprotection was the extent to which the situation or context of parent–child interaction warranted high levels of parental direction and affection. Rubin, Cheah, and Fox (2001) examined mothers' patterns of being physically close, warm, and controlling with their 4-year-old children in two contexts: in free play and in a structured teaching task that was quite difficult for children. Interestingly, mothers were not consistent in their displays of such "solicitous" behaviors across contexts. Mothers who were more solicitous during free play—when children could be expected to be calm and not need such actions—had preschoolers who were more reticent during interactions with peers. Conversely, mothers who used more of these same behaviors during the teaching task—when children might be challenged and distressed—had preschoolers who were less reticent, especially if children had relatively weak emotional self-regulation and thus greater need for maternal involvement during stressful tasks. Thus, the demands of a situation and the child's needs in that situation appear to define whether a given maternal response will be effective or detrimental in supporting a child's competent behavior and positive development.

Preschoolers' capacities for self-regulation of emotional arousal appear to affect the extent to which they might be influenced by parental socialization (Hastings & De, 2008). Well-regulated children respond to challenging social situations more appropriately and calmly, such that they are more likely to cope competently even without the benefit of effective socialization. Conversely, children who are relatively poor at self-regulation are more dependent upon external sources of support for effective regulation, such as appropriately supportive parenting, to develop comparable levels of positive functioning. They are also more susceptible to the adverse effects of psychological control, which places them at greater risk for shyness and withdrawal. Hastings, Sullivan, and colleagues (2008) examined this proposal using children's cardiac vagal tone as an indicator of their physiological capacity for self-regulation through parasympathetic control of autonomic arousal. Children with lower vagal tone (less parasympathetic self-regulation) were more reticent with peers only if they had more overprotective mothers. Furthermore, maternal socialization might even affect preschoolers' physiological capacity for self-regulation. Mothers who were more negative, critical, and restrictive had preschoolers who manifested lower vagal tone during play interactions with unfamiliar children (Hastings, Nuselovici, et al., 2008), which suggests that they responded to the situation as a threat rather than an opportunity for social engagement. This state of underregulated arousal could motivate children to withdraw from peers.

The adverse effects of mothers' psychological control of preschoolers also continue over time, contributing to children's shyness in the elementary school period. Paralleling what has been found over the transition from toddler to preschool age (Rubin et al., 2002), it has also been reported that socially withdrawn preschoolers with more oversolicitous mothers, 3 years later, are likely to be more shy and withdrawn compared to children with less solicitous mothers (Degnan, Henderson, Fox, & Rubin, 2008). Examining the links between parenting of preschoolers and social withdrawal in grades 1–6, Booth-LaForce and Oxford (2008) found that mothers who were more supportive and respectful of preschoolers' autonomy, and expressed less hostility, had children who were the least socially withdrawn throughout the elementary school years. Conversely, children who were highly withdrawn during the elementary school years were more likely to have experienced hostile and unsupportive maternal parenting in preschool that discouraged autonomy. These children were also more likely to be unpopular, excluded from peer activities, and lonely (Booth-LaForce & Oxford, 2008). Clearly, inappropriate maternal socialization in the preschool period can set the stage for lasting social difficulties and distress.

Childhood (6–10 Years)

Compared to the literature on younger children, there have been fewer studies of the links between shyness and parental socialization during childhood and beyond. Of course, as children proceed through elementary school and toward adolescence, other agents of socialization become increasingly involved in their lives. Children spend more time at school and in extracurricular activities that do not include parents. Peers and friends, teachers, and nonfamilial adults (e.g., coaches) all help to shape children's ongoing development. However, parents do not stop their involvement in their children's lives, and parental socialization continues to make important contributions to social and emotional functioning as children age.

Maternal parenting can affect the stability of children's earlier shy characteristics. Shyness and reticence in preschoolers were found to predict social withdrawal at 7 years only if children's mothers were more negatively controlling and showed less positive affect during interactions with their school-age children (Hane, Cheah, Rubin, & Fox, 2008). Control, warmth, and responsiveness are also concurrently associated with children's shyness. Compared to mothers of sociable children, mothers of highly withdrawn children use stronger imperatives and are less likely to respond to children's bids during interactions involving another child (Mills & Rubin, 1998). Similarly, mothers who issue more directives and are less warm when discussing solutions to hypothetical social problems have children who are lonely, and described by peers as sad, alone, and disliked, both concurrently and 1 year later (McDowell, Parke, & Wang, 2003). The quality of family relationships also continues to be important, as ambivalent attachment continues to be particularly characteristic of socially anxious children (Brumariu & Kerns, 2008), and socially withdrawn children's perceptions of their families as negative and emotionally distant increase their risk for depression (Gullone, Ollendick, & King, 2006).

Considering these studies, it would appear that the parenting experiences of shy and withdrawn children have changed by school age. There is less evidence that shy children continue to experience overly affectionate parenting, or intrusive control coupled with very high warmth. Rather than being oversolicitous, the mothers of shy school-age children appear to behave in a more "classically authoritarian" style, continuing to be very controlling but showing less warmth or positive affect toward their children. It might be the case that as children reach an age when most parents would expect more autonomy and competence, mothers of shy children become less accepting or patient with the continued neediness or distress of their children. This is a theme we return to when we examine the belief systems of parents of shy children.

Adolescence (11–16 Years)

There have been very few studies of adolescents in which the relations between parenting and shyness or withdrawal have been studied. However, some insight might be gleaned from the larger body of clinical studies that has examined the parenting experiences of adolescents with anxiety problems given that withdrawal is a symptom of social anxiety disorder. Hudson and Rapee (2001, 2002) studied children and youth with diagnosed anxiety disorders and their mothers during cognitively challenging tasks, and found that these mothers displayed more negativity and intrusive involvement than mothers of nonclinically diagnosed children. Normatively, one would expect maternal control to decrease from childhood to adolescence as children's capacity for autonomous activity increases. This developmental difference in maternal involvement was found only for the mothers of typical children; mothers of clinically anxious 12- to 15-year-old adolescents were likely to be just as intrusive and overinvolved as mothers of clinically anxious 7- to 11-year-old children (Hudson & Rapee, 2001). Furthermore, this pattern of parenting appeared to be more attributable to mothers' approach to childrearing than to anxious children's elicitation of overinvolvement, because these mothers were just as intrusive with the undiagnosed (typical) siblings of anxious children and adolescents (Hudson & Rapee, 2002). These studies support earlier retrospective studies that socially phobic adults remember their parents as overcontrolling and less affectionate than do nonphobic adults (e.g., Arrindell, Emmelkamp, Monsma, & Brilman, 1983).

Among nonclinical community samples Barber et al. (1994) found that maternal- and child-reported psychological control, incorporating overprotection, criticism, and love withdrawal, was related to self-reported internalizing difficulties in fifth, eighth, and tenth graders. McCabe, Clark, and Barnett (1999) reported a negative relation between maternally reported supportive behavior and teacher-reported social withdrawal and shyness in sixth graders. More recently, van Brakel, Muris, Bögels, and Thomassen (2006), found that for 11- to 15-year-olds identified as inhibited *and* insecure, parental control was significantly associated with anxiety. Finally, in a longitudinal study, Rubin, Chen, McDougall, and Bowker (1995) reported that more socially withdrawn 11-year-olds were, at age 14, more likely to report feeling insecure and disconnected from parents. Thus, similar to the research with shy children and anxious adolescents, the family contexts of shy and withdrawn youth appear to involve unsupportive, negative, and overcontrolling parents.

To date, there have been virtually no dedicated studies of the contributions of parenting in childhood to the development of shyness and withdrawal from childhood into adolescence. In a recent study of the transition from elementary to middle school, Kennedy Root and Rubin (2009) hypothesized that the stability of children's shyness from elementary school to middle school (early adolescence) would be moderated by children's experiences of intrusive or enmeshed parenting. Peers in the two school contexts reported on children's behaviors and, indeed, the stability of shyness was highest for children whose mothers were the most intrusive or enmeshed—and also for children whose mothers were the most punitive. Clearly, these findings are consistent with previous research (e.g., Hane et al., 2008) and support the conclusion that a continued pattern of intrusively overinvolved, restrictive, and negative parenting maintains or exacerbates the stability of shy and withdrawn behavior through childhood and into adolescence.

Fathering and Children's Shyness and Social Withdrawal

Although there have been far fewer investigations of paternal socialization, a small number of studies provide some insight into the associations between fathers' parenting and the development of children's shyness. Although some researchers have reported that paternal attachment and parenting are not associated with children's shyness (LaFrenière et al., 1992), more researchers have documented support for the potential importance of fathers' contributions to children's shyness. In general, the pattern of associations is consistent with those noted for maternal socialization.

As they reported for mothers, Park and colleagues (1997) found that fathers who were less supportive, less affectionate, and more negative and intrusive with their 18- and 30-month-old sons had boys who were less inhibited at 3 years, especially if the boys had been emotionally negative infants. This study stands in stark contrast to most research, but as the investigators acknowledged, this might have been due to the nature of their observational and coding procedures. What was characterized as being unresponsive and demanding might have "actually reflected a parent's sensitive awareness that a child was inhibited, which motivated the parent to 'push' or otherwise encourage the child to master his anxieties" (p. 225).

McShane and Hastings (2009) found that fathers who were more critical and less supportive had young children who were more anxious and isolated at preschool. The benefits of fathers' supportive parenting and the risks of fathers' psychological control for young children's reticent behavior were strongest for children with poor self-regulatory abilities (Hastings, Sullivan, et al., 2008). In both of these examinations, fathers' parenting added incrementally to the prediction of children's behavior, after accounting for maternal socialization. Thus, children's experiences of paternal socialization appear to be important for their development of shyness and social withdrawal.

Parke and colleagues (McDowell et al., 2003; Rah & Parke, 2008) have also found that school-age children who experience greater directive control or less responsive parenting from fathers are less liked by and involved with peers, and are less able to generate positive goals and effective strategies to resolve social dilemmas. Again, these paternal contributions were independent of any effects of maternal parenting. Finally, working with preadolescents, Miller, Murry, and Brody (2005) found that boys with fathers who were less responsive and supportive during discussions were shyer at school, whereas mothers' behavior was not associated with sons' shyness.

Overall, this small set of studies indicates that children's shyness is associated with fathers' parenting in ways that are similar to its link with mothers' parenting. There is less consistent evidence for the risk entailed by fathers' oversolicitousness (McShane & Hastings, 2009) than for derision and strict overcontrol, which might reflect differences between parents in their likelihood to shelter children (Parke & Buriel, 1998). Furthermore, it is clear that paternal socialization is not just a "by-product" of maternal childrearing. At least for children with both a mother and a father, fathers' parenting might be just as important as mothers' parenting for shaping children's social comfort and competence with peers (Parke, 1995). It is evident that more attention to the roles of fathers in the socialization of children's shyness is warranted.

Looking at the Parents of Shy Children

Parent Characteristics

Recognizing that research has documented consistent associations between specific patterns of parenting and children's likelihood of being shy, it is important to understand why some parents adopt the maladaptive socialization practices that put their children at risk. Some researchers have considered maternal personality and psychopathology. Mothers who are neurotic or easily psychologically distressed, or who themselves have anxiety or affective problems, are more likely to have inhibited, shy, or anxious children (Ellenbogen & Hodgins, 2004; Zahn-Waxler, Klimes-Dougan, & Slattery, 2000). While undoubtedly genetic commonalities contribute to mother and child similarity in social wariness, the socialization behaviors of anxiety-prone mothers might also convey risk for shyness to their children. Mothers who are shy, anxious, prone to psychological distress, or neurotic have been found to be more controlling, overprotective, and derisive in their parenting, and also less responsive (Bögels, van Oosten, Muris, & Smulders, 2001; Clark, Kochanska, & Ready, 2000; Coplan, Arbeau, & Armer, 2008; Mills et al., 2007), particularly if their children are shy (Coplan, Reichel, & Rowan, 2009). The links between maternal anxiety and children's anxiety have been found to be at least partly attributable to anxious mothers' greater use of overprotective parenting (Bayer et al., 2006).

Clearly, mothers with neurotic personalities or anxious tendencies appear likely to engage in socialization practices that inculcate anxiety or shyness in their own children. There are also other direct and indirect ways in which these maternal characteristics could affect children's social and emotional development. Neurotic or anxious mothers are likely to experience and to express more distress and negative affect in the context of parenting. Repeated exposure to maternal distress might undermine children's sense of security, and children might model mothers' maladaptive behaviors in their own social interactions with others. As well, anxious mothers might avoid social situations that they find stressful, such as playgroups, sporting teams, or public events, and thereby deny their children the opportunities to experience and to cope successfully with group activities. Additional research is needed to determine the extent to which such mechanisms contribute to the links between mothers' personal characteristics and children's likelihood of becoming shy.

Parental Beliefs

Considerable work has also gone into examining the parental belief systems, or parenting cognitions, that underlie socialization practices that inculcate shyness. Parental beliefs comprise the ways parents think and feel about their children, and about themselves as parents. This includes the causal explanations or attributions that parents make for children's behavior, the socialization goals they have while parenting, the strategies they consider appropriate to use with children, their sense of efficacy or competency as parents, and the emotions they experience in the context of childrearing. These dynamic belief systems contribute to how parents respond to children's behaviors during interactions, and to broader aspects of childrearing, such as the ways in which parents establish the home environment (Bugental & Goodnow, 1998). They are also contextually bound and malleable, as parental beliefs change adaptively across childrearing situations, and children's behaviors and characteristics contribute to parental beliefs (Hastings & Rubin, 1999).

When asked to think about their young children displaying shyness or social withdrawal, most mothers (and fathers) have reported that they would feel surprised or confused, that they expect the behavior to be a transient or passing stage, that they would want their children to feel better, and that they would avoid being overtly controlling by using indirect responses, such as planning future playdates (Hastings & Rubin, 1999; Mills & Rubin, 1990). However, mothers of socially withdrawn preschoolers respond quite differently when asked to think about their children being shy with peers. These mothers report more negative emotions, including disappointment and guilt, view the shy behavior as dispositional or characteristic of their children, and suggest becoming directly involved to change their children's immediate behavior (Rubin & Mills, 1990). These parental beliefs appear, at least in part, to be reactions to parents' experiences of raising inhibited or shy children. Indeed, more inhibited or fearful toddlers have mothers and fathers who become increasingly less encouraging of their children's independence over time (Rubin et. al., 1999), and mothers who are less confused by preschoolers' shyness and more likely to become directly involved by comforting and playing (Hastings & Rubin, 1999). Thus, although their actions are likely motivated by compassion and the desire to prevent their children's distress, parents appear to react to their young children's early displays of social difficulty in ways expected to exacerbate, rather than ameliorate, shyness.

This picture appears to change after the preschool period, however. Most parents know that social skills should improve with age, and they feel increasingly negatively about socially inappropriate behaviors from older children (Dix, 1991). Compared to mothers of socially competent elementary school-age children, mothers of withdrawn children report shyness as less surprising (probably due to their children's dispositional characteristics), and less amenable to change through parental efforts (Mills & Rubin, 1993). When mothers of highly withdrawn preschoolers were interviewed 2 years later, they saw their children as responsible for their shy behavior, which they expected to remain stable over time (Rubin & Mills, 1992). These studies suggest that mothers of shy children become more resigned or pessimistic over time, and less patient with their older children's social difficulties. This might contribute to the previously noted developmental shift in the associations of parenting with children's shyness, replacing the coddling oversolicitousness of preschoolers with critical authoritarian control of school-age and older children. Unfortunately, neither pattern of socialization is likely to help shy children cope better with their social wariness and develop greater social confidence and competence.

Contexts of Parenting: Culture and the Socialization of Shyness

From Bronfenbrenner's bioecological perspective, the surrounding community and culture serve as contexts of parenting and socialization. How parents of shy children think, feel, and act is shaped by their cultural milieus, and parents in turn transfer those cultural messages about shyness to their children (see Chen, Chapter 10, this volume). Although the majority of research on the socialization of shyness has been conducted in North America and Western Europe, the past decade has seen the emergence of interest in cross-cultural perspectives.

In Western culture, autonomy and assertiveness are valued, and shyness in children is considered socially immature, maladaptive, and undesirable (Rubin & Asendorpf, 1993). Conversely, the traditional Confucian and Taoist philosophies of China promote self-restraint and discourage individualism or self-promotion (King & Bond, 1985), and inhibited and wary behaviors in children are viewed as appropriate and valued (Chen, Rubin, & Sun, 1992). Research has shown that this difference in cultural values is reflected in parenting. Comparing mothers in Canada and Mainland China, Chen and colleagues (1998) found that Chinese mothers were more accepting and encouraging of achievement, and less controlling with more inhibited toddlers; Canadian mothers of inhibited toddlers were more controlling and protective, and less accepting and encouraging of achievement. Chinese mothers' more positive responses to inhibition might contribute to the more competent and socially accepted trajectories shown by shy Chinese children compared to their Western counterparts (Chen, Rubin, & Li, 1995).

Just like people, though, cultures can change as they develop, and there has been a rapid course of "Westernization" in contemporary Chinese society, such that shyness may now be viewed as less adaptive and beneficial. Examining the correlates of shyness in Chinese children over 12 years, Chen, Cen, Li, and He (2005) found that shyness was more strongly associated with social and academic achievement in a 1990 cohort than in a 1998 cohort and, by 2002, shyness was associated with peer rejection, school problems, and depression. Paralleling this, a more recent study of parenting and shyness in China shows that children's withdrawal, reticence, and solitary behaviors are associated with mothers' coercion, directiveness, overprotection, and shaming (Nelson, Hart, Wu, Roper, Jin, & Young, 2006).

South Korea's ties to Western cultures and values predate those of China, and research on shyness and parenting beliefs in Korea, China, and North America indicate several points of convergence and divergence across the three cultures (Cheah & Rubin, 2004; Cheah & Park, 2006). Although all mothers report negative emotional responses to withdrawal, Chinese and Korean mothers are more likely than European American mothers to attribute withdrawal to external causes. Conversely, both South Korean and European American mothers prioritize goals of making the child feel happy and more self-confident in response to social withdrawal, which they approach by trying to obtain the child's perspectives regarding his or her solitary behavior, whereas Chinese mothers seek to promote the child's functioning for the betterment of the peer group. These differences suggest that Chinese mothers still approach parenting from Confucian perspectives more strongly than do Korean mothers, who blend Eastern and Western values in their beliefs about shyness. These findings are augmented by a recent report by Park, Song, and Rubin (2008), who found that Korean toddlers' inhibition predicted their shyness and reticence at preschool age when their mothers had been more overprotective, mirroring findings in Western samples (Rubin et al., 2002).

The cultural perspectives on children and families in Southern Europe differ in many ways from those of Northern Europe and North America (Rubin et al., 2006). Luck or fate is seen as a dominant force in shaping development, and strong connections with extended family are favored over ties with peers, which might account for Italian mothers reporting less strong emotional responses to children's shyness than did English Canadian mothers, but more internal attributions (e.g., stable, hard to change) (Schneider, Attili, Vermigli, & Younger, 1997). However, it might also be the case that cultural beliefs around socialization vary not only between countries but even between communities within a country. Sicilian parents value assertiveness and sociability (Casiglia, LoCoco, & Zappulla, 1998), and report less acceptance and more authoritarian parenting of inhibited toddlers (Rubin et al., 2006). Analogously, differences between accepting versus protective responses to children's shyness have been noted in communities in Yucatan, Mexico that differ in their attributions about the sources of problems (Cervera & Méndez, 2006).

Taken together, these findings suggest that parents' approaches to the rearing of shy children are nested within the broader cultural context that dictates whether inhibited, withdrawn, and shy behaviors are seen as problematic, immature, and interfering with social success or as acceptable and conducive to group harmony. Culture is not static, however, and changes in the roles or characteristics that define success within a culture might lead to changes in parents' attitudes and behaviors toward shy children. Thus, cross-cultural research on socialization would benefit from the use of longitudinal designs and inclusion of parents' identification with the dominant values of their surrounding cultures.

CONCLUSIONS

In conclusion, the empirical research on parenting and children's development of shyness mirrors the tenets of transactional, bidirectional, and bioecological theories of development. Integrating the patterns of findings across studies, a developmental model of the socialization of shyness can be constructed. At least within Western cultures, it begins early in life, as emotionally reactive, distress-prone, or temperamentally inhibited infants and toddlers elicit maladaptive socialization responses from their parents, reflected in aspects of psychological control such as intrusive overcontrol, egregious physical affection, or derision, criticism, and rejection. Parents seem particularly prone to such responses if they themselves experience heightened anxiety or emotional distress. In parallel, temperamentally vulnerable or emotionally dysregulated infants and toddlers are most sensitive to the adverse effects of poor parenting, because their relatively poor self-regulatory capacities leave them more dependent upon external sources of support, specifically, parenting.

The interplay of young children's high neediness and parents' inappropriate caregiving undermines the development of secure attachment relationships, diminishing developing toddlers' preparedness to cope autonomously with social interactions with peers and nonfamilial adults. Encountering other children at day care, preschool, or the playground, these children become upset and withdraw from interactions. Their parents seek to prevent future distressing events by staying close to the children and micromanaging their social activities, or even by avoiding such activities to diminish the children's contacts with unfamiliar people and situations. However, these actions rob the children of opportunities to practice and develop their social skills, reinforce the pattern of avoiding or withdrawing from interactions, and thereby lead to stable patterns of shy behavior.

As their shy children move through the elementary school years, parents increasingly perceive their children's reticent behavior as an immutable and enduring characteristic. They also become increasingly dissatisfied and impatient with their children's shyness, because it violates their culturally based expectations for children's normative development of autonomy and independence, and their children's distress also acts as a chronic stressor on parents. Overt physical affection is replaced by negativity and authoritarian control, which maintain children's feelings of incompetence and insecurity, and their shyness and social isolation. Inhibited and withdrawn children with overprotective parents thereby develop into shy and reticent youth with authoritarian parents, with isolation, loneliness, and depression emerging as likely adverse outcomes of this unfortunate trajectory.

The empirical evidence for this model is not yet complete, of course, and we have inferred a series of temporal and causal links that have not been fully documented. Furthermore, in keeping with the tenets of developmental psychopathology, there are likely to be many points of departure from this stable pathway toward shyness. Sensitive, supportive, and positive parenting can help vulnerable children to develop social comfort and competence. Accepting peers and close friends, and nurturing teachers and other adults, might ameliorate some of the influences of maladaptive parental socialization. The luck of the genetic draw might lead to desirable maturational changes around puberty that increase children's acceptance by peers and their self-esteem. We contend, however, that parental socialization lies at the core of developing children's sense of self and ability to engage competently with others, as well as their receptiveness to positive influences by other socialization agents. Recognizing the critically central roles of parental socialization and parent–child relationships in children's development of shyness and social withdrawal is fundamental for understanding the challenges faced by shy children. In turn, this knowledge will be vital in efforts to design and implement effective interventions to help shy children overcome their reticence and attain comfort and confidence in the social world.

REFERENCES

Ainsworth, M. D. S., Blehar, M. C., Waters, E., & Wall, S. (1978). *Patterns of attachment*. Hillsdale, NJ: Erlbaum.

Arrindell, W. A., Emmelkamp, P. M., Monsma, A., & Brilman, E. (1983). The role of perceived parental rearing practices in the aetiology of phobic disorders: A controlled study. *British Journal of Psychiatry, 143,* 183–187.

Barber, B. K., & Harmon, E. L. (2002). Violating the self: Parental psychological control of children and adolescents. In B. K. Barker (Ed.), *Intrusive parenting: How psychological control affects children and adolescents* (pp. 15–52). Washington, DC: American Psychological Association.

Barber, B. K., Olsen, J. E., & Shagle, S. C. (1994). Associations between parental psychological and behavioral control and youth internalized and externalized behaviors. *Child Development, 65,* 1120–1136.

Baumrind, D. (1997). Necessary distinctions. *Psychological Inquiry, 8,* 176–229.

Bayer, J. K., Sanson, A. V., & Hemphill, S. A. (2006). Children's moods, fears, and worries: Development of an early childhood parent questionnaire. *Journal of Emotional and Behavioral Disorders, 14,* 41–49.

Becker, W. C. (1964). Consequence of different kinds of parenting disciplines. In L. Hoffman & L. W. Hoffman (Eds.), *Review of child development research* (Vol. 1, pp. 169–208). New York: Russell Sage Foundation.

Bell, R. Q. (1979). Parent, child, and reciprocal influences. *American Psychologist, 34,* 821–826.

Bögels, S. M., van Oosten, A., Muris, P., & Smulders, D. (2001). Familial correlates of social anxiety in children and adolescents. *Behaviour Research and Therapy, 39,* 273–287.

Booth-LaForce, C., & Oxford, M. L. (2008). Trajectories of social withdrawal from grades 1 to 6: Prediction from early parenting, attachment, and temperament. *Developmental Psychology, 44,* 1298–1313.

Bowlby, J. (1980). *Attachment and loss: Vol. 3. Loss: Sadness and Depression.* New York: Basic Books.

Bronfenbrenner, U., & Morris, P. A. (2006). The bioecological model of human development. In R. M. Lerner & W. Damon (Eds.), *Handbook of child psychology: Vol 1. Theoretical models of human development* (6th ed., pp 793–828). Hoboken, NJ: Wiley.

Brumariu, L. E., & Kerns, K. A. (2008). Mother–child attachment and social anxiety symptoms in middle childhood. *Journal of Applied Developmental Psychology,* 29, 393–402.

Bugental, D. B., & Goodnow, J. J. (1998). Socialization processes. In N. Eisenberg (Ed.), *Handbook of child psychology: Vol. 3. Social, emotional, and personality development* (pp. 389–414). New York: Wiley.

Calkins, S. D., & Fox, N. A. (1992). The relations among infant temperament, security of attachment, and behavioral inhibition at twenty-four months. *Child Development,* 63, 1456–1472.

Casiglia, A. C., LoCoco, A., & Zappulla, C. (1998). Aspects of social reputation and peer relationships in Italian children: A cross-cultural perspective. *Developmental Psychology,* 34, 723–730.

Cervera, M. D., & Méndez, R. M. (2006). Temperament and ecological context among Yucatec Mayan children. *International Journal of Behavioral Development,* 30, 326–337.

Cheah, C. S. L., & Park, S. (2006). South Korean mothers' beliefs regarding aggression and social withdrawal in preschoolers. *Early Childhood Research Quarterly,* 21, 61–75.

Cheah, C. S. L., & Rubin, K. H. (2004). European American and Mainland Chinese mothers' responses to aggression and social withdrawal in preschoolers. *International Journal of Behavioral Development,* 28, 83–94.

Chen, X., Cen, G., Li, D., & He, Y. (2005). Social functioning and adjustment in Chinese children: The imprint of historical time. *Child Development,* 76, 182–195.

Chen, X., Hastings, P. D., Rubin, K. H., Chen, H., Cen, G., & Stewart, S. L. (1998). Child-rearing attitudes and behavioral inhibition in Chinese and Canadian toddlers: A cross-cultural study. *Developmental Psychology,* 34, 677–686.

Chen, X., Rubin, K. H., & Li, B. (1995). Depressed mood in Chinese children: Relations with school performance and family environment. *Journal of Consulting and Clinical Psychology,* 63, 938–947.

Chen, X., Rubin, K. H., & Sun, Y. (1992). Social reputation and peer relationships in Chinese and Canadian children: A cross-cultural study. *Child Development,* 63, 1336–1343.

Clark, L. A., Kochanska, G., & Ready, R. (2000). Mothers' personality and its interaction with child temperament as predictors of parenting behavior. *Journal of Personality and Social Psychology,* 79, 274–285.

Clinton, H. R. (1996). *It takes a village and other lessons children teach us.* New York: Simon & Shuster.

Coplan, R. J., Arbeau, K. A., & Armer, M. (2008). Don't fret, be supportive!: Maternal characteristics linking child shyness to psychosocial and school adjustment in kindergarten. *Journal of Abnormal Child Psychology,* 36, 359–371.

Coplan, R. J., Findlay, L. C., & Nelson, L. J. (2004). Characteristics of preschoolers with lower perceived competence. *Journal of Abnormal Child Psychology,* 32, 399–408.

Coplan, R.J., Reichel, M., & Rowan, K. (2009). Exploring the associations between maternal personality, child temperament, and parenting: A focus on emotions. *Personality and Individual Differences,* 46, 241–246.

Cummings, E. M., Davies, P. T., & Campbell, S. B. (2000). *Developmental psycho-pathology and family process: Theory, research, and clinical implications.* New York: Guilford Press.

Degnan, K. A., & Fox, N. A. (2007). Behavioral inhibition and anxiety disorders: Multiple levels of a resilience process. *Development and Psychopathology, 19,* 729–746.

Degnan, K. A., Henderson, H. A., Fox, N. A., & Rubin, K. H. (2008). Predicting social wariness in middle childhood: The moderating roles of childcare history, maternal personality and maternal behavior. *Social Development, 17,* 471–487.

Denham, S. A. (1993). Maternal emotional responsiveness and toddlers' social–emotional competence. *Journal of Child Psychology and Psychiatry, 34,* 715–728.

Dix, T. (1991). The affective organization of parenting: Adaptive and maladaptive processes. *Psychological Bulletin, 110,* 3–25.

Dumas, J. E., LaFrenière, P. J., & Serketich, W. J. (1995). "Balance of power": A transactional analysis of control in mother–child dyads involving socially competent, aggressive, and anxious children. *Journal of Abnormal Psychology, 104,* 104–113.

Early, D. M., Rimm-Kaufman, S. E., Cox, M. J., Saluja, G., Pianta, R. C., Bradley, R. H., et al. (2002). Maternal sensitivity and child wariness in the transition to kindergarten. *Parenting: Science and Practice, 2,* 355–377.

Ellenbogen, M. A., & Hodgins, S. (2004). The impact of high neuroticism in parents on children's psychosocial functioning in a population at high risk for major affective disorder: A family–environmental pathway of intergenerational risk. *Development and Psychopathology, 16,* 113–136.

Erickson, M. F., Sroufe, L. A., & Egeland, B. (1985). The relationship between quality of attachment and behavior problems in preschool in a high-risk sample. *Monographs of the Society for Research in Child Development, 50*(1–2), 147–166.

Fox, N. A., Henderson, H. A., Marshall, P. J., Nichols, K. E., & Ghera, M. M. (2005). Behavioral inhibition: Linking biology and behavior within a developmental framework. *Annual Review of Psychology, 56,* 235–262.

Gullone, E., Ollendick, T. H., & King, N. J. (2006). The role of attachment representation in the relationship between depressive symptomatology and social withdrawal in middle childhood. *Journal of Child and Family Studies, 15,* 271–285.

Hane, A. A., Cheah, C., Rubin, K. H., & Fox, N. A. (2008). The role of maternal behavior in the relation between shyness and social reticence in early childhood and social withdrawal in middle childhood. *Social Development, 17*(4), 795–811.

Hastings, P. D., & De, I. (2008). Parasympathetic regulation and parental socialization of emotion: Biopsychosocial processes of adjustment in preschoolers. *Social Development, 17,* 211–238.

Hastings, P. D., Nuselovici, J. N., Utendale, W. T., Coutya, J., McShane, K. E., & Sullivan, C. (2008). Applying the polyvagal theory to children's emotion regulation: Social context, socialization, and adjustment. *Biological Psychology, 79,* 299–306.

Hastings, P. D., & Rubin, K. H. (1999). Predicting mothers' beliefs about preschool-aged children's social behavior: Evidence for maternal attitudes moderating child effects. *Child Development, 70,* 722–741.

Hastings, P. D., Sullivan, C., McShane, K. E., Coplan, R. J., Utendale, W. T., & Vyncke, J. D. (2008). Parental socialization, vagal regulation, and preschoolers' anxious difficulties: Direct mothers and moderated fathers. *Child Development, 79,* 45–64.

Hudson, J. L., & Rapee, R. M. (2001). Parent–child interactions and anxiety disorders: An observational study. *Behaviour Research and Therapy, 39,* 1411–1427.

Hudson, J. L., & Rapee, R. M. (2002). Parent–child interactions in clinically anxious children and their siblings. *Journal of Clinical Child and Adolescent Psychology, 31,* 548–555.

Kennedy Root, A., & Rubin, K. H. (2009, April). *The stability of shyness/withdrawal across the transition from elementary-to-middle school: The moderating role of parenting.* Paper presented at the Biennial Meeting of the Society for Research in Child Development, Denver, CO.

Kiang, L., Moreno, A. J., & Robinson, J. L. (2004). Maternal preconceptions about parenting predict child temperament, maternal sensitivity, and children's empathy. *Developmental Psychology, 40,* 1081–1092.

King, A. Y. C., & Bond, M. H. (1985). The Confucian paradigm of man: A sociological view. In W. S. Tsang & D. Wu (Eds.), *Chinese culture and mental health* (pp. 29–45). London: Academic Press.

Kochanska, G. (1998). Mother–child relationship, child fearfulness, and emerging attachment: A short-term longitudinal study. *Developmental Psychology, 34,* 480–490.

Kuczynski, L., & Parkin, C. M. (2007). Agency and bidirectionality in socialization: Interactions, transactions, and relational dialectics. In. J. E. Grusec & P. D. Hastings (Eds.), *Handbook of socialization: Theory and research* (pp. 259–283). New York: Guilford Press.

LaFrenière, P. J., Provost, M. A., & Dubeau, D. (1992). From an insecure base: Parent–child relations and internalizing behaviour in the pre-school. *Early Development and Parenting, 1,* 137–148.

Maccoby, E. E., & Martin, J. A. (1983). Socialization in the context of the family: Parent–child interaction. In E. M. Hetherington (Ed.), *Handbook of child psychology: Vol. 4. Socialization, personality, and social development* (4th ed., pp. 1–102). New York: Wiley.

Malatesta, C. Z., Culver, C., Tesman, J. R., & Shepard, B. (1989). The development of emotion expression during the first two years of life. *Monographs of the Society for Research in Child Development, 54*(1–2), 1–104.

Matas, L., Arend, R. A., & Sroufe, L. A. (1978). Continuity of adaptation in the second year: The relationship between quality of attachment and later competence. *Child Development, 49,* 547–556.

McCabe, K. M., Clark, R., & Barnett, D. (1999). Family protective factors among urban African American youth. *Journal of Clinical Child Psychology, 28,* 137–150.

McDowell, D. J., Parke, R. D., & Wang, S. J. (2003). Differences between mothers' and fathers' advice-giving style and content: Relations with social competence and psychological functioning in middle childhood. *Merrill–Palmer Quarterly, 49,* 55–76.

McLeod, B. D., Wood, J. J., & Weisz, J. R. (2007). Examining the association between parenting and childhood anxiety: A meta-analysis. *Clinical Psychology Review, 27,* 155–172.

McShane, K. E., & Hastings, P. D. (2009). Psychological control in parents of preschoolers: Implications for behavior in early child care settings. *International Journal of Behavioral Development, 33.* doi:10.1177/0165025409103874.

Miller, S. R., Murry, V. M., & Brody, G. H. (2005). Parents' problem solving with preadolescents and its association with social withdrawal at school: Considering parents' stress and child gender. *Fathering, 3,* 147–163.

Mills, R. S. L., Freeman, W. S., Clara, I. P., Elgar, F. J., Walling, B. R., & Mak, L. (2007). Parent proneness to shame and the use of psychological control. *Journal of Child and Family Studies, 16,* 359–374.

Mills, R. S., & Rubin, K. H. (1990). Parental beliefs about problematic social behaviors in early childhood. *Child Development, 61,* 138–151.

Mills, R. S. L., & Rubin, K. H. (1993). Socialization factors in the development of social withdrawal. In K. H. Rubin & J. B. Asendorpf (Eds.), *Social withdrawal, inhibition, and shyness in childhood* (pp. 117–148). Hillsdale, NJ: Erlbaum.

Mills, R. S. L., & Rubin, K. H. (1998). Are behavioural and psychological control both differentially associated with childhood aggression and social withdrawal? *Canadian Journal of Behavioural Science, 30,* 132–136.

Nelson, L. J., Hart, C. H., Wu, B., Roper, S. O., Jin, S., & Yang, C. (2006). Relations between Chinese mothers' parenting practices and social withdrawal in early childhood. *International Journal of Behavioral Development, 30,* 261–271.

Park, S., Belsky, J., Putnam, S., & Crnic, K. (1997). Infant emotionality, parenting, and 3-year inhibition: Exploring stability and lawful discontinuity in a male sample. *Developmental Psychology, 33,* 218–227.

Park, S.Y., Song, J. H., & Rubin, K. H. (2008). The heterogeneity of solitary behaviors in 4-year-old children as related to child inhibition and parenting behaviors. *Korean Journal of Child Studies, 29,* 97–113.

Parke, R. D. (1995). Fathers and families. In M. H. Bornstein (Ed.). *Handbook of parenting: Vol. 3. Status and social conditions of parenting* (pp. 27–63). Hillsdale, NJ: Erlbaum.

Parke, R. D., & Buriel, R. (1998). Socialization in the family: Ethnic and ecological perspectives. In W. Damon & N. Eisenberg (Eds.), *Handbook of child psychology: Vol 3. Social, emotional, and personality development* (5th ed., pp. 463–552). Hoboken, NJ: Wiley.

Rah, Y., & Parke, R. D. (2008). Pathways between parent–child interactions and peer acceptance: The role of children's social information processing. *Social Development, 17,* 341–357.

Renken, B., Egeland, B., Marvinney, D., Mangelsdorf, S., & Sroufe, L. A. (1989). Early childhood antecedents of aggression and passive-withdrawal in early elementary school. *Journal of Personality, 57,* 257–281.

Rubin, K. H., & Asendorpf, J. B. (1993). Social withdrawal, inhibition, and shyness in childhood: Conceptual and definitional issues. In K. H. Rubin & J. B. Asen-dorf (Eds.), *Social withdrawal, inhibition, and shyness in childhood* (pp. 3–17). Hillsdale, NJ: Erlbaum.

Rubin, K. H., Burgess, K. B., & Hastings, P. D. (2002). Stability and social-behavioral consequences of toddlers' inhibited temperament and parenting behaviors. *Child Development, 73,* 483–495.

Rubin, K. H., Cheah, C. S. L., & Fox, N. (2001). Emotion regulation, parenting and display of social reticence in preschoolers. *Early Education and Development, 12,* 97–115.

Rubin, K. H., Chen, X., McDougall, P., & Bowker, A. (1995). The Waterloo Longitudinal Project: Predicting internalizing and externalizing problems in adolescence. *Development and Psychopathology, 7,* 751–764.

Rubin, K. H., Hastings, P. D., Stewart, S. L., Henderson, H. A., & Chen, X. (1997). The consistency and concomitants of inhibition: Some of the children, all of the time. *Child Development, 68,* 467–483.

Rubin, K. H., Hemphill, S. A., Chen, X., Hastings, P. D., Sanson, A., LoCoco, A., et al. (2006). Parenting beliefs and behaviors: Initial findings from the International Consortium for the Study of Social and Emotional Development (ICSSED). In K. H. Rubin & O. B. Chung (Eds.), *Parenting beliefs, behaviors, and parent–child relations* (pp. 81–103). New York: Psychology Press.

Rubin, K. H., & Mills, R. S. L. (1990). Maternal beliefs about adaptive and maladaptive social behaviors in normal, aggressive, and withdrawn preschoolers. *Journal of Abnormal Child Psychology, 18,* 419–435.

Rubin, K. H., & Mills, R. S. L. (1992). Parents' thoughts about children's socially adaptive and maladaptive behaviors: Stability, change, and individual differences. In I. E. Sigel, A. V. McGillicuddy-DeLisi, & J. J. Goodnow (Eds.), *Parental belief systems: The psychological consequences for children* (2nd ed., pp. 41–69). Hillsdale, NJ: Erlbaum.

Rubin, K. H., Nelson, L. J., Hastings, P. D., & Asendorpf, J. (1999). The transaction between parents' perceptions of their children's shyness and their parenting styles. *International Journal of Behavioral Development, 23,* 937–958.

Sameroff, A. (1975). Transactional models of early social relations. *Human Development, 18,* 65–79.

Schaeffer, E. S. (1959). A circumplex model of maternal behavior. *Journal of Abnormal and Social Psychology, 59,* 226–235.

Schneider, B. H., Attili, G., Vermigli, P., & Younger, A. (1997). A comparison of middle class English-Canadian and Italian mothers' beliefs about children's peer-directed aggression and social withdrawal. *International Journal of Behavioral Development, 21,* 133–154.

Spangler, G., & Schieche, M. (1998). Emotional and adrenocortical responses of infants to the Strange Situation: The differential function of emotional expression. *International Journal of Behavioral Development, 22,* 681–706.

Thomasgard, M., & Metz, W. P. (1993). Parental overprotection revisited. *Child Psychiatry and Human Development, 24,* 67–80.

van Brakel, A. M. L., Muris, P., Bögels, S. M., & Thomassen, C. A. (2006). Multifactorial model for the etiology of anxiety in non-clinical adolescents: Main and interactive effects of behavioral inhibition, attachment and parental rearing. *Journal of Child and Family Studies, 15,* 569–579.

Zahn-Waxler, C., Klimes-Dougan, B., & Slattery, M. J. (2000). Internalizing problems of childhood and adolescence: Prospects, pitfalls, and progress in understanding the development of anxiety and depression. *Development and Psychopathology, 12,* 443–466.

7

Social Withdrawal in Childhood and Adolescence
Peer Relationships and Social Competence

KENNETH H. RUBIN
JULIE BOWKER
HEIDI GAZELLE

During the past three decades, the study of children's peer relationships and social skills has taken a prominent position in the fields of developmental and clinical psychology. This reflects, in part, a growing conviction that children who are socially skilled enjoy strong and positive relationships with their peers; in turn, those who are accepted by their peers and able to develop supportive friendships fare well in their social, emotional, and academic lives. It is also known that children who are socially unskilled often suffer from peer rejection and friendlessness that place them "at risk" for later socioemotional and academic difficulties (for relevant reviews, see Rubin, Bukowski, & Laursen, 2009). Why the latter group is at risk has not been well addressed from the perspective of a "grand theory" of peer interactions and relationships. Yet there is a good deal of consensus across diverse theoretical perspectives as to the many benefits of peer interactions and relationships in childhood and adolescence. In this chapter, we briefly review theories that suggest the significance of peer interactions and relationships for normal psychosocial adaptation. Thereafter, we review the empirical literature pertaining to one subgroup of children, many of whose members have been described as lacking in social competence and as having less than adequate relationships with their peers. Given the focus of this edited volume, it should not be too surprising that this group comprises those who are socially anxious and withdrawn.

RELEVANT THEORY

Piaget (1932), in his earliest writings, portrayed children's relationships with peers, unlike their relationships with adults, as being relatively balanced, egalitarian, and as falling along a more or less horizontal plane of power assertion and dominance. It was within this egalitarian context that Piaget believed children could experience opportunities to examine conflicting ideas and explanations, to negotiate and discuss multiple perspectives, and to decide to compromise with or to reject the notions held by peers. From such interactions, Piaget argued that children came to develop the capacity for sensitive "perspective taking," or the ability to understand the thoughts, feelings, and literal viewpoints of others, which in turn was thought to form the basis for socially competent behavior, and the development of meaningful and rich social relationships (for a review, see Rubin, Bukowski, & Parker, 2006).

Mead (1934) was another early theorist who asserted the significance of social interaction for normal development. Like Piaget, Mead emphasized the importance of the development of perspective taking through peer interaction. With participation in organized, rule-governed activities with others, especially peers, children were thought to learn to consider and coordinate the perspectives of multiple others with respect to the self. Such perspective-taking experiences led to the conceptualization of the "generalized other," or the organized perspective of the social group, which in turn led to the emergence of an organized sense of self.

The classic *personality theory* of Sullivan (1953) has served as a guide for much current research concerning children's peer relationships and social skills. Like Piaget, Sullivan believed that the concepts of mutual respect, equality, and reciprocity developed from peer relationships. Sullivan, however, emphasized the significance of chumships or *best*-friendships, for the emergence of these concepts. For example, Sullivan believed that the *intimacy* of children's same-sex chumships during the juvenile years and beyond promoted psychological well-being and identity development, and contributed to later successes in romantic relationships. Sullivan's theory has proved influential in terms of the contemporary study of children's friendships and romantic relationships (e.g., Furman, Simon, Shaffer, & Bouchey, 2002), as well as the understanding of loneliness as a significant motivational force in development and adjustment (e.g., Asher & Paquette, 2003).

Learning and *social learning theory* have also stimulated current research on children's peer relationships and social skills. It was originally suggested, and it is now known, that children learn about their social worlds, and how to behave within them, through direct peer tutelage, as well as by observing each other. In this regard, children punish or ignore non-normative social behavior and reward or reinforce positively those behaviors viewed as culturally appropriate and competent (e.g., see Chen & French, 2008, for a review).

In *ethological theory*, it is argued that there is a relation between biology and the ability to initiate, maintain, or disassemble social relationships. It is a central tenet of ethological theory that social behavior and organizational structure are limited by biological constraints, and that they serve an adaptive evolutionary function (Hawley, 2003; Hinde & Stevenson-Hinde, 1976). Taken together, these theories, and the data supportive of them, have led psychologists to conclude that peer interactions and relationships are important forces in the development of normal social relationships and social skills. But these theories are focused on the putative *benefits* of peer interactions and relationships. They "speak to" the development of competent behavioral styles and adaptive extrafamilial relationships. The theories offer little with regard to establishing how *insufficient* or *deficient* interactions and relationships can lead to maladaptive behavioral styles, or to nonexistent or dysfunctional extrafamilial relationships.

SOCIAL AND SOCIAL-COGNITIVE COMPETENCE

If peer interaction leads to the development of (1) social competence, (2) the understanding of the self in relation to others, (3) acceptance by the peer group, and (4) supportive friendships, it seems reasonable to think that children, who, for whatever reason, refrain from engaging in social interaction and avoid the company of their peers may be at risk for developmental difficulties in these areas. This premise "drives" much of the current research on social withdrawal. In the following section, we focus on the construct of social competence and examine the extant literature on the social cognitions, social behaviors, and social skills of socially withdrawn children and young adolescents.

Social Competence

Social competence may best be characterized as a "judgment call" based on an audience's view of an actor's skilled behavior repertoire (McFall, 1982). The consistent demonstration of friendly, cooperative, prosocial, successful, and socially acceptable behavior over time and across settings is likely to lead to the judgment of the actor as socially competent. Thus, the "socially competent child" is one whose behavior is judged positively by peers and

who is able to (1) become engaged in a peer group structure and participate in group-oriented activities; (2) become involved in satisfying relationships constructed upon balanced and reciprocal interactions; and (3) satisfy
individual goals and needs, and develop accurate and productive means of
understanding experiences with peers on both the group and dyadic levels
(Rubin & Rose-Krasnor, 1992). Several common properties are shared in
the aforementioned examples. First, there is reference to *effectiveness*. Second, there is the implication that the actor is able to guide the behaviors and
contingent responses of others to meet his or her own needs or goals. Given
these criteria, Rubin and Rose-Krasnor have defined "social competence" as
the ability to achieve personal goals in social interaction, while simultaneously maintaining positive relationships with others over time and across
situations. A significant feature of this definition is its implicit recognition
of the importance of balancing personal desires against social consequences.
This emphasis reflects the essential duality of self and other, placing the individual within a social and personal context.

Social Information Processing

Why are some children and young adolescents more socially competent than
others? Rubin and Rose-Krasnor (1992) have suggested that when a child is
faced with a social dilemma (e.g., how to make a new friend; how to join a
play group; how to gain access to an attractive object), the following goal-
oriented sequence applies: First, the child chooses a social goal. Second, he
or she examines the social context; this involves interpreting relevant social
cues. For example, who is in the room? Are they familiar to the child? Are
they younger or older than the child? Are they perceived to be more dominant or submissive to the child? These social features are likely to influence
the child's goal and strategy selection (Krasnor & Rubin, 1983). Third, the
child accesses and selects strategies that aid in achieving the perceived social
goal in the specific situation of concern. Fourth, the child enacts the strategy. Finally, the child evaluates the outcome of the strategy. Was the goal
achieved? Did the strategy fail? If the initial strategy is unsuccessful, the
child may repeat it, or he or she may select and enact a new strategy, or
abandon the situation entirely.

   Other relevant social cognitive models exist. For example, Crick and
Dodge (1994) proposed a six-sequence model that involves (1) the encoding
of social cues; (2) the interpretation of encoded cues; (3) the clarification
of goals; (4) the accessing and generation of potential responses; (5) the
evaluation and selection of responses; and (6) the enactment of the chosen
response. Recently, Lemerise and Arsenio (2000) integrated *emotional* experiences into Crick and Dodge's social information-processing model. The
inclusion of emotion into this model is important to the study of socially

withdrawn children, because it is likely that many withdrawn children react to negative social situations with fear and anxiety. These emotions, in turn, may influence the information that is attended to and the information that is recalled. And this mood-congruent information processing might reinforce withdrawn children's social schemas or "working models" that the social world is fear-inducing. Indeed, these emotional responses may explain, in part, why some children withdraw in social company.

Studies of Social Information Processing, Social Problem Solving, and Social Withdrawal

Rubin and colleagues have demonstrated that when socially withdrawn 5-year-olds are asked how they would go about obtaining an attractive object from another child, making a new friend, or obtaining help from another, they produce fewer alternative solutions, display more rigidity in generating alternative responses, and are more likely to suggest adult intervention to aid in the solution of hypothetical social problems compared to their more sociable agemates (e.g., Rubin, 1982; Rubin, Daniels-Beirness, & Bream, 1984). These findings are augmented by the discovery that social withdrawal in early childhood is associated with deficits in the ability to take the perspectives of others (LeMare & Rubin, 1987). Similar findings have been reported in a sample of anxious shy children ages 6–11 years (Banerjee & Henderson, 2001).

From a theoretical perspective, one may surmise that it is the lack of peer interaction that leads to such deficits in thinking about solving social problems and about others' thoughts, feelings, and perspectives. However, neither longitudinal nor experimental studies exist to address this issue of causality. And by mid- and late childhood, many socially withdrawn children do *not* have difficulty in proactively generating solutions to meet some social goals (e.g., object acquisition; making a new friend; seeking help from a peer) presented to them in hypothetical interpersonal dilemmas (Rubin, 1985). These findings may suggest that only minimal experiences in peer interaction or simply observing others solving their interpersonal dilemmas over time is required for the development of some adaptive ways of thinking about solutions to interpersonal problems.

But not all withdrawn children are able to generate positive and assertive social goals and strategies. And, as noted previously, it seems likely that such difficulties may be traced to socially withdrawn children's emotional *reactions* to problematic social situations that befall them and to the enactment phase of the social information-processing sequence (e.g., Stewart & Rubin, 1995). Indeed, researchers have speculated that social dilemmas may evoke emotionally dysregulated reactions in withdrawn children; their inability to regulate and overcome their wariness has been proposed to result in an unassertive, submissive, if not avoidant, social problem-solving style and in less than successful outcomes following their attempts to make their ways through the social world. Recent research supports these speculations. For example, it has been reported that when confronted with a hypothetical event resulting in negative consequences, socially withdrawn 10-year-olds were more likely than their typical agemates to react with anger to the negative social event, and to suggest solving the dilemma through social avoidance (Burgess, Wojslawowicz, Rubin, Rose-Krasnor, & Booth-LaForce, 2006).

Studies of Social Competence In Situ

In early observational research, Rubin and colleagues paired socially withdrawn and nonwithdrawn 4- and 5-year-olds with same-sex, same-age, nonwithdrawn play partners (e.g., Rubin & Borwick, 1984; Rubin et al., 1984) and coded their behaviors during free play. The data revealed that the distribution of children's goals, the means by which they attempted to meet these goals, and the success rates of these strategies varied between the two groups. Concerning *goals,* withdrawn children were more likely to attempt to gain their partners' attention and were less likely than their more sociable counterparts to attempt to gain access to objects or to elicit action. The attention-seeking goals, which comprised over 50% of the socially withdrawn children's goals, required that their targets simply glance momentarily at the requestor; object acquisition and elicit action goals required active compliance from the targets and, as such, could be considered more "costly" to the targets. Thus, the social goals of withdrawn children appeared to be "safer" or of lower "cost" to their play partners than those of their more sociable agemates. Given the high proportion of low-cost goals, one may have predicted that the requests of withdrawn children would have been more successful than those of the nonwithdrawn children. This was not the case. Success rates for withdrawn versus nonwithdrawn children were 54% and 65%, respectively.

Other between-groups differences were revealed for the total number of requests directed at targets (withdrawn children made fewer) and the proportion of direct requests (imperatives) produced (withdrawn children made fewer). Thus, withdrawn children were observed to be less sociable and less assertive than their nonwithdrawn agemates. Given that social interaction necessarily involves at least two partners, it is noteworthy that Rubin and colleagues found that the social goals, strategies, and outcomes for the play partners of the withdrawn and typical children varied by dyadic grouping. First, the goals of the partners of withdrawn children were more costly than those of the partners of nonwithdrawn children; second, the strategies directed to withdrawn children were more direct; third, the outcomes were more successful. These data confirm the emerging picture of the withdrawn child as an unassertive, compliant youngster whom agemates view as easily influenced and manipulated.

In a follow-up developmental study of 7- and 9-year-olds, Stewart and Rubin (1995) found that socially withdrawn children displayed fewer social initiations, produced fewer socially assertive strategies, and were less successful in their attempts compared to their more sociable agemates. Significantly, their typical agemates experienced fewer failures in meeting their social goals with increasing age, but withdrawn children did not. Furthermore, the discrepancy in failure rates for "high-cost" social goals between the two target groups increased with increasing age. Finally, the withdrawn children were less likely than typical children to reinitiate a social problem-solving attempt subsequent to failure.

Further support for this picture of social incompetence and failure is drawn from subsequent studies of the peer management attempts of withdrawn versus nonwithdrawn children. For example, Rubin and colleagues have examined the role relationships of children playing dyadically or in peer quartets (Nelson, Rubin, & Fox, 2005; Rubin, 1985). Typically, in these investigations, socially withdrawn and nonwithdrawn children have been observed interacting with other nonwithdrawn agemates. And data in these studies were coded so as to allow an analysis of the peer management attempts of the children; in short, it was noted each time a child requested (verbally or nonverbally) his or her playmate to perform or not to perform a behavior. Observers also coded when the child asserted his or her own rights, thus attempting to influence the behavior of the partner. Finally, the success or failure of each behavior management attempt was coded.

In a first study of 7-year-olds, withdrawn children were less likely to attempt to manage the behaviors of their partners; furthermore, their attempts were proportionally less likely to result in success than those of nonwithdrawn children (Rubin, 1985). In a subsequent longitudinal investigation, Nelson et al. (2005) speculated that the consistent experience of *in situ* failure to obtain peer compliance may well be interpreted by children as representing personal failure in, and rejection by, the peer group. In support, these researchers found that socially reticent behavior during early childhood (age 4 years) was negatively associated with observed peer compliance; in turn, this lack of peer acceptance/compliance predicted negative self-perceptions of social competence at age 7 years.

From Peer Failure to Social Cognition

Attribution theory provides a conceptual framework for understanding the link between social-cognitive processes and experiences with peers. The basic premise of attribution theory is that individuals' attributions about why events occur guide their behavior. Many researchers have applied attributional theory to the study of children's social behaviors. Goetz and Dweck (1980), for instance, explored the association between children's interpretations of an experience with peers (i.e., being rejected from joining a pen pal club) and their subsequent behavior. They found that children who attributed failure to be accepted into a pen pal club to *personal internal causes* were debilitated in later attempts to gain entry into the club.

With regard to social withdrawal, Rubin and Krasnor (1986) found that extremely withdrawn children tended to blame their social failures on personal, dispositional characteristics rather than on external events or circumstances. More recently, Wichmann, Coplan, and Daniels (2004) reported that when 9- to 13-year-old withdrawn children were presented with hypothetical social situations in which ambiguously caused negative events happened to them, they attributed the events to internal and stable "self-defeating" causes. Importantly, withdrawn children more than non-withdrawn children in the Wichmann et al. study indicated that when faced with such negative situations, they were more familiar with failure experiences, and withdrawn children reported that a preferred strategy would be to withdraw and escape (see also Burgess et al., 2006). Moreover, researchers have found that when children have anxious expectations of peer rejection, they become increasingly withdrawn over time (London, Downey, Bonica, & Paltin, 2007).

Taken together, these findings suggest that if children interpret social experiences negatively, inappropriately, and inaccurately, they may prove to be their own worst enemies. A "negative feedback loop" may evolve, wherein the initially fearful and withdrawn child comes to believe that his or her social failures are internally based, and these self-blaming beliefs are reinforced by not only the expectation of peer rejection but also the experience of failed social initiatives and peer noncompliance (e.g., Rubin, Bowker, & Kennedy, 2009). When confronted by the "real-life" social world, withdrawn children may be less able than their nonwithdrawn peers to meet their social goals, due to their self-blaming and negative social-cognitive tendencies. This "negative feedback loop" may account for the consistent finding that in the middle and later years of childhood, socially withdrawn children develop increasingly negative self-perceptions, poor self-esteem, and feelings of loneliness (e.g., Boivin & Hymel, 1997; Boivin, Hymel, & Bukowski, 1995).

Blaming the self for one's interpersonal difficulties, anxiously expecting peer rejection, experiencing failure in attempts to move successfully through the world of peers, and dealing with one's social problems through avoidance collectively can lead to a variety of negative outcomes, such as depression, low self-esteem, and increased withdrawal (e.g., Garnefski, Kraaij, &

van Etten, 2005; Reijntjes, Stegge, Terwogt, Kamphuis, & Telch, 2006). Thus, the aforementioned findings may help to explain longitudinal associations between childhood social withdrawal and adolescent internalizing problems (e.g., Bell-Dolan, Reaven, & Peterson, 1993; Boivin et al., 1995; Dill, Vernberg, & Fonagy, 2004; Hymel, Rubin, Rowden, & LeMare, 1990; NOlen-Hoeksema, Girgus, & Seligman, 1992; Rubin, Chen, Mcdougall, Bowker, & Mckinnon, 1995).

PEER ACCEPTANCE, REJECTION, EXCLUSION, AND VICTIMIZATION

Shy/withdrawn children were once believed to be, on average, sociometrically *neglected* by peers (neither much liked nor disliked; Coie & Kupersmidt, 1983; Dodge, 1983). More recent research widely indicates that shy/withdrawn children are, on average, more sociometrically *rejected* or actively disliked by peers than their nonwithdrawn agemates (Cillessen, van IJzendoorn, van Lieshout, & Hartup, 1992; Gazelle et al., 2005; Rubin, Chen, & Hymel, 1993). The discrepancy between earlier and later work is likely due, at least in part, to improvements in sociometric methodology (Terry, 2000) and an increased emphasis on examining not only different types of solitude (Rubin, Coplan, & Bowker, 2009), but also heterogeneity among shy/withdrawn children with regard to peer rejection (Gazelle, 2008).

Research on the peer relationships of shy/withdrawn children has examined not only peer rejection but also peer acceptance, exclusion, and victimization. The first two of these peer relations constructs—acceptance and rejection—are attitudinal variables. In other words, peer-reported acceptance (being well liked by peers) and rejection (being widely disliked by peers) indicate peers' preference (or lack thereof) for a child as a playmate or social partner, but do not indicate how peers actually treat or behave toward a child. In contrast, peer exclusion (being left out of peers' activities by being passively ignored or actively refused entry) and victimization (being mistreated by peers, including teasing, verbal put-downs, and physical harm) describe how a child is actually treated by peers. In many respects, the observational studies described in the previous section represent attempts to document acts of peer exclusion.

This distinction is important because, although peer attitudes and treatment are meaningfully correlated, and evidence suggests that attitudes contribute to exclusion and victimization, careful analyses reveal that these constructs play distinct roles in peer relations processes (Boivin, Hymel, & Hodges, 2001). Furthermore, it may be misleading to assume that the strength of the relation between anxious withdrawal and peer acceptance or rejection necessarily indicates the extent of peer mistreatment of withdrawn children. For instance, evidence appears to support a stronger association between shyness/withdrawal and peer exclusion than between shyness/withdrawal and peer rejection (Gazelle & Ladd, 2003; for behavioral evidence of exclusion as documented earlier, see also Rubin, 1985; Stewart & Rubin, 1995). This is likely because factors such as peer perceptions of shy/withdrawn children as vulnerable or as easy targets for exclusion, also may contribute to exclusion, above and beyond the effects of rejection (Gazelle, 2008; Rubin, Coplan, et al., 2009). Indeed, many investigators have described socially withdrawn children as "whipping boys" (Olweus, 1993), "easy marks" (Rubin, Wojslawowicz, et al., 2006), physically weak (Hodges, Malone, & Perry, 1997), and anxiously vulnerable (Gazelle & Ladd, 2003).

Realizing the full impact of peer exclusion for withdrawn children requires that exclusion be conceptualized as not only an outcome of withdrawal but also a factor that may change the course of withdrawal itself, as well as withdrawn children's social and emotional adjustment more broadly. Gazelle and Ladd (2003) found that only those anxious withdrawn children who were excluded by peers in early grade school displayed greater stability in anxious solitude and elevated levels of depression over the course of middle childhood. Similarly, Gazelle and Rudolph (2004) have shown that over the course of fifth and sixth grade, high exclusion by peers led anxious solitary youth to maintain or exacerbate the extent of their social avoidance and depression, whereas the experience of low exclusion predicted increased social approach and less depression. These findings support a "diathesis–stress model." which posits that individual vulnerability or diathesis (anxious solitude) is activated when accompanied by interpersonal adversity (peer mistreatment).

There is empirical support for connections between anxious withdrawal and being the target of not only peer exclusion but also peer victimization (e.g., Erath, Flanagan, & Bierman, 2007; Hanish & Guerra, 2004; Kochenderfer-Ladd, 2003). At the same time, there is also support for the reverse direction of effect: Regular exposure to bullying may lead to increased fear of classmates and further withdrawal from peer interaction and school-related activities (Hoglund & Leadbetter, 2007). Importantly, recent studies using growth curve modeling found that the experience of both peer exclusion and victimization accounted for significantly greater stability or increases in the behavioral expression of anxious withdrawal from childhood through early adolescence (Gazelle & Ladd, 2003; Oh et al., 2008). Taken together, these investigations suggest a reciprocal, mutually exacerbating relation between social withdrawal (individual vulnerability) and peer mistreatment (interpersonal/environmental adversity).

Developmental Timing of Peer Difficulties
in Shy/Withdrawn Children

Evidence about the timing of the onset of peer relations difficulties in shy/withdrawn children has evolved in recent years. Early work suggested that shy/withdrawn children were not sociometrically rejected by their peers in early childhood but came to be rejected by middle childhood (Rubin, Chen, & Hymel, 1993). Researchers proposed that the occurrence of late-onset rejection may be due to developmental changes in peer perceptions of shyness/social withdrawal (Bukowski, 1990; Younger, Gentile, & Burgess, 1993; see also Crozier & Burnham, 1990). Specifically, it was proposed that shy/withdrawn behavior was not as salient to young children as other forms of behavior that deviate from the norm (e.g., aggression), because it is less concrete and less likely to affect them directly. More recently, however, researchers using different methodologies have found that young children are reliable informants of shyness/withdrawal (Coplan, Girardi, Findlay, & Frohlick, 2007), and that teachers report peer rejection and mistreatment of withdrawn children as early as preschool and kindergarten (Coplan, Prakash, O'Neil, & Armer, 2004; Coplan, Arbeau, & Armer, 2008; Gazelle & Ladd, 2003; Gazelle & Spangler, 2007; Hart et al., 2000). This latter research coincides with findings that the observed display of socially reticent and withdrawn behavior in early childhood is associated with not only peer exclusion but also sociometric rejection (e.g., Hart et al., 2000; Nelson et al., 2005). Similarly, shy/withdrawn behavior, as identified by teachers and child care providers, is concurrently and predictively related to peer rejection and exclusion in kindergarten and first grade (Gazelle & Ladd, 2003; Gazelle & Spangler, 2007). Although it is difficult to establish temporal precedence of shyness/withdrawal and peer difficulties in early elementary school, because they co-occur rapidly upon school entry (Gazelle & Ladd, 2003), some evidence indicates that early childhood shyness/withdrawal predicts subsequent peer difficulties in first grade (Gazelle & Spangler, 2007).

The co-occurrence of shyness/withdrawal and peer exclusion in the early years of elementary school appears to have important implications for children's psychological adjustment in middle childhood, especially when these two conditions endure over time. Early exclusion of shy/withdrawn children predicts sustained elevation in depressive symptoms over the course of middle childhood (Gazelle & Ladd, 2003). Furthermore, similar patterns occur in the early adolescent period (Gazelle & Rudolph, 2004). For example, when compared with their nonexcluded counterparts, excluded shy/withdrawn fifth and sixth graders demonstrated heightened self-reported depressive symptoms and teacher-rated helpless social behavior over the course of a year, whereas their nonexcluded shy/withdrawn counterparts demonstrated improvements in not only these indicators of maladjustment but also in prosocial/approach-oriented social behavior (Gazelle & Rudolph, 2004). These patterns suggest that the co-occurrence of shyness/withdrawal and peer mistreatment constitutes a diathesis–stress process in which children who are characterized by the initial vulnerability or diathesis of social anxiety (e.g., being worried about how they will be treated by peers) develop more stable and persistent social and emotional problems when their worries are confirmed by stressful peer experiences (e.g., peer exclusion). However, in the absence of peer stress, these children appear better adjusted.

Heterogeneity among Shy/Withdrawn Children in Peer Relations, Emotion, and Behavior

In a departure from the traditional focus on average adjustment of withdrawn children, researchers have recently reported a great deal of diversity in the stability and longitudinal outcomes among socially withdrawn children (Gazelle & Ladd, 2003; Gazelle & Rudolph, 2004; Oh et al., 2008). Several individual factors may affect developmental trajectories for socially withdrawn children. One such factor is the sex of the child. Several studies have indicated that shy/withdrawn boys experience more peer adversity and emotional maladjustment than do girls (e.g., Coplan et al., 2004, 2008; Gazelle & Ladd, 2003; Morison & Masten, 1991). However, this appears to be a question of degree rather than the fundamental relation between shyness/withdrawal and risk for social and emotional difficulties. Shy/withdrawn girls are clearly at risk for peer rejection and victimization (e.g., Gazelle et al., 2005). Furthermore, patterns are dependent upon age and outcome of interest. For instance, in a sample of young adolescents, shy/withdrawn girls and boys were equally likely to be excluded, but exclusion in shy/withdrawn girls predicted earlier and more sustained elevation in self-reported depressive symptoms than it did for boys (Gazelle & Rudolph, 2004).

Another individual factor that may influence trajectories of social withdrawal and the experience of peer rejection and exclusion is the inability to regulate negative emotions. In their research on the stability and consequences of behavioral inhibition (a putative precursor of shy/anxious behavior; Rubin, Coplan, et al., 2009), Fox, Rubin, and colleagues have reported that behaviorally inhibited toddlers who demonstrate physiologically and behaviorally assessed emotion dysregulation are at higher risk for subsequent social reticence (and, as described earlier, for peer exclusion; Nelson et al., 2005) at 4 years than their more emotionally regulated agemates (e.g., Fox, Henderson, Rubin, Calkins, & Schmidt, 2001; Rubin, Burgess, & Hastings, 2002; see also Fox and Reeb-Sutherland, Chapter 5, this volume).

Two recent studies suggest that highly emotional or emotionally dys-regulated shy/withdrawn elementary school-age children are at greater risk for peer difficulties and for a pattern of more stable, if not increasing, shy-ness/withdrawal and internalizing problems (Bowker, Rubin, Rose-Krasnor, & Booth-LaForce, 2008; Booth-LaForce & Oxford, 2008). For example, Bowker and colleagues (2008) found that the expression of internalizing emotions moderated the initial and longitudinal associations between with-drawn behavior and peer exclusion. Withdrawn children who frequently displayed internalizing emotions were more likely than their well-regulated withdrawn counterparts to experience peer exclusion. Taken together, there appear to be emotional, perhaps dispositional characteristics that may help to explain variations in the extent to which withdrawn children experience peer exclusion.

Other recent work indicates that heterogeneity in peer treatment among withdrawn children is related to additional social behavior characteristics that co-occur with withdrawal. Gazelle (2008) identified several subgroups of shy/withdrawn children who differed significantly from one another in the extent to which they were agreeable, attention seeking, externaliz-ing, or behaviorally normative. Members of these groups were identified by peers as frequently playing alone, engaging in onlooking behavior, and appearing shy and nervous around peers. Agreeable shy/withdrawn chil-dren were nonetheless perceived by peers as responsive to others' initiations and cooperative. Normative shy/withdrawn children were not perceived as displaying behaviors that deviated from the norm (except for shyness/withdrawal). Attention-seeking shy/withdrawn children were perceived by peers as seeking attention from peers via annoying or immature (but not aggressive) behavior. Externalizing shy/withdrawn children were perceived to be aggressive (physically, verbally, and/or relationally) or hyperactive or distractible (many of these children also scored high on attention-seeking behaviors). Agreeable shy/withdrawn children demonstrated positive social adjustment, whereas normative, attention-seeking, and externalizing shy/withdrawn children demonstrated successively greater degrees of peer rela-tions difficulties. Moreover, there were differences in the type of peer adver-sity experienced by different subgroups. For instance, attention-seeking shy/withdrawn children were observed to be the most ignored/excluded at recess, whereas externalizing shy/withdrawn children were the most victimized.

Summary

In this section, we have indicated that, in general, children and young ado-lescents who are shy and withdrawn are at risk for experiencing peer rejec-tion, exclusion, and victimization. And it is known that the experience of peer rejection and exclusion is likely to have important implications for their concurrent and future social and emotional development (Parker, Rubin, Erath, Wojslawowicz, & Buskirk, 2006; Rubin, Bukowski, et al., 2006). Socially withdrawn children who are mistreated by peers are at risk for subsequent consequences, such as loneliness, negative self-regard, rejection sensitivity, anxiety, and depression.

Nevertheless, a substantial number of socially withdrawn children do not experience peer rejection, exclusion, and victimization. A child × environment model of adjustment would suggest that when children who demonstrate social withdrawal (individual vulnerability) encounter peer exclusion and victimization (environmental stressors), they move further away from their peers and experience increased psychosocial difficulties (Gazelle & Ladd, 2003; Gazelle & Rudolph, 2004). Conversely, their withdrawn counterparts who do not encounter rejection and exclusion become less withdrawn over time and experience fewer adjustment problems (Oh et al., 2008).

Research is now required to explore the factors that may buffer shy, withdrawn children from experiencing rejection. Some of these factors include temperament, emotion dysregulation, multifaceted behavioral profiles, and the family environment. Chapters in this volume by Fox and Reeb-Sutherland (Chapter 5), Schmidt and Buss (Chapter 2), and Hastings, Nuselovici, Rubin, and Cheah (Chapter 6) explore these factors in depth.

FRIENDSHIP

Definitions, Functions, and Provisions

Friendships in childhood and early adolescence can perhaps best be thought of as reciprocal dyadic relationships, most often between same-age and same-sex individuals (Rubin, Bukowski, et al., 2006). The characterization of friendship as a *reciprocal* relationship means that *both* individuals must view each other as a friend. In contrast to parent–child relationships, "friendships" are considered *voluntary,* such that individuals choose to become involved in these relationships. This also means that friendships can "break up" or dissolve over time. Finally, friendships are characterized by *mutual* affection. Both individuals in a friendship should share an affection or liking for one another. Based on this definition, the assessment of friendship during any developmental period should involve two steps: (1) Individuals should first be asked to nominate or name their friends, and (2) only mutual friendship nominations should subsequently be considered (Parker et al., 2006; Rubin, Bukowski, et al., 2006).

Friendships in childhood serve to provide (1) support, self-esteem enhancement, and positive self-evaluation; (2) emotional security; (3) affection and opportunities for intimate disclosure; and (4) instrumental and informational assistance. Friendships also (5) offer consensual validation of interests, hopes, and fears; (6) promote the growth of interpersonal sensitivity; and (7) offer prototypes for later romantic, marital, and parental relationships (Newcomb & Bagwell, 1995). In the last 30 years, the psychosocial benefits of having friends and being involved in friendships have been well-documented (e.g., Bagwell, Newcomb, & Bukowski, 1998; Ladd, Kochenderfer, & Coleman, 1996). For example, investigators have shown that children with friends report less psychological distress and higher self-esteem than do children without friends (e.g., Berndt & Keefe, 1995). Additionally, positive friendship quality has been associated with higher levels of global self-worth, more positive perceptions of social competence, and lower levels of internalizing problems (e.g., Rubin, Dwyer, Booth-LaForce, Burgess, & Rose-Krasnor, 2004; Fordham & Stevenson-Hinde, 1999; Keefe & Berndt, 1996). Given these putative benefits of friendship, it appears important to consider the friendship experiences of socially withdrawn children. Developmentally, friendships take on special significance during middle to late childhood, when friendships become more intimate and influential (e.g., Urberg, 1992; Sullivan, 1953). Accordingly, in the next section, our review focuses on the friendships of children during middle to late childhood and early adolescence.

The Friendships of Socially Withdrawn Children and Young Adolescents

Most children have at least one mutual "good" or "best" friend. For example, Parker and Asher (1993) reported that approximately 78% of children in the third, fourth, and fifth grades had at least one mutual friendship (as determined by mutual nominations of "friend"), and 55% had a mutual *best* friendship (as determined by mutual nominations of "very best" friend). Once friendships are formed, the majority of children's friendships are maintained or stable for at least 1 school year (Cillessen, Jiang, West, & Laszkowski, 2005). And children's friendships become increasingly stable with age. Berndt and Hoyle (1985), for instance, found that 50% of 5-year-olds' friendships were stable for 1 school year, compared to a 75% stability rate for 10-year-olds' friendships.

Friendship Prevalence and Social Withdrawal

Because friendship involvement has been positively associated with social competence (Buhrmester, 1990; Gest, Graham-Bermann, & Hartup,

2001), it might be expected that many socially withdrawn children are unable to form friendships. Yet this is not the case; instead, it has been shown that the majority of socially withdrawn children have at least one stable, mutual best friendship (Rubin et al., 2006). This appears to be true in both early (e.g., Ladd & Burgess, 1999) and middle to late childhood (e.g., Rubin, Wojslawowicz, et al., 2006; Schneider, 1999). For example, Rubin, Wojslawowicz, et al. (2006) found that approximately 65% of socially withdrawn 10-year-olds had a mutual best friendship, and approximately 70% of these best friendships were maintained across the academic year; these friendship involvement and stability percentages were nearly identical to those of nonwithdrawn 10-year-olds. Despite little difficulty forming at least *one* friendship, however, it is the case that anxious withdrawal has been found to predict negatively the *number* of mutual friendships during middle childhood (Pedersen, Vitaro, Barker, & Borge, 2007).

Friendship Homophily and Social Withdrawal

What might explain socially withdrawn children's apparent ease in forming a best friendship? It is known that children are initially attracted to those who are similar to them with regard to observable characteristics (race, sex) and behavioral preferences (e.g., Rubin, Lynch, Coplan, Rose-Krasnor, & Booth, 1994). And like factors associated with interpersonal attraction, "surface" characteristics, such as sex, race, and ethnicity (Aboud & Mendelson, 1996), and behaviors such as prosocial behavior, and aggressive and risk-taking behaviors (e.g., Popp, Laursen, Kerr, Stattin, & Burk, 2008; Vitaro, Tremblay, Kerr, Pagani, & Bukowski, 1997) are associated with friendship formation and maintenance.

Importantly, "friendship homophily" applies to shy and socially withdrawn behavior, as well as to internalizing distress (Haselager, Hartup, van Lieshout, & Riksen-Walraven, 1998; Hogue & Sternberg, 1995). Rubin, Wojslawowicz, et al. (2006) reported that both socially withdrawn children and their mutual best friends are more victimized than nonwithdrawn children and their mutual best friends during late childhood. Since many children may actively select similar peers as their friends, it may be that similarity in psychosocial difficulties helps to draw socially withdrawn children into friendships despite their lack of social skills. Of course, not all withdrawn children form friendships with similarly withdrawn and victimized children (e.g., Guroglu, van Lieshout, Haselager, & Scholte, 2007). Yet very little attention has been paid to the significance of variability in the characteristics of socially withdrawn children's friends (for one notable exception, see Oh et al., 2008, described below).

Friendship Quality and Social Withdrawal

It is well-known that children who are socially competent are likely to become involved in friendships of positive relationship quality (e.g., Cillessen et al., 2005). Thus, it may not be too surprising that the friendships of socially withdrawn children appear to be relatively poor in relationship quality (Rubin, Wojslawowicz, et al., 2006; Schneider, 1999). In one study, withdrawn young adolescents rated their best friendships as lacking in helpfulness, guidance, and intimate disclosure; the best friends of these withdrawn young adolescents rated their friendships as involving less fun, help, and guidance than did the best friends of nonwithdrawn young adolescents (Rubin, Wojslawowicz, et al., 2006). Results from an observational study of withdrawn fifth graders and their mutual friends indicated that withdrawn children tend to be relatively restricted in verbal communication with their friends (Schneider, 1999). Due to their experiences with interpersonal failure and their social anxieties, it may be that socially withdrawn children fail to engage in the *mutual* "give and take" that is necessary for positive friendship experiences. Support for this notion is drawn from a recent study of socially withdrawn and anxious young adolescents' conceptions of their friendships (Schneider & Tessier, 2007). Socially withdrawn young adolescents were more likely than nonwithdrawn young adolescents to discuss their *own* needs when thinking about their friendships, and were more likely to cite their friendships as a source of help (Schneider & Tessier, 2007). Alternatively, Rubin, Wojslawowicz, et al. (2006) have argued that a "misery loves company" scenario may exist for socially withdrawn children and their best friends. The similarities between socially withdrawn children and their best friends may draw them together, but the friendships may be characterized by mutual misery and anxiety, and ineffective coping.

Despite the fact that withdrawn children tend to form friendships with similarly withdrawn and victimized children, and that their friendships are relatively poor in relationship quality, some evidence suggests that their friendships do contribute positively to their adjustment and psychological well-being. For example, in one study, socially withdrawn children with a mutual best friendship were perceived by peers as more sociable and popular than socially withdrawn children without a mutual best friendship (Rubin, Wojslawowicz, et al., 2006). Moreover, in a study of how socially withdrawn children interpret hypothetical negative social scenarios involving unfamiliar peers and good friends, Burgess and colleagues (2006) found that socially withdrawn children's tendencies to blame themselves for their social difficulties were diminished when scenarios involved a good friend. And results from a recent study indicate that the presence of a high-quality friendship protects socially withdrawn children from developing internalizing problems during adolescence (Bowker & Rubin, 2008). Taken together, these results suggest that the presence of friendships, particularly those that are of high quality, provide socially withdrawn children with positive social experiences that may in turn improve their standing within the larger peer group and help to alleviate their social anxieties.

The absence of friendship, the presence of unstable friendships, and having a withdrawn friend have been identified as friendship "risk" factors for socially withdrawn children. For instance, Oh et al. (2008) identified three distinct social withdrawal growth trajectories across a 4-year period (fifth through eighth grade): (1) low stable withdrawal, (2) increasing withdrawal, and (3) decreasing withdrawal. A number of friendship factors predicted initial class membership and/or growth within each class. For example, the absence of a mutual friendship and the presence of unstable best friendships further exacerbated social withdrawal for children in the increasing withdrawal trajectory. Furthermore, children with socially withdrawn friends at the start of the study (fall of the fifth-grade school year) showed higher levels of initial social withdrawal, and having a socially withdrawn friend after the transition from elementary school into middle school (fall of the sixth-grade school year) appeared to increase children's social withdrawal over time.

Summary

Most socially withdrawn children are involved in at least one best friendship. But recent research has shown that these friendships are with others who share the salient characteristics of the socially withdrawn child; that is, the best friends are often withdrawn themselves and likewise experience victimization in the peer group. Furthermore, although research suggests that a high-quality friendship may help socially withdrawn children, many of the friendships of withdrawn children in the middle to late childhood and early adolescence appear qualitatively impoverished relative to those of their non-withdrawn agemates. Taken together, the friendships of socially withdrawn children do not augur well for them, unless those friendships happen to be with nonwithdrawn, nonexcluded, socially supportive individuals (e.g., Oh et al., 2008). How socially anxious and withdrawn children can make themselves attractive to socially competent, kind, and generous peers is certainly a question worth asking in future years. And in keeping with the position that not all socially withdrawn children are at risk for peer rejection, exclusion, and negative internalizing outcomes, researchers would do well to examine the concomitants and consequences of socially withdrawn children who demonstrate greater or lesser friendship skills.

SUMMARY, CONCLUSIONS, AND FUTURE DIRECTIONS

In this chapter, we have examined the peer relationships and friendships of socially withdrawn children. By and large, it has been reported that many socially withdrawn children experience peer rejection and exclusion, as well as victimization. This alone should place socially withdrawn children at risk for negative psychosocial outcomes. However, recent research has also shown that the friendships of socially withdrawn children may contribute significantly to their risk status.

Importantly, there has emerged evidence that the developmental course of social withdrawal from early childhood through the adolescent period may best be described as demonstrating the "principle of multifinality," which suggests that similar initial conditions may lead to dissimilar outcomes. As Rubin and colleagues have surmised in their developing conceptual model of the precursors and outcomes of social withdrawal (e.g., Rubin, Coplan, et al., 2009), factors that may prove influential in plotting varying trajectories include biology and genetics (e.g., Calkins, Fox, & Marshall, 1996; Hariri et al., 2002), parenting and parent–child relationship experiences (e.g., Rubin et al., 2002), and contextual factors (school, neighborhood, culture; e.g., Chang, 2003; Chen, Cen, Li, & He, 2005; Gazelle, 2006; Schneider, Richard, Younger, & Freeman, 2000). In these regards, a comprehensive model of the development of shyness/withdrawal must consider many seemingly independent factors and the dynamic ways in which they interact to create a variety of developmental outcomes. This being the case, progress in the next decade of research on the peer relations of shy/withdrawn children and adolescents requires addressing the dynamic interaction of multiple levels of both individuals and their environments.

And, finally, in keeping with the view that varying factors may be responsible for the negative outcomes experienced by some socially anxious and withdrawn children, it seems timely to suggest that attention be paid to developing prevention and intervention programs. Thus far, the intervention literature has proved slim indeed (see Mychailyszyn, Cohen, Edmunds, Crawley, and Kendall [Chapter 14] and Rapee [Chapter 13], this volume); the prevention literature is practically nonexistent. Clearly, those children who demonstrate early signs of anxious withdrawn behavior (behavioral inhibition during the toddler period; social reticence in early childhood) deserve to evoke the attention of those who develop programs of prevention and intervention.

ACKNOWLEDGMENTS

Preparation of this chapter was supported in part by Grant No. R01-MH58116 from the National Institute of Mental Health to Kenneth H. Rubin and by Grant No. 1K01-MH076237-01A1 from the National Institute of Mental Health to Heidi Gazelle.

REFERENCES

Aboud, F., & Mendelson, M. (1996). Determinants of friendship selection and quality: Developmental perspectives. In W. Bukowski & A. Newcomb (Eds.), *The company they keep: Friendship in childhood and adolescence* (pp. 87–112). New York: Cambridge University Press.

Asher, S., & Paquette, J. (2003). Loneliness and peer relations in childhood. *Current Directions in Psychological Science, 12*(3), 75–78.

Bagwell, C., Newcomb, A., & Bukowski, W. (1998). Preadolescent friendship and peer rejection as predictors of adult adjustment. *Child Development, 69,* 140–153.

Banerjee, R., & Henderson, L. (2001). Social-cognitive factors in childhood social anxiety: A preliminary investigation. *Social Development, 10,* 558–572.

Bell-Dolan, D., Reaven, N., & Petersen, L. (1993). Child depression and social functioning: A multidimensional study of the linkages. *Journal of Clinical Child Psychology, 22,* 306–315.

Berndt, T., & Hoyle, S. (1985). Stability and change in childhood and adolescent friendships. *Developmental Psychology, 21,* 1007–1015.

Berndt, T., & Keefe, K. (1995). Friends' influence on adolescents' adjustment to school. *Child Development, 66,* 1313–1329.

Boivin, M., & Hymel, S. (1997). Peer experiences and social self-perceptions: A sequential model. *Developmental Psychology, 33,* 135–145.

Boivin, M., Bukowski, W., & Hymel, S. (1995). The roles of social withdrawal, peer rejection, and victimization by peers in predicting loneliness and depressed mood in childhood. *Development and Psychopathology, 7,* 765–785.

Boivin, M., Hymel, S., & Hodges, E. (2001). Toward a process view of peer rejection and harassment. In S. Graham & J. Juvonen (Eds.), *Peer harassment in school: The plight of the vulnerable and victimized* (pp. 265–289). New York: Guilford Press.

Booth-LaForce, C., & Oxford, M. (2008). Trajectories of social withdrawal from grades 1 to 6: Prediction from early parenting, attachment, and temperament. *Developmental Psychology, 44,* 1298–1313.

Bowker, J., & Rubin, K. (2008, July). *Predicting adolescent social withdrawal and internalizing problems: The moderating role of friendship quality.* In K. Rubin & J. Bowker (Cochairs), Individual differences in peer relationships and adjustment during childhood and adolescence: The consideration of individual, relationships, and cultural factors. Paper presented at the biennial meetings of the International Society for the Study of Behavioral Development, Wurzburg, Germany.

Bowker, J., Rubin, K., Rose-Krasnor, L., & Booth-LaForce, C. (2008). *Social withdrawal, negative emotion, and peer difficulties during late childhood.* Unpublished manuscript.

Bukowski, W. (1990). Age differences in children's memory of information about aggressive, socially withdrawn, and prosociable boys and girls. *Child Development, 61*(5), 1326–1332.

Buhrmester, D. (1990). Intimacy of friendship, interpersonal competence, and adjustment during preadolescence and adolescence. *Child Development, 61*, 1101–1111.

Burgess, K., Wojslawowicz, J., Rubin, K., Rose-Krasnor, L., & Booth-LaForce, C. (2006). Social information processing and coping styles of shy/withdrawn and aggressive children: Does friendship matter? *Child Development, 77*, 371–383.

Calkins, S., Fox, N., & Marshall, T. (1996). Behavioral and physiological antecedents of inhibition in infancy. *Child Development, 67*, 523–540.

Chang, L. (2003). Variable effects of children's aggression, social withdrawal, and prosocial leadership as functions of teacher beliefs and behaviors. *Child Development, 74*(2), 535–548.

Chen, X., Cen, G., Li. D., & He, Y. (2005). Social functioning and adjustment in Chinese children: The imprint of historical time. *Child Development, 76*, 182–195.

Chen, X., & French, D. (2008). Children's social competence in cultural context. *Annual Review of Psychology, 59*, 591–616.

Cillessen, A., Jiang, X., West, T., & Laszkowski, D. (2005). Predictors of dyadic friendship quality in adolescence. *International Journal of Behavioral Development, 29*, 165–172.

Cillessen, A., van IJzendoorn, H., Van Lieshout, C., & Hartup, W. (1992). Heterogeneity among peer-rejected boys: Subtypes and stabilities. *Child Development, 63*(4), 893–905.

Coie, J., & Kupersmidt, J. (1983). A behavioral analysis of emerging social status in boys' groups. *Child Development, 54*(6), 1400–1416.

Coplan, R. J., Arbeau, K. A., & Armer, M. (2008). Don't fret, be supportive!: Maternal characteristics linking child shyness to psychosocial and school adjustment in kindergarten. *Journal of Abnormal Child Psychology, 36*, 359–371.

Coplan, R. J., Girardi, A., Findlay, L., & Frohlick, S. (2007). Understanding solitude: Young children's attitudes and responses towards hypothetical socially withdrawn peers. *Social Development, 16*, 390–409.

Coplan, R. J., Prakash, K., O'Neil, K., & Armer, M. (2004). Do you "want" to play?: Distinguishing between conflicted-shyness and social disinterest in early childhood. *Developmental Psychology, 40*, 244–258.

Crick, N., & Dodge, K. (1994). A review and reformulation of social information processing in children's social adjustment. *Psychological Bulletin, 115*, 74–101.

Crozier, W., & Burnham, M. (1990). Age-related differences in children's understanding of shyness. *British Journal of Developmental Psychology, 8*(2), 179–185.

Dill, E., Vernberg, E., & Fonagy, P. (2004). Negative affect in victimized children:

The roles of social withdrawal, peer rejection, and attitudes toward bullying. *Journal of Abnormal Child Psychology, 32,* 159–173.

Dodge, K. (1983). Behavioral antecedents of peer social status. *Child Development, 54*(6), 1386–1399.

Erath, S., Flanagan, K., & Bierman, K. (2007). Social anxiety and peer relations in early adolescence: Behavioral and cognitive factors. *Journal of Abnormal Child Psychology, 35*(3), 405–416.

Fordham, K., & Stevenson-Hinde, J. (1999). Shyness, friendship quality, and adjustment during middle childhood. *Journal of Child Psychology and Psychiatry, 40*(5), 757–768.

Fox, N., Henderson, H., Rubin, K., Calkins, S., & Schmidt, L. (2001). Continuity and discontinuity of behavioral inhibition and exuberance: Psychophysiological and behavioral influences across the first four years of life. *Child Development, 72,* 1–21.

Furman, W., Simon, V., Shaffer, L., & Bouchey, H. (2002). Adolescents' working models and styles for relationships with parents, friends, and romantic partners. *Child Development, 73*(1), 241–255.

Garnefski, N., Kraaij, V., & van Etten, M. (2005). Specificity of relations between adolescents' cognitive emotion regulation strategies and internalizing and externalizing psychopathology. *Journal of Adolescence, 28,* 619–631.

Gazelle, H. (2008). Behavioral profiles of anxious solitary children and heterogeneity in peer relations. *Developmental Psychology, 44*(6), 1604–1624.

Gazelle, H. (2006). Class climate moderates peer relations and emotional adjustment in children with an early childhood history of anxious solitude: A child × environment model. *Developmental Psychology, 42,* 1179–1192.

Gazelle, H., & Ladd, G. (2003). Anxious solitude and peer exclusion: A diathesis–stress model of internalizing trajectories in childhood. *Child Development, 74*(1), 257–278.

Gazelle, H., Putallaz, M., Li, Y., Grimes, C., Kupersmidt, J., & Coie, J. (2005). Anxious solitude across contexts: Girls' interactions with familiar and unfamiliar peers. *Child Development, 76*(1), 227–246.

Gazelle, H., & Rudolph, K. (2004). Moving toward and away from the world: Social approach and avoidance trajectories in anxious solitary youth. *Child Development, 75*(3), 829–849.

Gazelle, H., & Spangler, T. (2007). Early childhood anxious solitude and subsequent peer relationships: Maternal and cognitive moderators [Special issue: New findings from secondary data analysis: Results from the NIHCD Study of Early Child Care and Youth Development]. *Journal of Applied Developmental Psychology, 28,* 515–535.

Gest, S., Graham-Bermann, S., & Hartup, W. (2001). Peer experience: Common and unique features of number of friendships, social network centrality, and sociometric status. *Social Development, 10,* 23–40.

Goetz, T., & Dweck, C. (1980). Learned helplessness in social situations. *Journal of Personality and Social Psychology, 39,* 246–255.

Guroglu, B., van Lieshout, C., Haselager, G., & Scholte, R. (2007). Similarity and complementary of behavioral profiles of friendship types and types of friends:

Friendships and psychosocial adjustment. *Journal of Research on Adolescence, 17*(2), 357–386.

Hariri, A., Mattay, V., Tessitore, A., Kolachana, B., Fera, F., Goldman, D., et al. (2002). Serotonin transporter genetic variation and the response of the human amygdala. *Science, 297,* 400–403.

Hanish, L., & Guerra, N. (2004). Aggressive victims, passive victims, and bullies: Developmental continuity or developmental change. *Merrill–Palmer Quarterly, 50,* 17–38.

Hart, C., Yang, C., Nelson, L., Robinson, C., Olsen, J., Nelson, D., et al. (2000). Peer acceptance in early childhood and subtypes of socially withdrawn behaviour in China, Russia and the United States. *International Journal of Behavioral Development, 24*(1), 73–81.

Haselager, G., Hartup, W., van Lieshout, C., & Riksen-Walraven, J. (1998). Similarities between friends and nonfriends in middle childhood. *Child Development, 69*(4), 1198–1208.

Hawley, P. (2003). Strategies of control, aggression and morality in preschoolers: An evolutionary perspective. *Journal of Experimental Child Psychology, 85*(3), 213–235.

Hinde, R., & Stevenson-Hinde, J. (1976). Toward understanding relationships: Dynamic stability. In P. Bateson & R. Hinde (Eds.), *Growing points in ethology* (pp. 451–479). Cambridge, UK: Cambridge University Press.

Hodges, E., Malone, M., & Perry, D. (1997). Individual risk and social risk as interacting determinants of victimization in the peer group. *Developmental Psychology, 33,* 1032–1039.

Hoglund, W., & Leadbetter, B. (2007). School functioning in early adolescence: Gender-linked responses to peer victimization. *Journal of Educational Psychology, 99*(4), 683–699.

Hogue, A., & Steinberg, L. (1995). Homophily of internalized distress in adolescent peer groups. *Developmental Psychology, 31,* 897–906.

Hymel, S., Rubin, K., Rowden, L., & LeMare, L. (1990). Children's peer relationships: Longitudinal prediction of internalizing and externalizing problems from middle to late childhood. *Child Development, 61*(6), 2004–2021.

Keefe, K., & Berndt, T. (1996). Relations of friendship quality to self-esteem in early adolescence. *Journal of Early Adolescence, 16*(1), 110–129.

Kochenderfer-Ladd, B. (2003). Identification of aggressive and asocial victims and the stability of their peer victimization. *Merrill–Palmer Quarterly, 49*(4), 401–425.

Krasnor, L., & Rubin, K. (1983). Preschool social problem-solving: Attempts and outcomes in naturalistic interaction. *Child Development, 54,* 1545–1558.

Ladd, G., & Burgess, K. (1999). Charting the relationship trajectories of aggressive, withdrawn, and aggressive/withdrawn children during early grade school. *Child Development, 70,* 910–929.

Ladd, G., Kochenderfer, B., & Coleman, C. (1996). Friendship quality as a predictor of young children's early school adjustment. *Child Development, 67,* 1103–1118.

LeMare, L., & Rubin, K. (1987). Perspective taking and peer interaction: Structural and developmental analyses. *Child Development, 58*(2), 306–315.

Lemerise, E., & Arsenio, W. (2000). An integrated model of emotion processes and cognition in social information processing. *Child Development, 71*, 107–118.

London, B., Downey, G., Bonica, C., & Paltin, I. (2007). Social causes and consequences of rejection-sensitivity. *Journal of Research on Adolescence, 17*(3), 481–506.

McFall, R. (1982). A review and reformulation of the concept of social skills. *Behavioral Assessment, 4*(1), 1–33.

Mead, G. (1934). *Mind, self, and society: From the standpoint of a social behaviorist.* Oxford, UK: University of Chicago Press.

Morison, P., & Masten, A. S. (1991). Peer reputation in middle childhood as a predictor of adaptation in adolescence: A seven-year follow-up. *Child Development, 62*(5), 991–1007.

Nelson, L., Rubin, K., & Fox, N. (2005). Social and nonsocial behaviors and peer acceptance: A longitudinal model of the development of self-perceptions in children ages 4 to 7 years. *Early Education and Development, 20*, 185–200.

Newcomb, A., & Bagwell, C. (1995). Children's friendship relations: A meta-analytic review. *Psychological Bulletin, 117*, 306–347.

Nolen-Hoeksema, S., Girgus, J., & Seligman, M. (1992). Predictors and consequences of childhood depressive symptoms: A 5-year longitudinal study. *Journal of Abnormal Psychology, 101*(3), 405–422.

Oh, W., Rubin, K., Bowker, J., Booth-LaForce, C., Rose-Krasnor, L., & Laursen, B. (2008). Trajectories of social withdrawal middle childhood to early adolescence. *Journal of Abnormal Child Psychology, 36*(4), 553–566.

Olweus, D. (1993). Victimization by peers: Antecedents and long-term outcomes. In K. H. Rubin & J. B. Asendorpf (Eds.), *Social withdrawal, inhibition and shyness in childhood* (pp. 315–341). Mahwah, NJ: Erlbaum.

Parker, J., & Asher, S. (1993). Friendship and friendship quality in middle childhood: Links with peer group acceptance and feelings of loneliness and social dissatisfaction. *Developmental Psychology, 29*, 611–621.

Parker, J., Rubin, K., Erath, S., Wojslawowicz, J., & Buskirk, A. (2006). Peer relationships, child development, and adjustment: A developmental psychopathology perspective. In D. Cicchetti (Ed.), *Developmental psychopathology: Vol. 2. Risk, disorder, and adaptation* (pp. 419–493). New York: Wiley.

Pedersen, S., Vitaro, F., Barker, E., & Borge, A. (2007). The timing of middle-childhood peer rejection and friendship: Linking early behavior to early-adolescent adjustment. *Child Development, 78*(4), 1037–1051.

Piaget, J. (1932). *The moral judgment of the child.* Glencoe, IL: Free Press.

Popp, D., Laursen, B., Kerr, M., Stattin, H., & Burk, W. (2008). Modeling homophily over time with an actor–parent interdependence model. *Developmental Psychology, 44*(4), 1028–1039.

Reijntjes, A., Stegge, H., Terwogt, M., Kamphuis, J., & Telch, M. (2006). Emotion regulation and its effects on mood improvement in response to *in vivo* peer rejection challenge. *Emotion, 6*, 543–552.

Rubin, K. (1982). Social and social-cognitive developmental characteristics of young isolate, normal and sociable children. In K. H. Rubin & H. S. Ross (Eds.), *Peer relationships and social skills in childhood* (pp. 353–374). New York: Springer-Verlag.

Rubin, K. (1985). Socially withdrawn children: An "at risk" population? In B. Schneider, K. H. Rubin, & J. Ledingham (Eds.), *Children's peer relations: Issues in assessment and intervention* (pp. 125–139). New York: Springer-Verlag.

Rubin, K., & Borwick, D. (1984). The communication skills of children who vary with regard to sociability. In H. Sypher & J. Applegates (Eds.), *Social cognition and communication* (pp. 152–170). Hillsdale, NJ: Erlbaum.

Rubin, K., Bowker, J., & Kennedy, A. (2009). Avoiding and withdrawing from the peer group in middle childhood and early adolescence. In K. H. Rubin, W. Bukowski, & B. Laursen (Eds.), *Handbook of peer interactions, relationships, and groups* (pp. 303–321). New York: Guilford Press.

Rubin, K., Bukowski, W., & Laursen, B. (Eds.). (2009). *Handbook of peer interactions, relationships, and groups.* New York: Guilford Press.

Rubin, K., Bukowski, W., & Parker, J. G. (2006). Peer interactions, relationships, and groups. In W. Damon, R. M. Lerner, & N. Eisenberg (Eds.), *Handbook of child psychology: Vol. 3. Social, emotional, and personality development* (6th ed., pp. 571–645). New York: Wiley.

Rubin, K., Burgess, K., & Hastings, P. (2002). Stability and social-behavioral consequences of toddlers' inhibited temperament and parenting behaviors. *Child Development, 73,* 483–495.

Rubin, K., Chen, X., & Hymel, S. (1993). The socio-emotional characteristics of extremely aggressive and extremely withdrawn children. *Merrill–Palmer Quarterly, 39,* 518–534.

Rubin, K., Chen, X., McDougall, P., Bowker, A., & McKinnon, J. (1995). The Waterloo Longitudinal Project: Predicting adolescent internalizing and externalizing problems from early and mid-childhood. *Development and Psychopathology, 7,* 751–764.

Rubin, K., Coplan, R., & Bowker, J. (2009). Social withdrawal and shyness in childhood and adolescence. *Annual Review of Psychology, 60,* 141–171.

Rubin, K., Daniels-Beirness, T., & Bream, L. (1984). Social isolation and social problem solving: A longitudinal study. *Journal of Consulting and Clinical Psychology, 52,* 17–25.

Rubin, K., Dwyer, K., Booth-LaForce, C., Kim, A., Burgess, K., & Rose-Krasnor, L. (2004). Attachment, friendship, and psychosocial functioning in early adolescence, *Journal of Early Adolescence, 24,* 326–356.

Rubin, K., & Krasnor, L.(1986). Social-cognitive and social behavioral perspectives on problem solving. In M. Perlmutter (Ed.), *Cognitive perspectives on children's social and behavioral development: The Minnesota Symposia on Child Psychology* (Vol. 18, pp. 1–68). Hillsdale, NJ: Erlbaum.

Rubin, K., Lynch, D., Coplan, R., Rose-Krasnor, L., & Booth, C. (1994). "Birds of a feather … ": Behavioral concordances and preferential personal attraction in children. *Child Development, 65,* 1778–1785.

Rubin, K., & Rose-Krasnor, L. (1992). Interpersonal problem solving. In V. B. Van Hasselt & M. Hersen (Eds.), *Handbook of social development* (pp. 283–323). New York: Plenum Press.

Rubin, K., Wojslawowicz, J., Burgess, K., Rose-Krasnor, L., & Booth-LaForce, C. L. (2006). The friendships of socially withdrawn and competent young adolescents. *Journal of Abnormal Child Psychology, 34,* 139–153.

Schneider, B. (1999). A multi-method exploration of the friendships of children considered socially withdrawn by their peers. *Journal of Abnormal Psychology, 27*, 115–123.

Schneider, B., Richard, J., Younger, A., & Freeman, P. (2000). A longitudinal exploration of the continuity of children's social participation and social withdrawal across socioeconomic status levels and social settings. *European Journal of Social Psychology, 30*, 497–519.

Schneider, B., & Tessier, N. (2007). Close friendship as understood by socially withdrawn, anxious early adolescents. *Child Psychiatry and Human Development, 38*(4), 339–351.

Stewart, S., & Rubin, K. (1995). The social problem solving skills of anxious-withdrawn children. *Development and Psychopathology, 7*, 323–336.

Sullivan, H. (1953). *The interpersonal theory of psychiatry.* New York: Norton.

Terry, R. (2000). Recent advances in measurement theory and the use of sociometric techniques. In A. H. N. Cillessen & W. M. Bukowski (Eds.), *Recent advances in the measurement of acceptance and rejection in the peer system* (pp. 27–53). San Francisco: Jossey-Bass.

Urberg, K. (1992). Locus of peer influence: Social crowd and best friend. *Journal of Youth and Adolescence, 21*, 439–450.

Vitaro, F., Tremblay, R., Kerr, M., Pagani, L., & Bukwoski, W. (1997). Disruptiveness, friends' characteristics, and delinquency in early adolescence: A test of two competing models of development. *Child Development, 68*, 676–689.

Wichmann, C., Coplan, R., & Daniels, T. (2004). The social cognitions of socially withdrawn children. *Social Development, 13*, 377–392.

Younger, A., Gentile, C., & Burgess, K. (1993). Children's perceptions of social withdrawal: Changes across age. In K. H. Rubin & J. B. Asendorpf (Eds.), *Social withdrawal, inhibition, and shyness in childhood* (pp. 215–235). Hillsdale, NJ: Erlbaum.

8

Long-Term Development of Shyness

Looking Forward and Looking Backward

JENS B. ASENDORPF

In developmental psychology, "shyness" in infants and young children refers to (1) an affective state in social situations, characterized by transient shy behavior and underlying physiological reactions, that may vary from bold disinhibition to a totally inhibiting phobic reaction, or (2) a temporarily stable personality trait that may vary from boldness to social phobia. This chapter focuses on the development of trait shyness.

INHIBITION AND SHYNESS IN EARLY CHILDHOOD

Around 8 months of age, nearly every infant starts reacting shyly to adult strangers once in a while, and later, most children react shyly from time to time in specific situations. Both extreme shyness and the complete absence of shyness indicate problems with socioemotional adaptation. However, interindividual differences in shyness to strangers do not show sufficient temporal stability over the first 18 months to be considered a personality trait. Only later can a first form of trait shyness be observed. This phenomenon is often referred to as "behavioral inhibition to the unfamiliar." Researchers have established that, at this age, interindividual differences in inhibited behavior are consistent between novel social situations (e.g., facing an adult stranger) and nonsocial situations (e.g., facing unfamiliar toys; Garcia-Coll, Kagan, & Reznick, 1984; Kagan, Reznick, Clarke, Snidman, & Garcia-Coll, 1984). These authors have also studied the concurrent and predictive correlates of high versus low inhibition (often defined as the upper and lower 15% of the distribution of a normal sample) in considerable detail (see Kagan & Snidman, 2004, for a review).

However, it would be overly simplistic to reduce shyness in childhood only to this temperamental trait. Asendorpf (1990) used the Munich Longitudinal Study on the Genesis of Individual Competencies (LOGIC; Weinert & Schneider, 1999) to study the consistency of inhibited behavior across unfamiliar and familiar situations (confrontation with an adult stranger; dyadic play with an unfamiliar peer in the laboratory vs. with a familiar peer in the familiar preschool setting; inhibition during free play over 3 years of preschool/kindergarten; see Asendorpf, 1993, for a detailed description). Multiple measures within settings confirmed that inhibition was highly consistent between adult and peer strangers but less consistent with inhibition in the classroom, and not at all consistent with inhibition toward a familiar peer. Other studies found a rather low consistency of inhibition across familiar and unfamiliar situations. This pattern of findings suggests that factors other than inhibited temperament contribute to individual differences in shy behavior in familiar situations.

Indeed, longitudinal analyses of classroom data have shown that the influence of observed instances of peer neglect or rejection on inhibition increase over time, independent of the level of inhibition toward strangers. Asendorpf (1990, 1993) interpreted these findings to represent the increasing influence of social-evaluative concerns on inhibition in the classroom. Follow-ups of extreme groups comparing stable inhibition toward strangers and stable inhibition in the more familiar peer group in the second and third year in preschool have revealed that stable, high inhibition toward strangers is unrelated to self-esteem up to age 12, whereas stable high inhibition in the familiar peer group significantly predicts low social self-esteem between 8 and 12 years of age (Asendorpf & van Aken, 1994). Thus, inhibition in the familiar peer group, which is probably due to social-evaluative concerns, is a risk factor for internalizing problems over the childhood years; the same is not the case for inhibition with strangers. In support of this finding, a more recent longitudinal study showed that teacher-assessed anxious solitude became associated with peer exclusion soon after entry into kindergarten, and that early peer exclusion in anxious–solitary children increased the risk of developing stable inhibition and depression (Gazelle & Ladd, 2003).

These findings suggest that shyness in the peer group might be particularly important for the development of adult shyness, because it can be due to the temperamental factors of inhibition toward the unfamiliar and negative experiences with peers, factors of individual differences that are partly independent of each other but become associated later on. Because temperament is more likely stable than peer neglect or rejection across different peer groups, the relation between inhibition toward the unfamiliar and social-evaluative anxiety is expected to increase with age due to the continuous effect of temperament on the experience of neglect or rejection. This hypothesis has been supported in a longitudinal study by Gest (1997), who found that inhibition toward the unfamiliar was not correlated with negative peer relationships in late childhood (ages 8–11), but it was in early adulthood (ages 17–24).

TWO- AND THREE-FACTOR MODELS OF SHYNESS

Asendorpf (1990) has interpreted these findings in terms of a two-factor model of shy behavior based on the theory of Gray (1982). Drawing upon animal and psychopharmacological research, Gray proposed the existence of a behavioral inhibition system (BIS) at the neurophysiological level that mediates responses to three kinds of stimuli: novel stimuli, conditioned cues for punishment, and conditioned cues for frustrating nonreward. According to Gray, any such stimulus evokes behavioral inhibition, increased physiological arousal, and increased attention. Interindividual differences arise due to a different sensitivity ("strength") of this BIS and to interindividual differences in learning history (how many and which stimuli become cues for punishment or frustrating nonreward through conditioning). Asendorpf (1989, 1990) noted that this temperamental theory nicely explains the fact that both strangers (novel cues) and situational cues for being rejected or ignored by others (cues for punishment or frustrating nonreward) lead to inhibitory tendencies in both adults and children (see Figure 8.1). A few other studies have also linked the BIS and the behavioral activation system (BAS) to socioemotional functioning in childhood (e.g., Blair, 2003). It should be noted that more recent versions of Gray's theory (e.g., reinforcement sensitivity theory; Corr, 2008; Smillie, 2008) also provide an even stronger neuroscientific basis for this two-factor model of shy behavior.

When this model of shy behavior is applied to trait shyness, a child may react shyly to a particular person because of a temperamental disposition that may be genetically based or due to early caregiving, *or* because the child has often been rejected or ignored by this person (a parent, a sibling, or a familiar peer). Because the second "experiential source" of shyness also triggers the BIS, it interacts with the temperamental source in a predictable way (amplification of response). Thus, a child with a "weak" BIS who is often rejected by parents, may nonetheless not become shy, whereas a child with a "strong" BIS, who is moderately rejected or ignored by the parents, may nonetheless become shy in their presence. Such interactions between

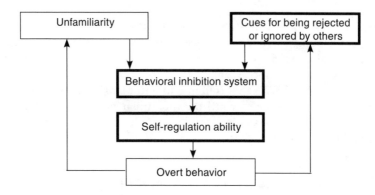

FIGURE 8.1. A three-factor model of shyness. Bold lines indicate sources of inter-individual differences. From Asendorpf (2008a, Figure 1). Copyright by Elsevier. Reprinted by permission.

temperament and social experiences have been explored in numerous studies (e.g., Coplan, Arbeau, & Armer, 2008; Gazelle, 2006; Rubin, Burgess, & Hastings, 2002).

More recently, Asendorpf (2008a) extended this earlier two-factor view of shyness to a three-factor model that includes effortful control: Whether the inhibitory tendencies result in shy behavior depends on the child's self-regulatory abilities (see Figure 8.1). Asendorpf (2008a) referred to research by Eisenberg and colleagues (2001), who took up the hypothesis originally put forward by Rothbart and Bates (1998) that the development of *effortful self-regulation* leads to important changes in children's temperament-based reactions. "Effortful control" is commonly defined as the efficiency of executive attention. It involves abilities to focus or shift attention as needed, and to activate or inhibit behavior as needed. Eisenberg et al. distinguished effortful control from "reactive control" that is less under voluntary control; as an example, inhibition may be an immediate reaction to unfamiliarity or social-evaluative concerns. They found some evidence that effortful control fosters the skills needed to get along with others and to engage in socially constructive behaviors. More specifically, effortful control helps children disposed to high inhibitory tendencies, due either to inhibition with strangers or social-evaluative anxiety, to self-regulate their initially inhibited response (Eisenberg et al., 2001).

Relatedly, Asendorpf (1994) found that for children in the LOGIC study, social competence, as judged by preschool teachers, and general intelligence, as assessed by standard IQ tests, both moderated the long-term outcomes of preschool inhibition: More competent and more intelligent children were better able to overcome inhibition in both laboratory and school settings. There is good evidence that more socially competent and more intelligent children are better able to self-regulate their reactivity (Eisenberg et al., 2001); therefore, Asendorpf's finding may be interpreted in terms of the enhanced self-regulation ability of the more competent children.

As noted earlier, shy behavior is shown by not only children who react in an inhibited fashion but also by children who act in a reserved, modest, unassuming way in the presence of others, without signs of fear or anxiety. As the model in Figure 8.1 suggests, such modest behavior can be an outcome of self-regulated inhibition. Importantly, this may not always be the case; children may be socialized to behave in a modest way. Cultural norms for modesty may determine the outcomes of self-regulated inhibition (see Chen, Chapter 10, this volume, for a relevant discussion).

CULTURAL INFLUENCES

This cultural influence on shyness first became obvious to developmental psychologists in a cross-cultural study by Chen, Rubin, and Sun (1992). These researchers compared the peer reputations of shy–sensitive Canadian and Chinese children. Whereas shy–sensitive children were less popular among their peers in Canada, they were above average in popularity and showed superior school adjustment in China. The authors interpreted this result as the influence of the Confucian norms for modesty in China at the threshold of Westernization. In line with this interpretation, studies carried out 8 and 12 years later could not replicate the original findings; instead, shy–sensitive Chinese children in large cities today are as low in peer popularity and school adjustment as they are in Western cultures (Chen, Cen, Li, & He, 2005).

These findings highlight the problem that shy behavior may be due not only to inhibition but also to self-regulation according to cultural norms favoring modesty, without underlying inhibition. The bottom line is that three different types of shyness in children can be distinguished: inhibition with strangers, social-evaluative anxiety, and modesty.

LOOKING FORWARD:
LONG-TERM OUTCOME OF EARLY SHYNESS

The earliest study on the long-term outcome of early shyness was the Fels Longitudinal Study (Kagan & Moss, 1962), in which two measures of observed anxiety in unfamiliar social situations at ages 3–6 were both significantly correlated with social anxiety in adulthood. Interestingly, later, extensive studies of temperamental inhibition by Kagan and associates did not (yet) result in reports about significant predictions from early inhibition toward the unfamiliar to adulthood personality or socioemotional adaptation. The only significant prediction was reported by Schwartz, Wright, Shin, Kagan, and Rauch (2003), who found that observed high versus low inhibition at ages 2–3 predicted recorded high versus low magnetic resonance imaging (MRI) responses to novel faces compared to familiar faces at age 22. However, only a small number of children were followed into adulthood (e.g., the MRI data were based on only 22 participants), such that firm conclusions about nonpredictions from early temperamental inhibition cannot be drawn. Another limitation of these studies by Kagan and associates is that they often rely on comparisons between extremely inhibited and extremely uninhibited children (in most cases the upper and lower 15% of the distribution); therefore, it is not clear whether correlates of inhibition are due mainly to uninhibition or to inhibition.

Much better evidence for the long-term outcome of early inhibition is provided by the Dunedin Longitudinal Study, which follows a large, representative New Zealand birth cohort ($N = 1,037$) into adulthood (Caspi & Silva, 1995). Based on behavioral observations in various situations, 8% of the sample as classified as inhibited at age 3 and followed up until age 26. Compared to a control group of well-adjusted children (40% of the sample), the inhibited children reported more harm avoidance and less social potency and positive emotionality at both age 18 and 26, and at age 26 were described by informants as lower in extraversion but *not* higher in neuroticism (Caspi et al., 2003). The psychiatric interviews at age 21 showed that the inhibited children were *not* more likely to have anxiety disorders of various kinds, including social phobia, but were more often depressed and had more often attempted suicide (Caspi, Moffitt, Newman, & Silva, 1996). Thus, the evidence for internalizing disorders in adulthood for formerly extremely inhibited children was mixed. Importantly, social phobia was not related to early inhibition, nor am I aware of any other prospective longitudinal study that has shown this, contrary to frequent claims in the clinical literature based on retrospective reports (e.g., Stemberger, Turner, Beidel, & Calhoun, 1995).

With regard to life course sequelae of childhood inhibition, two longitudinal studies reported delays in social transitions for children classified as inhibited in middle childhood. In their reanalysis of the Berkeley Guidance Study, Caspi, Bem, and Elder (1988) found such delays only for inhibited boys at ages 8–10 years. These inhibited boys married 3 years later, became fathers 4 years later, and entered a stable occupational career 3 years later than the remaining boys. No such delays were found for the inhibited girls; instead, these girls became women who spent less time in the labor force and married men with higher occupational status. This should not be attributed to instability of female inhibition, because "Q"-sort ratings of inhibition based on two clinical interviews at ages 30 and 40 correlated significantly with both boys' and girls' inhibition. The strong sex difference in the outcomes can be attributed to the traditional gender roles for this 1928 birth cohort that required action and the assertive establishment of social contacts, particularly from men.

In an attempt to replicate these life course patterns in a 1955–1958 Swedish cohort, Kerr, Lambert, and Bem (1996) studied children who were rated by their mothers as shy with unfamiliar people at ages 8–10 years, when they were 25 and 35 years old. Self-judgments of inhibition at age 35 correlated significantly with childhood inhibition for females but not at all for males. Inhibited boys married 4 years later than controls and became fathers 3 years later; shy girls were educational underachievers (i.e., reached a lower educational level after researchers controlled for IQ). No effects on the number of job changes or monthly income were observed. Thus, this study replicated the delays for inhibited boys regarding marriage and parenthood, as well as the absence of this effect for girls; unfortunately, age at beginning a stable career was not recorded.

In a recent follow-up of the LOGIC study, Asendorpf, Denissen, and van Aken (2008) replicated the findings of delayed social transitions into adulthood for both boys and girls, and also found a low stability of shyness between early childhood and adulthood. In this 19-year longitudinal study, the 15% most inhibited children at ages 4–6 years were targeted by preschool teacher Q-sort judgments and compared at age 23 with controls who were below average in preschool inhibition. This asymmetrical extreme group procedure avoids the problem in the earlier studies by Kagan and associates and in correlational studies of not being able to separate effects of high inhibition and low inhibition from one another. The asymmetrical extreme group procedure (that was already applied by Asendorpf & van Aken, 1994) is more sensitive to effects of high scorers than to effects of low scorers. Because the teacher judgments were based mainly on observations of the children in their preschool peer group, inhibition refers in this study mainly to social-evaluative anxiety and its effortful regulation. Table 8.1 presents the main findings of this forward prediction.

The inhibited participants reported as many peer relationships as controls and interacted with both same- and opposite-sex peers *more* frequently, had nonromantic relationships with opposite-sex peers who were 2.4 years younger on average, had half as often a stable romantic partner at the time of testing, and got involved in such a relationship 8 months later. This overall pattern suggests that inhibited participants avoided age-appropriate contact with potential romantic partners of their age (Connolly & Goldberg, 1999) and instead invested in nonromantic relationships with same-sex and relatively immature opposite-sex peers (a kind of downward orientation to

TABLE 8.1. Outcome of Inhibited Preschool Children at Age 23

Outcome at age 23 years	Inhibited ($n = 19$)		Controls ($n = 77$)		Difference	
	M	SD	M	SD	d^a	p^a
Parental judgment of shyness	3.46	1.20	2.75	0.77	0.81	.01
Currently has romantic partner (yes/no)	0.32	0.48	0.64	0.48	0.64	.01
Latency to first partnership (years)[b]	1.42	1.44	0.74	1.13	0.51	.02
Latency to first full-time job (years)[b]	3.43	1.92	2.57	1.61	0.51	.02
Contact frequency with same-sex peers	4.32	0.89	3.83	0.91	0.54	.04
Contact frequency with opposite-sex peers	3.37	0.92	2.70	1.08	0.63	.04
Age of opposite-sex peers (years)	20.63	1.55	23.04	2.18	1.02	.001
Age at testing (years)	23.09	0.44	22.67	0.41	0.91	.001

[a] t-test for group difference, one-tailed for first four rows.

[b] After 18th birthday.

Note. Adapted from Asendorpf, Denissen, and van Aken (2008, Table 1). Copyright 2008 by the American Psychological Association. Adapted by permission.

the opposite sex). Thus, regarding the age-appropriate transition to a stable romantic partnership, it seems that inhibited participants spent more time in the preceding phase of nonromantic peer relationships and unstable dating relationships. The delay in forming stable romantic relationships squares nicely with the finding of delayed marriage in inhibited boys in earlier studies (Caspi et al., 1988; Kerr et al., 1996).

Inhibited participants also showed a delay of 10 months in the transition to first full-time job. Because this transition is delayed by higher education, particularly a university education, it was important to control for educational level. However, inhibition was unrelated to educational level; therefore, the delay in the transition to the first full-time job remained unaffected by educational level. This finding may foreshadow a delayed transition into a stable career, with resulting occupational underachievement, as found by Caspi et al. (1988) for shy boys at midlife.

One of the most important findings of the study was that the delayed transitions were shown by not only inhibited males, as in earlier studies, but also inhibited females. This lack of sex differentiation in developmental transitions was to be expected, because of the erosion of traditional sex roles in Germany after the 1950s (Germany ranked second in the cross-cultural study of egalitarian gender roles carried out by Williams & Best, 1990). In the present 1980 birth cohort, no sex × inhibition interactions with regard to delayed transitions were found, nor sex × inhibition interactions in any other respect. It seems that the longitudinal paths for inhibited children have lost their earlier sex-specific bias in current German culture (and perhaps in other Western countries as well).

Curiously, inhibited participants showed another unexpected delay. They visited the laboratory for the age 23 testing 8 months later than expected (the timing of the invitation to the laboratory was based on their birthdays). According to the staff responsible for the invitation and testing, they had difficulties in persuading some participants to undergo follow-up testing, and in making sure they kept their promises. Indeed, the assessments at this age were completed more than 6 months later than originally expected because of such problematic cases. It seems that inhibited participants were overrepresented among them. Their hesitations concerning testing may be just another example of a general tendency of shy adults to avoid unfamiliar and evaluative situations (Asendorpf, 1989).

Sometimes zero findings are as important as significant differences. The result that the formerly inhibited children did not consider themselves as inhibited and did not show any internalizing difficulties in adulthood, such as neuroticism, low self-esteem, and loneliness, was such an important zero finding. It is important because self-perceived shyness and social anxiety in older children, adolescents, and adults are regularly accompanied by lower social self-esteem (e.g., Cheek & Melchior, 1990). This study was no exception: Self-rated shyness at age 23 correlated −.70 with social self-esteem with opposite-sex peers and −.50 with global self-worth.

The lack of internalizing problems at age 23 in the early inhibited group seems to be contradicted by the fact that the parents judged this group as significantly more inhibited than the control group. However, it should be noted that parents likely acquired a view that their child was inhibited in early childhood and may have preserved this view into adulthood even if the child's inhibition showed marked changes. In addition, the parents may have given more weight to observable behavior in adulthood, such as the delayed development of stable romantic relationships, than did the participants themselves, who may have based their self-judgment of inhibition more on private experiences of internalizing problems such as low social self-esteem. A relatively low correlation of .33 between parental judgments, and self-judgments of inhibition was consistent with both interpretations.

When only the top 8% of the distribution in inhibition was targeted (using the same criteria as applied to the inhibited group in the Dunedin Longitudinal Study), these children did show a tendency toward internalizing difficulties, with effect sizes similar to those found in the Dunedin Longitudinal Study. However, due to the much smaller number of extremely inhibited children in the LOGIC sample, deviations from the control group were not significant, except for low social self-esteem. Together these findings suggest that early inhibition (even when observed in the familiar peer group in which children face the risk of becoming excluded) is not a serious risk for internalizing problems in adulthood, except for an extremely inhibited subgroup.

These results were backed up by analyses that excluded the lowest 15% of the distribution in the control group. These analyses were done to make sure the effects could not be attributed to the groups with extremely *low* scores. This procedure reduced somewhat the power for finding significant differences, resulting in slightly higher *p* values. However, the effect sizes were only minimally affected and sometimes even increased.

Together with the observed delays in social transitions, the results of these prospective longitudinal studies suggest that inhibited children develop into cautious, reserved adults, but with few signs of internalizing problems. These problems seem to be due to later-appearing factors, such as problems with love relationships in adolescence.

LOOKING BACKWARD: ANTECEDENTS OF ADULT SHYNESS

In order to capture such influences on adult shyness intermediate between early childhood and adulthood, it is useful to complement the traditional forward predictions of the last section by backward retrodictions: What are the antecedents of adult shyness in later childhood and adolescence? Most studies aimed at retrodicting antecedents of adult shyness are cross-sectional: Shy adults or their parents are asked to recall earlier events, relationships, or personality characteristics, and these reports are compared to those of a control group low in shyness; group differences are then interpreted as evidence for antecedents of shyness. These studies, however, are plagued by retrospective biases: The currently shy members of the shy group may more cautiously remember certain events, may judge certain relationships or personality traits in the past less extremely, or may remember more shy behavior in the past than there was in reality. For example, cross-sectional studies of antecedents of adult social phobia often find that adults with social phobias recall more shy or anxious behaviors in childhood than do controls (Stemberger et al., 1995), whereas there is no evidence from prospective studies that childhood shyness or social anxiety is a risk factor for adult social phobia (see review in the last section of this chapter). This discrepancy is very likely the result of retrospective biases in the adults with social phobias.

In contrast, prospective longitudinal studies, such as LOGIC, allow for retrodictions of antecedents of adult shyness that are not threatened by retrospective biases, because the antecedents were concurrently assessed rather than recalled. Just as the predictive power of prospective studies is increased by using more reliable predictors that are aggregated across different assessments (inhibition in early childhood was aggregated across 2 or 3 years of assessment), the power of retrodictive studies is increased by aggregation, too. Because shyness in adults was assessed at only one point in time (age 23), aggregation across time was not possible. Instead, I capitalized on the fact that concurrent reports of shyness and inhibition at age 23 were available from the LOGIC participants themselves, and from at least one of their parents (most often from both mother and father). Because self-view and parent view present quite different perspectives on the participant's shyness, as shown by the significant but rather low correlation of .33 between self-reported and parent-reported shyness (the mean of the mother's and the father's report, allowing for a missing score for one of them), it seemed more appropriate to target high shyness in terms of consensually high shyness from both perspectives rather than by the average of self- and parent-rated shyness.

Therefore, I targeted a group of consensually shy adults (scores above 67th percentile in both self- and parent-rated shyness), resulting in 19 consensually shy participants (thus, in an extreme group of the same size as the early inhibited group, see Table 8.1). This consensually shy group was compared with a control group comprising participants with consensually lower scores (scores below the 67th percentile for both self- and parent-rated shyness), resulting in 56 controls. The main significant antecedents of consensually high adult shyness resulting from this backward prediction are presented in Table 8.2, grouped by age range. To further increase retrodictive power, all antecedents were aggregated as much as possible across measures and years of assessment.

As one might expect from the forward predictions, the teacher Q-sort measure of inhibition observed mainly in class was *not* a significant predictor of consensual shyness in adulthood, because this measure predicted parent-rated but not self-rated adult shyness. But the early parental judgment of shyness *and* observed shy behavior to strangers in the laboratory (both aggregated across 3 years of assessment) did predict consensual shyness in adulthood (see Table 8.2). To exclude the possibility that the retrodiction of consensual shyness on observed shy behavior was only mediated by parental judgment (which may overestimate retrodiction because of an insensitivity of the parents to changes in their child's shyness), I additionally retrodicted early observed shyness to strangers from the top 15% of the distribution of self-rated shyness, comparing this self-rated shy group ($n = 20$) with a control group below the median in self-rated shyness ($n = 67$). This self-rated shy group also had longer latencies to strangers in early childhood than the controls ($M = 0.31$ vs. $M = -0.22$; $d = 0.56$; $p < .05$, one-tailed test). Thus, inhibition with strangers was an antecedent of not only consensual shyness

TABLE 8.2. Antecedents of Consensual Shyness at Age 23

Antecedents	Shy ($n = 19$) M	SD	Controls ($n = 56$) M	SD	Difference d[a]	p[a]
Early childhood (ages 4, 5, 6 years)						
Parental judgment of shyness	3.90	1.65	2.97	0.91	0.71	.05
Latency to approach stranger[b]	0.39	0.67	–0.33	0.83	0.76	.05
Late childhood (ages 10 and 12 years)						
Parental judgment of						
Shyness	3.66	1.13	2.88	0.87	0.72	.01
Extraversion	3.59	0.71	3.98	0.68	0.50	.05
Adolescence (age 17 years)						
Parental judgment of						
Shyness	3.48	0.76	2.35	0.59	1.60	.001
Extraversion	3.46	0.57	4.02	0.62	0.84	.001
Emotional stability	3.47	0.62	3.74	0.43	0.51	.05
Self-judgment of						
Shyness	4.07	0.79	2.92	0.85	1.22	.001
Extraversion	3.53	0.72	4.19	0.56	0.97	.001
Emotional stability	3.40	0.50	3.82	0.52	0.72	.005
Global self-worth	3.76	0.79	4.27	0.47	0.79	.001
Self-worth with opposite-sex peers	3.65	0.80	3.97	0.52	0.47	.05
Loneliness	1.76	0.76	1.45	0.45	0.50	.05

[a] *t*-test for group difference.

[b] Aggregate of *z*-transformed latencies to an adult stranger and an unfamiliar peer.

but also self-rated shyness alone. Furthermore, analyses showed that this relation was not even significantly mediated by the parental judgments of shyness in childhood or adulthood.

Is early inhibition with strangers also an antecedent of internalizing difficulties in adulthood? To test this possibility, I aggregated the four available indicators of internalizing difficulties at age 23 (self-rated neuroticism, loneliness, general self-worth, and self-worth with opposite-sex peers), retrodicting early observed shyness with strangers from the top 15% of the distribution versus the lower half of the distribution of this aggregated index of internalizing difficulties. The group high in internalizing problems at age 23 did *not* have longer latencies to strangers in early childhood and was *not* rated higher in shyness with strangers by their parents at this age compared to the controls (in both cases, $t < 1.2$, $p > .25$). Thus, inhibition with strangers was an antecedent of shyness but not of internalizing difficulties.

Table 8.2 also shows that only parent-rated shyness and introversion were significant late childhood antecedents of consensual adult shyness. In stark contrast, in adolescence (age 17) both the parent- and the self-judgments showed full-blown internalizing difficulties as significant antecedents of consensual adult shyness: parent- and self-judgments of emotional instability (neuroticism), low global self-worth and low self-worth with opposite-sex peers (but *not* with same-sex peers), and loneliness. Similar assessments had already been carried out at age 12 for emotional instability and even earlier for global and social self-esteem and loneliness, but the assessments at these ages were not significantly related to consensual adult shyness.

This picture did not change much when adolescent internalizing difficulties were used to predict high versus below average self-rated adult shyness (operationalized as before for the analyses of behavioral inhibition) instead of consensual adult shyness. The main difference was that the parent-judged antecedents were not always significant anymore, and the self-rated antecedents became somewhat stronger—expected effects due to shared versus nonshared method variance. Although self-rated shyness and emotional instability at age 12 were already significant antecedents of adult self-rated shyness, the remaining indicators of internalizing difficulties at age 12 (global and peer-related self-esteem and loneliness) were not significantly related to self-rated adult shyness. Together these results suggest that the close relation between shyness and internalizing difficulties observed in adulthood (e.g., a correlation of $-.70$ between self-rated shyness and social self-esteem at age 23 in the LOGIC study) emerges not before early adolescence.

PUTTING THE PIECES TOGETHER

To interpret the overall, complex pattern of results on the long-term development of shyness as it is presented in the preceding two sections, it is helpful to distinguish clearly between the three types of shyness described in the first section of this chapter. The first type is rooted in behavioral inhibition to the unfamiliar, which emerges as a relatively stable behavioral trait during the second half of the second year of life. This behavioral trait is likely due primarily to interindividual differences in the strength of the BIS, as described by Gray (1982), and in more recent revisions by Gray and McNaughton (2000) and Corr (2008), and may be fully described at the neuroscience level in the future. These interindividual differences may be caused by genetic or early environmental differences and may be quite stable over development; in terms of self-regulation theory, they are part of the reactivity component of shyness. In terms of McCrae and Costa's (1999) personality theory, they are "basic tendencies." Children with a strong BIS cautiously approach novel situations and therefore show delays in major developmental transitions, such as entry into preschool (Asendorpf, 1990), engaging in the first stable romantic relationships in adolescence (Asendorpf et al., 2008), entry into university (Asendorpf & Wilpers, 1998), entry into the first job (Asendorpf et al., 2008; Caspi et al., 1988), and marrying and becoming parents (Caspi et al., 1988). This basic tendency, or "core personality trait" (Asendorpf & van Aken, 2003), may be as life course–persistent as the life-course-persistent tendency to show antisocial behavior (Moffitt, 1993).

In addition, shy behavior is influenced by acquired social-evaluative anxiety because of anticipated rejection or neglect by significant others—parents, siblings, peers, and perhaps even strangers—through excessive generalizations of expectations to become rejected or neglected in the future (Asendorpf, 1989, 1990). These interindividual differences are in early childhood rather independent of differences in the strength of the BIS and therefore show distinctive effects on internalizing problems for several years (Asendorpf & van Aken, 1994). However, because the social network of significant others, and the evaluations by these significant others, may change more than the strength of the BIS in the long run, mainly due to changes in the family of origin, important peer groups, and the families of destination, this second source of trait shyness is less stable; it is part of the reactivity component of shyness and a "characteristic adaptation" in terms of McCrae and Costa (1999), or a "surface characteristic" of personality in terms of Asendorpf and van Aken (2003).

Therefore, it is not surprising that in the LOGIC Study, early inhibition with strangers was an antecedent of adult shyness but not of adult internalizing difficulties—the same result that Asendorpf and van Aken (1994) reported for internalizing difficulties in childhood. They could trace back these difficulties to rejection or neglect in the early peer group but not to early inhibition with strangers. In adolescence, it seems to be rejection or neglect by potential romantic partners rather than rejection or neglect by peers in general that gives rise to social-evaluative anxiety and internalizing difficulties. This would explain why early inhibition predicted problems with opposite-sex peers rather than same-sex peers (see Table 8.1) and why low self-worth with opposite-sex peers (but not with same-sex peers) was an antecedent of adult shyness (see Table 8.2). Opposite-sex peers are here equated with potential romantic partners, because this applies to the large majority of adolescents with a heterosexual orientation. More precisely, however, it is the less familiar sex for both homo- and heterosexually oriented adolescents that is a source for romantic partners (Bem, 1996).

Why is the evaluation of the less familiar sex so important in adolescence and young adulthood? From an evolutionary perspective, the answer is that successful dating and mating is the most important developmental task in adolescence and young adulthood; therefore, selection pressures in all sexually replicating species have favored the evolution of proximate mechanisms that make sure that attention and energy is directed to mastering this task; consequently, we are particularly vigilant to cues of acceptance, neglect, and rejection by potential dating and mating partners (see Kirkpatrick & Ellis, 2004).

Viewed from Gray's (1982) perspective and more recent theories of reinforcement sensitivity, those with a high BIS are particularly disposed to high inhibition in encounters with possible dates and mates, not only because they are more sensitive to cues of punishment and frustrating nonreward in general, and therefore also to evaluations by others as being sexually unattractive, but also because these others are members of the less familiar sex that additionally triggers the BIS (an argument similar to Bem's in 1996). Consequently, shyness and internalizing difficulties become particularly closely coupled in adolescence—more closely than in childhood, during which peer rejection and neglect are less related to the familiarity of the peers.

According to this developmental two-factor view, early inhibition with strangers does not predict internalizing difficulties before this particularly close coupling between shyness and internalizing difficulties occurs (thus, not before adolescence), but it is predictive later on. In addition, it is continuously predictive of a cautious attitude toward novel situations that is perceived by parents as shyness and introversion even before adolescence.

A remaining, not yet satisfactorily resolved issue is the influence of the assumed third component of shyness: shyness due to modesty. Evidence for this self-regulatory component of shy behavior is stronger in the previously noted cross-cultural comparisons than in attempts to assess directly interindividual differences in self-regulation (Eisenberg et al., 2001), or in the study by Asendorpf (1994), who provided indirect evidence for such interindividual differences by showing moderating effects of early social competence and IQ on the long-term individual trajectories of shyness. Cascade models that simultaneously analyze different domains of development (Masten, Burt, & Coatsworth, 2006; Burt, Obradovic, Long, & Masten, 2008) are particularly suited to find spillover effects of various types of social competence, from self-regulation ability to long-term changes in trait shyness.

SUMMARY AND CONCLUSIONS

It is helpful to distinguish clearly between three types of shyness. The first one is rooted in behavioral inhibition to the unfamiliar, as it emerges as a relatively stable behavioral trait during the second half of the second year of life. This behavioral trait is likely due primarily to interindividual differences in the strength of the BIS, as described by Gray (1982), and in more recent revisions of his theory, and may be fully described at the neuroscience level in the future. These interindividual differences may be caused by genetic or early environmental differences, and may be quite stable over development. In terms of self-regulation theory, they are part of the reactivity component of shyness; in terms of McCrae and Costa's (1999) personality theory, they are "basic tendencies."

In addition, shy behavior is influenced by acquired social-evaluative anxiety because of anticipated rejection or neglect by significant others through excessive generalizations of expectations to become rejected or neglected in the future. These interindividual differences are in early child-hood rather independent of differences in the strength of the BIS, and there-fore show distinctive effects on internalizing problems for several years. Because the social network of significant others and evaluations by these significant others change more than the strength of the BIS in the long run, this second source of trait shyness is less stable; it is part of the reactivity component of shyness and a "characteristic adaptation" in terms of McCrae and Costa (1999).

Those with a high BIS are particularly disposed to high inhibition in encounters with possible dates and mates, not only because they are more sensitive to cues of punishment and frustrating nonreward in general, and therefore also to evaluations by others as being sexually unattractive, but also because these others are members of the less familiar sex that addi-tionally triggers the BIS. Consequently, shyness and internalizing difficulties become particularly closely coupled in adolescence—more closely than in childhood, during which peer rejection and neglect are less related to the familiarity of the peers.

Not yet sufficiently understood is the third component of shyness: shy-ness due to modesty. Evidence for this self-regulatory component of shy behavior is stronger in cross-cultural comparisons than in within-culture studies. Future studies of the distinctive role of this component in shy behav-ior and its development are needed to better understand shyness and its long-term development between early childhood and early adulthood.

ACKNOWLEDGMENTS

Parts of this chapter are adopted from Asendorpf (2008a, 2008b) and Asendorpf, Denissen, and van Aken (2008). I thank Marcel A. G. van Aken and Jaap J. A. Denissen for comments on an earlier draft.

REFERENCES

Asendorpf, J. B. (1989). Shyness as a final common pathway for two different kinds of inhibition. *Journal of Personality and Social Psychology, 57,* 481–492.
Asendorpf, J. B. (1990). Development of inhibition during childhood: Evidence for

situational specificity and a two-factor model. *Developmental Psychology, 26,* 721–730.

Asendorpf, J. B. (1993). Beyond temperament: A two-factorial coping model of the development of inhibition during childhood. In K. H. Rubin & J. B. Asendorpf (Eds.), *Social withdrawal, inhibition and shyness in childhood* (pp. 265–289). Hillsdale, NJ: Erlbaum.

Asendorpf, J. B. (1994). The malleability of behavioural inhibition: A study of individual developmental functions. *Developmental Psychology, 30,* 912–919.

Asendorpf, J. B. (2008a). Shyness. In M. M. Haith & J. B. Benson (Eds.), *Encyclopedia of infant and childhood development* (pp. 146–153). San Diego: Elsevier.

Asendorpf, J. B. (2008b). Developmental perspectives. In G. J. Boyle, G. Matthews, & D. H. Saklofske (Eds.), *Handbook of personality theory and testing: Vol. 1. Personality theories and models* (pp. 101–123). London: Sage.

Asendorpf, J. B., Denissen, J. J. A., & van Aken, M. A. G. (2008). Inhibited and aggressive preschool children at 23 years of age: Personality and social transitions into adulthood. *Developmental Psychology, 44,* 997–1011.

Asendorpf, J. B., & van Aken, M. A. G. (1994). Traits and relationship status. *Child Development, 65,* 1786–1798.

Asendorpf, J. B., & van Aken, M. A. G. (2003). Personality–relationship transaction in adolescence: Core versus surface personality characteristics. *Journal of Personality, 71,* 629–666.

Asendorpf, J. B., & Wilpers, S. (1998). Personality effects on social relationships. *Journal of Personality and Social Psychology, 74,* 1531–1544.

Bem, D. J. (1996). Exotic becomes erotic: A developmental theory of sexual orientation. *Psychological Review, 103,* 320–335.

Blair, C. (2003). Behavioural inhibition and behavioural activation in young children: Relations with self-regulation and adaptation to preschool in children attending head start. *Developmental Psychobiology, 42,* 301–311.

Burt, K. B., Obradovic, J., Long, J. D., & Masten, A. S. (2008). The interplay of social competence and psychopathology over 20 years: Testing transactional and cascade models. *Child Development, 79,* 359–374.

Caspi, A., Bem, D. J., & Elder, G. H. (1988). Moving away from the world: Life-course patterns of shy children. *Developmental Psychology, 24,* 824–831.

Caspi, A., Harrington, H., Milne, B., Amell, J. W., Theodore, R. F., & Moffitt, T. E. (2003). Children's behavioral styles at age 3 are linked to their adult personality traits at age 26. *Journal of Personality, 71,* 495–513.

Caspi, A., Moffitt, T. E., Newman, D. L., & Silva, P. A. (1996). Behavioral observations at age 3 years predict adult psychiatric disorders. *Archives of General Psychiatry, 53,* 1033–1039.

Caspi, A., & Silva, P. A. (1995). Temperamental qualities at age three predict personality traits in young adulthood: Longitudinal evidence from a birth cohort. *Child Development, 66,* 486–498.

Cheek, J. M., & Melchior, L. A. (1990). Shyness, self-esteem, and self-consciousness. In H. Leitenberg (Ed.), *Handbook of social and evaluation anxiety* (pp. 47–82). New York: Plenum Press.

Chen, X., Cen, G., Li, D., & Ile, Y. (2005). Social functioning and adjustment in

Chinese children: The imprint of historical time. *Child Development, 76,* 182–195.

Chen, X., Rubin, K. H., & Sun, Y. (1992). Social reputation and peer relationships in Chinese and Canadian children: A cross-cultural study. *Child Development, 63,* 1336–1343.

Connolly, J., & Goldberg, A. (1999). Romantic relationships in adolescence: The role of friends and peers in their emergence and development. In W. Furman, B. B. Brown, & C. Feiring (Eds.), *The development of romantic relationships in adolescence* (pp. 266–290). Cambridge, MA: Cambridge University Press.

Coplan, R. J., Arbeau, K. A., & Armer, M. (2008). Don't fret, be supportive: Maternal characteristics linking child shyness to psychosocial and school adjustment in kindergarten. *Journal of Abnormal Child Psychology, 36,* 359–371.

Corr, P.J. (2008). *The reinforcement sensitivity theory of personality.* Cambridge, UK: Cambridge University Press.

Eisenberg, N. Cumberland, A., Spinrad, T. L., Fabes, R. A., Shepard, S. A., Reiser, M., et al. (2001). The relations of regulation and emotionality to children's externalizing and internalizing problem behavior. *Child Development, 72,* 1112–1134.

Garcia-Coll, C., Kagan, J., & Reznick, J. S. (1984). Behavioral inhibition in young children. *Child Development, 55,* 1005–1019.

Gazelle, H. (2006). Class climate moderates peer relations and emotional adjustment in children with an early history of anxious solitude: A child × environment model. *Developmental Psychology, 42,* 1179–1192.

Gazelle, H., & Ladd, G. W. (2003). Anxious solitude and peer exclusion: A diathesis–stress model of internalizing trajectories in childhood. *Child Development, 74,* 257–278.

Gest, S. D. (1997). Behavioral inhibition: Stability and associations with adaptation from childhood to early adulthood. *Journal of Personality and Social Psychology, 72,* 467–475.

Gray, J. A. (1982). *The neuropsychology of anxiety: An inquiry into the functions of the septo-hippocampal system.* Oxford, UK: Oxford University Press.

Gray, J. A., & McNaughton, N. (2000). *The neuropsychology of anxiety: An inquiry into the functions of the septo-hippocampal system* (2nd ed.). Oxford, UK: Oxford University Press.

Kagan, J., & Moss, H. A. (1962). *Birth to maturity: A study of psychological development.* New York: Wiley.

Kagan, J., Reznick, J. S., Clarke, C., Snidman, N., & Garcia-Coll, C. (1984). Behavioral inhibition to the unfamiliar. *Child Development, 55,* 2212–2225.

Kagan, J., & Snidman, N. (2004). *The long shadow of temperament.* Cambridge, MA: Harvard University Press.

Kerr, M., Lambert, W. W., & Bem, D. J. (1996). Life course sequelae of childhood shyness in Sweden: Comparison with the United States. *Developmental Psychology, 32,* 1100–1105.

Kirkpatrick, L. A., & Ellis, B. J. (2004). An evolutionary–psychological approach to self-esteem: Multiple domains and multiple functions. In M. B. Brewer & M. Hewstone (Eds.), *Self and identity* (pp. 52–77). Malden, MA: Blackwell.

Masten, A. S., Burt, K. B., & Coatsworth, J. D . (2006). Competence and psychopathology in development. In D. Cicchetti & D. J. Cohen (Eds.), *Developmental psychopathology* (2nd ed., Vol. 3, pp. 696–738). New York: Wiley.

McCrae, R. R., & Costa, P. T., Jr. (1999). A five-factor theory of personality. In L. Pervin & O. P. John (Eds.), *Handbook of personality: Theory and research* (2nd ed., pp. 139–153). New York: Guilford Press.

Rothbart, M. K., & Bates, J. E. (1998). Temperament. In N. Eisenberg (Ed.), *Handbook of child psychology: Vol. 3. Social, emotional, and personality development* (pp. 105–176). New York: Wiley.

Rubin, K. H., Burgess, K. B., & Hastings, P. D. (2002). Stability and social-behavioral consequences of toddlers' inhibited temperament and parenting behaviors. *Child Development, 73,* 483–495.

Schwartz, C. E., Wright, C. I., Shin, L. M., Kagan, J., & Rauch, S. L. (2003). Inhibited and uninhibited infants "grown up": Adult amygdalar response to novelty. *Science, 300,* 1952–1953.

Smillie, L. D. (2008). What is reinforcement sensitivity: Neuroscience paradigms for approach–avoidance process theories of personality (Target article in *European Personality Reviews 2008*). *European Journal of Personality, 22,* 359–384.

Stemberger, R. T., Turner, S. M., Beidel, D. C., & Calhoun, K. S. (1995). Social phobia: An analysis of possible developmental factors. *Journal of Abnormal Psychology, 104,* 526–531.

Weinert, F. E., & Schneider, W. (1999). *Individual development from 3 to 12: Findings from the Munich Longitudinal Study.* Cambridge, UK: Cambridge University Press.

Williams, J. E., & Best, D. L. (1990). *Sex and psyche: Gender and self viewed cross-culturally.* Newbury Park, CA: Sage.

PART IV

CONTEXTS

9

Language Performance, Academic Performance, and Signs of Shyness
A Comprehensive Review

MARY ANN EVANS

The primary purpose of this review is to examine whether children and adolescents evidencing signs of shyness have less well-developed language and academic skills than their nondesignated peers, and as such to synthesize aspects of emotional and cognitive development. The secondary purpose is to apply the findings from both to inform parent and teacher interactions, and to provide directions for future research.

A number of terms used to describe children are relevant to this review. One set falls under the broader umbrella of temperament, entailing a biologically based behavioral tendency that is both relatively stable across time and context, and appears early in life. These include "behavioral inhibition," or fear and avoidance in the face of social and nonsocial novelty (e.g., Kagan, Resnick, & Snidman, 1986) and approach–withdrawal on temperament scales (e.g., Prior et al., 2008). These behavioral tendencies, most often studied in young children, and in longitudinal follow-ups of them, have been linked to anxiety disorders in older children (Kagan et al., 1986; Kagan, Snidman, Zentner, & Peterson, 1999; Prior, Smart, & Sanson, 2000), constituting diagnostic categories defined in the DSM-IV (American Psychiatric Association, 1994). "Social anxiety disorder" (formerly referred to as overanxious disorder and avoidant disorder of childhood), also called "social phobia," is described as a marked and persistent fear of social or performance situations in which embarrassment may occur such that there is marked distress that interferes with daily relationships (American Psychiatric Association, 1994, p. 411). "Avoidant personality disorder" entails a pervasive pattern of social inhibition, feelings of inadequacy, and hypersensitivity to negative evaluation that begins by early adulthood and is present in a variety of contexts (p. 662). "Selective mutism" (formerly elective mutism), often comorbid with or earlier occurring with social anxiety disorder, is characterized in the DSM-IV by consistent failure to speak in specific situations, despite speaking in others, that cannot be attributed to primary communication deficits, developmental disorder, or lack of language required for the situation. Several researchers have observed that these children are most often shy and withdrawn (Ford, Sladeczek, Carlson, & Kratochwill, 1998; Steinhausen & Juzi, 1996; Wright, 1968) and were slow to warm up or behaviorally inhibited in infancy or early childhood (Dummit et al., 1997).

Another set is more strongly connected to interpersonal interactions. Children are referred to as "socially withdrawn" (e.g., Rubin & Borwick, 1984) or "isolated" (e.g., Rubin, Daniels-Beirness, & Bream, 1982), "anxious–withdrawn" (e.g., Normandeau & Guay, 1998), "sensitive–isolated" (Masten, Morison, & Pellegrini, 1985), "fearfully shy" (Buss & Plomin, 1984), "reticent in their speech" (e.g., Evans, 1996; Van Kleeck & Street, 1982), "anxious–solitary" (Gazelle, 2006), and "shy" (e.g., Coplan & Armer, 2005). There is likely a large overlap in these concepts. For example, Crozier and Hostettler (2003) found that teacher ratings of five shyness items from the Emotionality, Activity, and Sociability (EAS) Temperament Survey and the four reticence items of Evans (1996) all loaded on one factor. Whereas Kagan (1994) views shyness and inhibition to the unfamiliar as equivalent, for Asendorpf (1990) shyness is a particular type of social withdrawal, entailing both a desire to approach and engage in interaction and a fear of doing so due to social-evaluative concerns. This has also been referred to as "conflicted shyness" by Coplan, Prakash, O'Neil, and Armer (2004). Although shyness is generally regarded as less severe than social anxiety disorder, studies have shown that those diagnosed with a social anxiety disorder or elective mutism are often reported to have been shy in earlier childhood (Black & Uhde, 1995; Hadley, 1994; Leonard & Topol, 1993). Shyness too, then, is linked both conceptually and longitudinally to the previously mentioned diagnosed disorders.

Finally, within the field of communication there is the concept of "communication apprehension," defined as the experience of anxiety associated with real or anticipated oral interaction with others (McCroskey, 1970). Although often thought of as relevant to school and workplace interactions, measures of communication apprehension span social interactions, making this literature relevant to this review.

Common to all of these is the notion that individuals so designated are fearful, anxious, wary, and reluctant to undertake social and verbal interactions in certain contexts that may be broad ranging or more constrained, and entail uncertainty, novelty, and real or perceived evaluation by others. For simplicity, I use the words "shy" and "shyness" in this review when making generalizations across studies and proposing conclusions.

LANGUAGE PERFORMANCE

With respect to the pragmatic aspects of language, shy individuals perceive making small talk, asking questions at school and work, talking with authority figures, and entering and engaging in conversation to be difficult. Difficulties with more fundamental aspects of expressive vocabulary and grammar might be a contributing factor. But there are other, more compelling reasons for hypothesizing that children with signs of shyness will have less developed skills in the semantic and syntactic aspects of language, as well as the pragmatic application. First, developmental scientists have maintained that the child is an active participant in the process of learning language (Cross, Nienhuys, & Kirkman, 1983; Nelson, 1988), and that practice facilitates the development of language and communication skills (Cazden, 1972; Gleason & Weintraub, 1978; Hoff-Ginsberg, 1991; Snyder-McLean & McLean, 1978). Speaking less is the most consistent marker of shyness. For example, results from numerous studies demonstrate that shy children spend less time in conversation (e.g., Asendorpf & Meier, 1993), are more silent within conversations (Asendorpf & Meier, 1993; Crozier & Badawood, 2009; Daly, 1978; Evans, 1987; McIness, Fung, Manassis, Fliksenbaum, & Tannock, 2004; Rubin et al., 1982), and have longer latencies to speak in conversation (e.g., Evans, 1987). (More detail on quantity of speech is provided later in this chapter in Table 9.1.) Moreover, shy children are more likely to have like parents (e.g., Daniels & Plomin, 1985), leading to the suggestion that there may be less conversation on the part of both the child and the parent to allow the child the same experience with language as children in other families. It has also been found that shy children are less successful in their communicative attempts with their peers and, after such failures, are less likely than their peers to make a second attempt (Stewart & Rubin, 1995). The interpretation put forward is that the negative emotions shy children experience after such social failures are less easily regulated by them, and as such are more likely to interfere with effective social problem solving, including verbal behavior. This more limited experience with different ways of going about social language may constrain language development. With negative social experiences, shy children may come to doubt themselves. There is substantial research documenting an association by age 7 between lower self-esteem and shy behavior (see, e.g., Boivin & Hymel, 1997; Rubin & Mills, 1988; Nelson, Rubin, & Fox, 2005), and it might be expected that lower confidence, sense of self-efficacy, and self-esteem might hamper participation in environments that foster language development.

In addition, child × environment models (e.g., Cairns, Elder, & Costello, 1996; Magnusson & Hakan, 1998; Sameroff, 1993) provide a framework for the notion that children may produce different reactions in their environment that affect their development. For example, they may elicit different verbal stimulation from others. Evans (1987) observed the interaction of kindergarten children who were reticent in their speech during classroom sharing time or "Show and Tell," rarely participating and speaking little when they did so. These children received proportionally more questions from their teacher, many with a simple choice response format. Infants with positive affect generate more verbal interaction with their caregivers (Lee, Chang-Song, & Choi, 2007), and such children show more advanced language at 20 months of age (Dixon & Shore, 1997; Dixon & Smith, 2000). The anxious child may also avoid novel contexts or be protected by parents from situations where different communication styles and opportunities would be afforded (Kagan, 1994; Prior et al., 2000). If it is the case that anxious children have poorer language skills, then, as proposed by Evans (1993, 1996), shyness and language skills may exist in a dynamic interplay, in which the shy child with less well-developed language skills may refrain from interaction, thus compromising language development, increasing or maintaining wariness in social interactions, and limiting opportunities for growth.

Despite these theoretical mechanisms that may contribute to less well-developed language in shy children, it must also be acknowledged at the outset that one could argue that any language differences one might see may not necessarily be a reflection of what shy children know or can do, but rather of what they do (i.e., their performance in whatever assessment context is used to measure their language skills). Some of the same mechanisms that might be thought to hinder language development, such as lower self-confidence, reluctance to take risks, or less perseverance, could also be argued to compromise the language behavior of shy children in research studies.

To what extent does empirical research show poorer language performance in shy children and adolescents? To address this question, I searched the research literature for studies with the key words "language/language development/ability" in combination with each of the terms introduced earlier. Reference lists in these articles were reviewed for additional relevant articles. I also included articles known to me in which language findings were secondary to the main focus. I excluded three groups of studies in an attempt to arrive at research with more "pure" measures of language skill. Studies in which verbal and nonverbal ability had been collapsed into a composite score confounded verbal and nonverbal ability. Studies using tests of verbal intelligence were also excluded. While vocabulary is often assessed as a part of verbal ability, verbal analogical reasoning, factual knowledge (including numeracy), understanding of societal conventions, and detection of verbal absurdities are also a part of verbal intelligence composites. Studies of social problem solving that collapsed across children's action and speech to arrive at a dependent variable also were not considered. Finally, studies with participants identified broadly as having internalizing difficulties were not considered, because this includes not only social withdrawal and anxiety but also depression, nor were studies of behavior problems that collapsed across externalizing and internalizing difficulties.

Forty-eight research papers are summarized in Table 9.1. The table most certainly does not comprise all research studies that have been conducted, if only because of the file drawer problem of studies with statistically nonsignificant findings not being published. However, several of the studies included assessments of abilities other than language to reduce this concern somewhat, and I feel that the studies presented provide a reasonable basis for evaluating the question. For each study the number of participants, age of participants, and instrument used to index shyness are noted. In the last column, the relevant findings, including the name of the assessment instruments for operationalizing the dependent variables, are listed. In studies in which shyness was treated as a continuous variable, concurrent and predictive correlations with the various test measures are presented, and where available, results from regression and structural equation modeling analyses. In the case of categorical treatment of data in which a shy group has been compared with another group, the comparison is with non-shy controls, unless otherwise stated. Finally, the studies have been grouped according to the term used to describe the target group. Within each group, studies are listed beginning with the youngest participants. These include studies of temperament/behavioral inhibition, proceeding through to studies of social anxiety and communication apprehension in middle childhood and adolescence, and within these groupings by date of publication. The exceptions here are the studies of selective mutism, which often have a wide range of ages within the samples (from 4 years through adolescence); hence, these studies are listed by date of publication. As much detail as is reasonable for a table has been included to help readers draw their own conclusions.

First, we see that associations between language development and shy temperament are apparent in infancy, with behaviorally inhibited infants as early as four months of age making fewer spontaneous vocalizations than uninhibited children (Rezendes, Snidman, Kagan, & Gibbons, 1993). Moreover, shyness is modestly negatively correlated with language production and expressive vocabulary at age 2 (Prior et al., 2008). Although there is the occasional null finding, this association holds through the preschool and primary school years in terms of expressive and receptive vocabulary,

TABLE 9.1. Research with Findings on Language and Shyness

Study	Participants	Descriptor and methodology notes	Findings (correlations, group differences, predictions)
Rezendes et al. (1993)	$n = 44$; age 14 months; retrospective to 4 and 9 months; follow-up at 20, 32, 48, and 66 months	Behaviorly inhibited versus uninhibited: observations	Less spontaneous speech at 14, 20, 32, 48, and 66 months in free play and lab interaction Fewer spontaneous vocalizations at 4 and 9 months (retrospective unpublished data in Rezendes et al.)
Broberg et al. (1990)	$n = 84$; ages 11–24 months; follow-up at 12 and 24 months; Sweden	Inhibition at 40 months: mothers' ratings on Infant Behavior Questionnaire[b]	r –.20 language subscale of the Griffiths Developmental Scale at 24 months; –.34 at 40 months
Kagan et al. (1999)	$n = 164$; 14 months; follow-up at 4 years	High reactivity to novelty versus low reactivity: observations	Fewer spontaneous comments and less smiling at age 4
Prior et al. (2008)	$n = 1,760$; ages 7–10 months	Temperament: Short Infant and Toddler Temperament Questionnaire at 12 and 24 months: shyness and low sociability	n.s. for shyness with MacArthur–Bates Communicative Development at 12 and 24 months (no value reported) Shy, less sociable on Communication Symbolic Behavior Scales at 24 months; shyness at 24 months is modest negative predictor of expressive vocabulary at 24 months
Gewirtz (1948)	$n = 38$, ages 5–6 years	Social apprehensiveness: teacher ratings on Fels Child Behavior Scales	r –.53 producing rhymes, –.33 alliterations; –.46 "things in the"; –.25 child names; –.47 adults names; –.50 things names—all word association tests r –.50 disarranged sentences; –.30 types; –.39 tokens— vocabulary diversity
Kemple et al. (1996)	$n = 64$; ages 4–5 years	Shyness: mothers' and teachers ratings on the Emotionality, Activity, Sociability Temperament Scale (EAS)	r n.s. for Peabody Picture Vocabulary Test (PPVT-R) (no value reported)

Study	Sample	Temperament measure	Language outcome
Slomkowski et al. (1992)[a]	n = 229; age 2 years; follow-up at ages 3 (n = 212) and 7 years (n = 164)	Affect–extraversion: composite of interest in persons, cooperativeness, fear, and happiness on Infant Behavior Record[b]	r .33 receptive and expressive scales of Sequenced Inventory of Communication Development receptive language at age 2; .27 and .31 at age 3; r .16–.23 with vocabulary and comprehension of the Wechsler Intelligence Scale for Children—Revised (WISC-R), Processing Word and Sentence Structure and Sentence Imitation, Clinical Evaluation of Language Fundamentals (CELF), and Token Test for Children at age 7
Spere et al. (2004)	n = 44 (from 400); age 4 years	Shyness: by mothers' ratings on Colorado Child Temperament Inventory (CCTI)	Lower vocabulary in the PPVT-R; Lower phonological awareness on the Test of Auditory Analysis Skills
Normandeau & Guay (1998)[a]	n = 291; age 5 years; follow-up at age 6 years; French Canada	Anxious–withdrawn: kindergarten teacher ratings on Questionnaire d'Évaluation des Comportements Préscolaires	r –.26 vocabulary of the PPVT (French version); r –.19 Test of Nonverbal Intelligence–2 at age 6
Rudasill et al. (2006)	n = 99; ages 4–5 years	Shyness: teacher ratings on Children's Behavior Questionnaire (CBQ)	r .13 mean length of utterance (MLU) in words and morphemes in play with researcher
Ting (2008)[a]	n = 55; age 5 years; Hong Kong with Cantonese as first language	Shyness: Revised Cheek–Buss Shyness Scale	r –.29 vocabulary of the PPVT (Chinese); –.30 PPVT (English); r –.13 Raven's Progressive Colored Matrices (RPCM) Predicted 9.7 and 7.2% of PPVT variance after controlling for parent education, socioeconomic status, and RPCM

(continued)

185

TABLE 9.1. (*continued*)

Spere et al. (2008)	$n = 67$ (from 105); age 4 years	Shyness: mothers' ratings on CCTI versus nonshy and middle groups; parallel forms of vocabulary tests given at home by mother and at school by tester	Fewer utterances than verbal and middle group discussing picture with mother in home n.s. sentence imitation for test of Language Development Primary–III and Comprehensive Receptive and Expressive Vocabulary Test n.s. for block design Wechsler Preschool and Primary Intelligence Scale–III (WPPSI) Scores from school higher than from home for expressive vocabulary; n.s. for receptive vocabulary
Rydell, Bohlin, & Thorell (2005)	$n = 112$; age 5 years; follow-up at age 6; Sweden	Behavioral inhibition: parent's rating on EAS	r –.20 vocabulary of PPVT
Crozier & Perkins (2002)	$n = 40$; ages 5–9 years	Shyness: teacher nomination, and rated on shy items of Buss–Plomin Temperament Scale, versus nonshy	Lower score on the British Picture Vocabulary Scale Fewer words spoken, different words, roots words and shorter MLU when telling narrative to pictures
Spere & Evans (2009)[a]	$n = 89$; age 5 years; from 142; follow-up at ages 6 and 7	Shyness: mother's rating on CCTI versus nonshy	r –.26 Receptive One-Word Picture Vocabulary Test, age 6 r –.31 Expressive One-Word Picture Vocabulary Test (EOWPVT), age 6 r –.11 word structure and –.13 sentence structure of the CELF, age 6 r –.19 alliteration awareness Prereading Inventory of Phonological Awareness (PIPA), age 6 r –.08 Expressive Vocabulary Test (EVT), age 7 r –.14 syntactic sentences of the Illinois Test of Psycholinguistic Abilities–3 and –.20 verbal fluency word associations of the CELF-IV, age 7 r –.21 Test of Phonological Awareness, age 7

Study	Sample	Measure	Findings
Reynolds & Evans (2009)	n = 40; age 5 years (selected from 117)	Shyness: mother's rating on CBQ; told the story Frog, Where Are You? to mother in home	Fewer words, different modifiers, incomplete utterances, story units; n.s. MLU, total utterances, modifiers, mental state verbs
Asendorpf & Meier (1993)	n = 41; second graders from sample of 140; Germany	High shy versus low shy, with sociability as second factor; by maternal report	Less speech in school situations—at school entry, at school recess, at school exit, for early lessons, and for late lessons; Less speech in unfamiliar situations and situations of medium familiarity; n.s. in familiar situations at home
Engfer (1993)	n = 39; 43 months; followed-up at 6 years; Germany	Shyness: mother's ratings on CBQ	Lower scores on vocabulary of WISC-R; n.s. block design of the Hamburg Wechsler Intelligence Scale
Coplan & Armer (2005)	n = 82; age 6 years	Shyness: maternal ratings of Child Social Preference Scale (CSPS)	r .08 vocabulary of the EOWPVT-R
Crozier & Badawood (2009)	n = 108; ages 52–71 months; Saudi Arabia	Shyness: teachers chose shy versus nonshy; created shy, nonshy, and mismatch groups by parent and teacher ratings on EAS	Shorter MLU (Show and Tell and free play); lower vocabulary in the PPVT (Arabic); More silent intervals (Show and Tell and free play)
Coplan & Weeks (2009)	n = 167; ages 6–7 years	Shyness: maternal ratings on CSPS	r −.25 pragmatic judgment of Comprehensive Assessment of Spoken Language in midyear; pragmatic language associated with a decrease in shyness across year in boys but not girls
Bzdrya, Evans, & Spooner (2002)	n = 108; ages 10–12 years	Shyness: self-ratings on Children's Shyness Questionnaire	n.s. Vocabulary in EVT; word associations in CELF; recreating sentences on Test of Language Competence—Expanded; Lower self-ratings on Children's Assertiveness Inventory; EVT mediated relation between shyness and assertiveness

(continued)

TABLE 9.1. (*continued*)

Crozier & Hostettler (2003)[a]	n = 240; age 10 years	Shyness: Two girls and two boys per class nominated as most shy by teacher versus nonshy controls; assigned to test conditions	Lower scores on Crichton Vocabulary Scales (expressive definitions) in one-to-one oral, not written, group condition
Rubin et al. (1982)	n = 52; age 5 years	Isolated: observations in play	r –.45 utterances, –.46 direct requests, –.27 indirect requests
Rubin (1982)	n = 123; age 4 years	Onlooker behavior: observations of play	r –.18 vocabulary PPVT
Rubin & Krasnor (1986)	n = 48; ages 5–6 years	Isolated: observations of play average and sociable	n.s. vocabulary PPVT
Rubin & Borwick (1984)	n = 5; dyads in each of preschool and kindergarten	Isolated: observations of play versus neutral play partner	Fewer requests to elicit action, and indirect request to acquire objects More low-cost requests for attention
Landon & Sommers (1979)	n = 40; verbal ages 36–74 months	Quiet versus chatterboxes: teacher nominations	Lower scores on expressive morphology in the Illinois Test of Psycholinguistic Ability; receptive syntax of the Northwestern Syntax Screening Test; Deep Test of Articulation More errors on Menyuk Sentence Repetition Test
Van Kleeck & Street (1982)	n = 4, age 3 years	Reticent versus talkative: teacher report	Shorter MLU, lower vocabulary PPVT; fewer complex utterances, and less variety of vocabulary in free play
Evans (1987)	n = 14, age 5 years	Reticent: least frequently speaking in 15 sessions of Show and Tell versus classmate; all variables collected in Show and Tell	Shorter MLU; longer latency to speech; number of comments, words volunteered, utterances per topic, topics per turn, more descriptions of present objects; fewer descriptions of absent object, narratives Fewer replies to teacher low-power remarks

Study	Sample	Measure	Findings
Vriniotis & Evans (1988)	n = 28; in each of grades, 2, 4, and 6	Reticent: teacher ratings of classroom participation versus controls	Lower scores on vocabulary of WISC-R, word associations of CELF; Fewer ways of phrasing communicative intents; fewer communicative intents to scenarios
Evans & Ellis (1992)	n = 8 dyads; age 6 years	Reticent: stably very quiet across kindergarten observed with nominated friend	More low-cost requests, nonverbal requests, information requests in the here and now
Evans (1996)	n = 128; age 5 years	Reticent: stably very quiet across kindergarten versus verbal and mixed controls by teacher ratings of verbal participation	Lower scores on vocabulary of EVT, processing composite of CELF, production composite of CELF, parent ratings of Verbal Communication Scale; n.s. vocabulary of PPVT, geometric design and block design of WISC; pattern analysis of Stanford–Binet–4
Stewart & Rubin (1995)	n = 145 across grades K, 2, and 4	Withdrawn–internalizing: 11, 8, and 11 in grades K, 2, and 4, respectively; versus average children	More indirect requests; fewer commands
Jones & Gerig (1994)[a]	n = 101; sixth graders	Silent: classroom observations using Brophy–Good Teacher–Child Observation Instrument, versus nonsilent	Fewer responses to open questions, initiated comments in class; n.s. response to direct questions
Lloyd & Howe, (2003)	n = 72; ages 4–5 years	Reticent: observations in free play (onlooker, unoccupied, wandering)	r −.31 vocabulary on PPVT-R; −.26 with divergent thinking (and higher r for reticent than solitary–passive and solitary–active children); r −.25 picture completion in WPPSI
Kolvin & Fundudis (1981)	n = 24; ages 6–8 years	Selective mutism (SM); 8 compared to 102 controls	45% of SM showed delayed speech development

(continued)

TABLE 9.1. *(continued)*

Black & Uhde (1995)	*n* = 30; ages 5–12 years	SM; no comparison group	10% of children with SM had history of delayed language development
Ford et al. (1998)	*n* = 153; 96 under age 12 years; 23 ages 12–20; 12 age 21 or older	SM; no comparison group; survey	23% reported working with a speech and language clinician on expressive or receptive language or articulation; an additional 35% worked on social skills or talking in small groups
Steinhausen & Juzi (1996)	*n* = 100; age 8 years	SM; no comparison group	20% had articulation disorder; 28% had expressive language disorder
Kristensen (2000)	*n* = 54; ages 3–16 years; Norway	SM versus controls	29% mixed expressive–receptive or expressive language disorder versus 2% controls; 43% phonological disorder versus 10% controls
McInnes et al. (2004)	*n* = 14; ages 7–14 years	SM versus social phobia; retold stories to mothers at home; small *n* of 7 in each group	Fewer details; less speech; lower grammatic complexity; fewer settings, initiation events, internal responses on Strong Narrative Assessment Procedure Trend to lower scores on phonological awareness of Lindamood Auditory Conceptualization Test (LACT) n.s. vocabulary of PPVT-III, WISC-III Performance IQ, finger windows of Wide Range Assessment of Memory and Learning
Kristensen & Oerbeck (2006)	*n* = 94; ages 6–17 years	SM	Lower scores on PPVT-III
Manassis et al. (2007)	*n* = 63; ages 6–10 years	SM versus normal controls and anxiety disorders	Scored lower than anxious and controls on vocabulary PPVT-III, phonological awareness of LACT, and on Test of Reception of Grammar Lower than anxious and controls on spatial working memory of WISC-III-PI and Visual Patterns Test n.s. finger windows forward and backward

190

Nowakowski et al. (2009)[a]	$n = 57$; ages 7–9 years	SM versus controls (and mixed anxiety)	Scored lower on vocabulary PPVT for girls; n.s. for boys
McCarthy (1929)	$n = 31$; ages 2–4 years	Introversion–extraversion: observations on Marsten Rating Scale[b]	r −.51 with talkativeness during play; n.s. with mean length of response
Kristensen & Torgersen (2008)	$n = 150$ from 2,568; ages 11–12 years; Norway	Social Anxiety versus attention-deficit/hyperactivity disorder, other disorder, no disorder	More mothers reporting language delay in child than other disorder or no-disorder groups

Note. [a] in column 1 indicates that study appears in Tables 9.1 and 9.2; [b] in column 3 indicates that direction of scale has been changed for these tables so that high scores = high shyness; subtest names in column 4 begin with lowercase letters, followed by test battery beginning with uppercase letters, for which some acronyms appear in first mention; n.s., not significant.

phonological awareness, morphology, syntax, verbal fluency, and pragmatics (e.g., requestive strategies and narrative skill). Very few studies of older children were located, and most pertained to children diagnosed with selective mutism and social anxiety disorder. Samples for these children revealed that between 28 and 48% of the children evidenced delayed language development, an incidence rate higher than nondiagnosed controls or population norms. However, these samples also often include a wide age range of participants, and it is not known whether weaker language skills spanned the age range or were localized to younger participants. There is clearly a need for more studies of older children and of advanced language skills to determine whether the associations observed in childhood are also observed among adolescents, and whether they might be attenuated through the verbal stimulation and experience gained through reading. Finally, it is noteworthy that numerous studies have used the Peabody Picture Vocabulary Test (PPVT), because this test requires children simply to point to their answer and make no verbal response. Children with selective mutism obtained lower scores than children with no diagnosed disorder, and similar relationships were found in less severe forms of shyness in studies elsewhere in Table 9.1.

Overall, the results across studies suggest that there is a negative association between shyness and language performance, but of a modest magnitude. Many of the studies do not proide standardized scores for the language measures, but among those that do, the average scores presented for the shy children often fall close to 100, the population mean. Thus, shyness is not to be associated necessarily with delayed language skills but with less developed language skills. However, given the fast pace of spoken discourse, especially among more verbally competent children and adults, less developed language skills may contribute to shy behavior and reduced social skill in children. In fact, two recent studies (Crozier & Badawood, 2009; Coplan & Weeks, 2009) and three earlier studies (Asendorpf, 1994; Bzydra, Evans, & Spooner, 1992; Coplan & Armer, 2005) have shown that vocabulary, pragmatic language skills, and verbal intelligence moderated the adjustment/assertiveness of shy schoolchildren and appear to act as protective factors.

In summary, these studies provide an affirmative answer to the question of whether shy/anxious children have less well-developed language skills, and a rationale has been presented for why this might exacerbate children's shyness. However, there are major methodological issues to be tackled to sort out whether the differences observed are in competence or performance. Some might argue that this distinction is irrelevant—that there is no clear way to test competence except by performance. Regardless, it is valuable to determine whether children's scores are artificially lowered by the anxiety that shy children experience in the presence of unfamiliar researchers and play partners, and under conditions of evaluation. A few of these studies have attempted this by assessing children in ways that should minimize their potential discomfort.

Evans and Ellis (1992) asked reticent children to nominate a friend in the classroom with whom they would like to play to form play dyads of reticent and nonreticent children. Compared to verbal children, who were paired with a play partner they did not nominate, shy children made more simple requests—low-cost requests, nonverbal requests, and information requests pertaining to the here and now. Spere, Evans, Hendry, and Mansell (2008) observed children interacting with their mothers at home around a set of pictures and found differences in the verbal behavior of shy and nonshy children, as did McInnes et al. (2004) when comparing children with selective mutism retelling stories to their mothers at home. Spere et al. (2008) also administered parallel forms of receptive and expressive vocabulary tests, one form by a researcher at school and the other by the mother at home, with the experimenter in the background to record responses and to indicate when the ceiling had been reached. Children's test scores were not lower at school, suggesting that the unfamiliarity of being assessed by an examiner at school does not negatively affect vocabulary scores among 4-year-olds.

As well, Crozier and Hostettler (2003) required 10-year-old children who could write to give definitions to words, and assigned them to three different testing conditions, with presumed decreasing degrees of anxiety: standard one-to-one oral testing; one-to-one testing with oral questions, but a written response; and group testing with written questions and answers. Shy children obtained lower scores in the one-to-one condition than did children in the group testing condition. However, they also found the same modest negative relation seen in other studies in the correlation between shyness and scores on the group-administered National Foundation for Education Research (NFER) Progress in English tests given as part of the school curriculum. In the end, Crozier and Hostettler concluded that their findings supported both the notion that the language of shy children is less developed, and that their performance is negatively affected by anxiety stemming from being the focus of attention in one-to-one testing. It should be noted, however, that their participants were older than those in most other studies of shy children, and that social-evaluative concerns may play a greater role in the scores of the older participants than in those of younger children.

Finally, if anxiety is the only factor in shy children's lower language scores, one should see consistency of poorer performance, including nonverbal tests, across studies. Several studies in Table 9.1 found no group differences rather than group differences, or slightly lower shyness correlations within the same sample on tests of nonverbal reasoning (e.g., Raven's Progressive Colored Matrices, Block Design and Geometric Design of the Wechsler Intelligence Scale for Children—Revised [WISC-R] and Wechsler

Preschool and Primary Scale of Intelligence [WPPSI], and Pattern Analysis of the Stanford–Binet–4) and nonverbal short-term memory (e.g., Finger Windows of the Wide Range Assessment of Memory and Leaning). This further undermines the speculation that the poorer language scores of shy children are entirely anxiety and performance based. More studies using both verbal and nonverbal measures are warranted to explore this further.

ACADEMIC PERFORMANCE

There are two reasons why shy children might fare as well as their peers or even better than very nonshy children in academic skills. Shy children are seen as compliant and nondisruptive in class and, at least on the surface, attentive to classroom demands. They might also be more "studious," retreating to academics, applying themselves to homework, and reading voraciously. Countering this are reasons for speculating that there may be a negative association between shyness and academic skills, as well as language skills. Asking questions and discussing concepts both in class and in peer situations may assist children to acquire, restructure, and consolidate knowledge. At least one study (Rimm-Kaufman et al., 2002) has shown that shy children talk less to and direct fewer requests to teachers, and many more studies (see Table 9.1) have shown reduced speech of shy children with their peers when at play and in class. Learning also sometimes involves taking risks, such as embracing new academic challenges and guessing when uncertain to then confirm the response, or to have it confirmed by others. This is something that shy children may be less willing to do (Levin & Hart, 2003; Spere, Evans, Mansell, & Hendry, 2007). Their "good behavior" may lead them to be overlooked somewhat or to have their difficulties discounted to some degree by teachers with demanding classroom loads (e.g., Keogh, 2003). Conversely, as I discuss later, negative biases in teacher perceptions of their competence could contribute to lower teacher expectations. Finally, shy children's anxiety over negative evaluation may interfere with learning, in that despite outward behavior, their attention might be divided between the task at hand and these evaluative concerns (Saranson, 1972; Wine, 1971). If these concerns are more pronounced among older children, then this might be especially true in the middle school and secondary school years. On the other hand, a concern over negative evaluation might encourage the individual to study harder.

Table 9.2 summarizes research findings on the association of standardized tests and academic grades with shyness. I did not consider studies using teacher ratings of performance to avoid significant findings that might be due to bias in teacher perceptions and shared variance that may be associated with the same informant rating both shyness and academic performance.

(The issues of temperament and perceptions of competence are discussed later in this review.) There are fewer studies (26) of academic performance than of language performance and, not surprisingly, proportionately fewer studies still (just nine across all the different shyness constructs) of children ages 5–8 years on tests of academic readiness and academic skills.

A review of Table 9.2 reveals considerable consistency in the findings, in that virtually all values are negative, dispelling the suggestion that shyness might be an asset in academic pursuits. However, the association, when found, is generally modest, with correlations indicating between 5 and 12% shared variance in the domains of both literacy and mathematics when these domains have been reported separately. Among these studies, only three have reported the findings for boys and girls separately. In their study of selectively mute children, Nowakowski et al. (2009) found that both boys and girls with selective mutism obtained lower mathematics scores than controls; in contrast, only girls with selective mutism obtained lower vocabulary scores. Kohn and Rosman (1972) also examined their data for preschool children by sex and determined that the negative association between apathy–withdrawal and achievement in grades 1 and 2 held equally for boys and girls. Finally, Dobbs, Doctoroff, Fisher, and Arnold (2006) conducted separate regressions for girls and boys, and found that the negative association between teacher ratings of withdrawal and scores on the tests of early mathematics achievement did not differ significantly for boys and girls. Thus, from these two studies, there appears to be little differentiation in achievement by sex among shy children.

On the whole then, it may be that there is a negative relation between academics and shyness that is genuinely modest. As noted earlier, shy children may not be as engaged in classroom activities, may be more prone to withdrawal and low task persistence when difficulty is encountered, may be less likely to take academic risks, and may less quickly receive intervention—all of which might affect their academic progress. It may also be that when participants are collapsed across classroom, uncontrolled curriculum effects in the mastery of academic skills attenuate the modest relation seen, such that some classroom environments (e.g., those with more structure) may be more enabling than others.

The relation may also be attenuated by effects of varying teacher–child relationships on shy children's learning. Children with higher-quality relationships with their teachers participate more and are more engaged in the classroom (Ladd, Birch, & Buhs, 1999), which would be expected to facilitate learning. In fact, several studies have shown that children with higher-quality teacher relationships have higher levels of academic achievement (e.g., Birch & Ladd, 1997; Furrer & Skinner, 2003; Hamre & Pianta, 2001; Pianta, Nimetz, & Bennet, 1997), perhaps because these teachers are better able to communicate with children and provide a secure base for approach-

TABLE 9.2. Research with Findings on Academics and Shyness

Study	Participants	Descriptor and methodology notes	Findings (correlations, group differences, predictions)
Ting (2008)[a]	$n = 55$; age 5 years; Cantonese as first language; Hong Kong	Shyness: Revised Cheek–Buss Shyness Scale (high score = high shy)	r .16 Chinese character/word reading
Kohn & Rosman (1972)	$n = 323$ preschoolers; follow-up at grade 1 and grade 2 ($n = 287$)	Apathy withdrawal: Kohn Social Competence Scale and Symptom Checklist	r –.37 Metropolitan Readiness Test in grade 1 r –.26 reading Metropolitan Achievement Test (MAT) in grade 2 Correlations held after partialing out maternal education, family income, minority group status, and occupational status of household head
Normandeau & Guay (1998)[a]	$n = 291$; age 5 years; follow-up at age 6; French Canada	Anxious withdrawn: teacher ratings on Questionnaire d'Évaluation des Comportements Préscolaires	r –.37 with mathematics; –.32 with French in grade 1 Structural equation modeling showed direct link (10% of variance) with school achievement
Bub, McCartney, & Willett (1972)	$n = 882$; age 24 months; follow-up at age 6	Internalizing: mothers' ratings on Child Behavior Checklist/2–3	Latent growth curve modeling showed negative prediction to letter–word, word attack, and applied math problems composite of Woodcock Psychoeducational Battery
Slomkowski et al. (1992)[a]	$n = 164$; age 2 years; follow-up at 7 years	Affect–Extraversion: composite of interest in persons, cooperativeness, fear, and happiness on Infant Behavior Record[b]	r –.12 reading recognition on Peabody Individual Achievement Test (PIAT) at age 7
Egeland et al. (1990)	$n = 28$ preschoolers; follow-up at grades 1, 2, and 3	Socially withdrawn: teacher ratings on Preschool Behavior Questionnaire and Behavior Problem Scale	Lower PIAT composite in grades 1 and 2; approached significance in grade 3
Dobbs et al. (2006)	$n = 108$; age 4–5 years	Withdrawal: teacher ratings on Child Behavior Checklist (CBCL)	r –.37 Test of Early Mathematics Achievement–2

196

Study	Sample	Measure	Findings
Spere & Evans (2009)[a]	n = 89; age 5 years; from 142; follow-up at age 6 and 7	Shyness: mothers' ratings on Colorado Child Temperament Inventory versus nonshy	r −.10 composite with letter-sound knowledge of Prereading Inventory of Phonological Awareness, and word identification and word attack on the Woodcock Reading Mastery Test—Revised (WRMT-R), age 6 r −.01 word identification and word attack composite on WRMT-R, age 7 r −.21 Test of Phonological Awareness, age 7
Broberg et al. (1997)	n = 123; age 40 months; follow-up at age 86 months; Sweden	Inhibition at 40 months by mothers' ratings on California Child Q-Set; at 40 and 86 months by teachers' ratings on Preschool Behavior Q-Sort[b]	n.s. word recognition, sentence reading, and reading comprehension composite (Broberg et al. referred to this as verbal ability); n.s. mathematical ability at 86 months When entered with previously tested mathematical abilities, day care quality, inhibition predicted 3.5% (negative) variance in mathematics
Green et al. (1980)	n = 116; age 9 years	Socially withdrawn: classroom observations of being alone and on task	r −.21 composite of reading, mathematics and language arts on the MAT
Lerner et al. (1985)	n = 194; age 10 years	Adaptability/approach–withdrawal: teacher and self-ratings on Dimensions of Temperament Survey[b]	r −.19 Comprehensive Test of Basic Skills composite n.s. word/paragraph reading on Stanford Achievement Test (SAT)
Crozier & Hostettler (2003)[a]	n = 240; age 10 years	Shyness: two girls and two boys per class nominated as most shy by teacher versus nonshy controls	r −.26 with National Foundation for Educational Research (NFER) Progress in English, −.32 NFER Progress in Mathematics
Masten et al. (1985)	n = 612; grades 3–6	Sensitive–isolated: peer nominations on Revised Class Play	r −.49 PIAT r −.39 academic achievement from records
Ludwig & Lazarus (1983)	n = 103; grades 4 and 5	Shy and least shy by teacher nomination	n.s. stanine on language of SAT, n.s. grade point average

(continued)

TABLE 9.2. (continued)

Jones & Gerig (1994)[a]	$n = 101$; sixth graders	Silent, identified through classroom observations using Brophy–Good Teacher–Child Observation Instrument, versus nonsilent	n.s. in proportion of silent and nonsilent in quartiles of California Achievement Test
Maziade et al. (1986)	$n = 42$; age 7 years; selected from 980; follow-up at age 12; French Canada	Temperament: Difficult, by ratings on the French version of Thomas, Chess, and Korn's Parent Temperament Questionnaire versus nondifficult controls[b]	Achievement index = number of terms above or below class average from grades 1–6 r –.39, adaptability with mathematics index; r .21 with reading index r –.39 approach–withdrawal with mathematics index; r .38 with reading index
Ialongo et al. (1995)	$n = 884$; age 6 years; follow-up at grade 5	Anxious: Self-report on the Children's Manifest Anxiety Scale—Revised	Children in top third of anxious group in grade 1 were about 10 times more likely to be in bottom third of California Achievement Test in grade 5
Chen et al. (1997)	$n = 582$; ages 9 and 12; follow-up at 2 years; China	Shyness inhibition: Teacher–Child Rating Scale	r .12 scores on academic examinations conducted by school
Rapport et al. (2001)	$n = 325$; ages 7–15 years; 3- to 4-year follow-up	Socially withdrawn: teacher ratings on CBL	r –.24 concurrent academic success on the Academic Performance Rating Scale r –.19, –.21, and –.11 on language, mathematics, reading, respectively, on SAT Indirect negative effect of withdrawal on achievement through classroom performance; effects on current academic behavior mediated relation of internalizing features to later achievement
Cunningham et al. (2004)	$n = 104$; age 7 years	Selective mutism (SM) versus controls; testing done at home	n.s. arithmetic and word recognition on Wide Range Achievement Test n.s. teacher ratings in math, reading, and academics overall, and general performance at school

198

Study	Sample	Measure	Results
Nowakowski et al. (2009)[a]	$n = 30$ with SM; age 8 years, 8 months; 46 with mixed anxiety age 9; 27 controls, age 7	SM versus mixed anxiety and controls	Lower mathematics scores on the PIAT n.s. reading and spelling on PIAT
Comadena & Comadena (1984)	$n = 48$; age 7 years, 8 months	Communication apprehension (CA): self-ratings on Measure of Elementary Communication Apprehension	r .16 mathematics on SAT r .06 reading on SAT
Watson & Monroe (1990)	$n = 203$; ages 8–12 years	CA: self-ratings on Communication Apprehension Behavior Inventory	r −.26 Comprehensive Test of Basic Skills
Comadena & Prusank (1988)	$n = 1,053$; grades 2, 4, 6, 7, and 8	CA: self-ratings on Measure of Elementary Communication Apprehension; divided into six levels of CA	High CA had lowest scores on mathematics, reading, and language of SAT; students low in CA performed 23% better than those high in CA in mathematics
Hurt & Preiss (1978)	$n = 118$; grades 7, 8, and 9	CA: self-report on Personal Report of Communication Apprehension	r −.25 with school grades controlling for attitude to school
Davis & Scott (1978)	$n = 429$; grades 9–12	CA: self-report on Personal Report of Communication Apprehension and Personal Report of Communication Fear	r −.27 Science Research Associates Achievement Test r −.22 grade point average

Note. [a] in column 1 indicates that study appears in Tables 9.1 and 9.2; [b] in column 3 indicates that direction of scale has been changed for these tables so that high scores = high shyness; subtest names in column 4 begin with lowercase letters, followed by test battery beginning with uppercase letters, for which some acronyms appear in first mention; n.s., not significant.

ing novel and challenging tasks. With respect to withdrawn children, Chang (2003) found that in classrooms where teachers were empathetic and warm, withdrawn children felt more socially competent and more positive about themselves in social interactions. Regrettably, however, shy children seem to be less able to form close relationships and more likely to form a dependent relationship with their teachers (e.g., Birch & Ladd, 1997; Rudasill, Rimm-Kaufman, Justice, & Pence, 2006; Rydell, Bohlin, & Thorell, 2005), and this may be particularly true in some classrooms.

Added to this is the potential effect of less positive appraisals of shy children by others. Previous research has shown that teachers are more likely to underestimate the intelligence of inhibited/withdrawn/communication apprehensive children (Martin & Holbrook, 1985) and to perceive these children as less intelligent and less academically competent (Coplan, Gavinski-Molina, Lagacé-Séguin, & Wichmann, 2001; Gordon & Thomas, 1967; McCroskey & Daly, 1976; but see Prakash & Coplan, 2007, for null finding in a sample of children in private school in India), and as less ready for school (McBryde, Ziviani, & Cuskelly, 2004). As noted in the review by Evans (2001), a main factor in these less positive appraisals is likely the children's restricted verbal behavior itself, with less speech or impaired speech interpreted as indicating less intelligence. While such perceptions might operate to make teachers more vigilant about a child's academic progress, they also may lead to less optimistic expectations for academic achievement and greater passivity over academic difficulties. In short, considerable classroom and teacher variation may contribute to the academic results in Table 9.2.

SUGGESTIONS FOR PARENTS AND TEACHERS

Despite the modest size of the relation between shyness and academic achievement, the overall negative associations and complete absence of positive associations, as with language skills, are enough to lead one to consider what parents and teachers might do to reduce the effects of shyness on language and academics to near zero. The reader is referred to reviews by Evans (2001) and Coplan and Arbeau (2008), which include suggestions for parents and teachers that I underscore and add to here.

Although it has been noted that teachers minimize the seriousness of shyness in comparison with aggressive behavior (e.g., Kashdan & Herbert, 2001; Nungesser & Watkins, 2005) and think children will grow out of their shyness (HoganBruen, Clauss-Ehlers, Nelson, & Faenza, 2003), recent research has shown that they have considerable concern over these children and a desire to help them (e.g., Arbeau & Coplan, 2007; Thijs, Koomen, & van der Leij, 2006). Moreover, they have offered many good suggestions for working with shy children that mesh nicely with what research has revealed about shyness. For example, Brophy and McCaslin (1992) and Evans (2001) found that the most common strategies cited by teachers include minimizing embarrassment and stress, making it clear that it is OK to make mistakes, supporting and encouraging children, praising their accomplishments, and reassuring them of their competence. These strategies should serve to enhance motivation and persistence, factors that are positively related to academic achievement (Bramlett, Scott, & Rowell, 2000; Martin & Holbrook, 1985; Schoen & Nagle, 1994). Paget, Nagle, and Martin (1984) and Paulsen, Bru, and Murberg (2006) found that teachers were especially attentive to and supportive of withdrawn children, and that their attention was more likely to involve praise, something to which withdrawn children are particularly responsive (Kennedy & Willcutt, 1964). However, it should be noted that praise is thought to be most effective for shy children when given inconspicuously. In addition, Chang (2003) found that when teachers were more empathetic towards withdrawn children, these children felt more socially competent and more positive about themselves in social interactions, and were more accepted by their peers. In fact, Gazelle (2006) has shown that a conflictual, disruptive, and chaotic classroom climate is particularly detrimental to the adjustment of anxious children.

Teachers also cite indirectly and gently pressuring shy children to change. The last part is important to avoid dependent and overprotective relationships with shy children (see review by Burgess, Rubin, Cheah, & Nelson, 2005) that may work against shy children learning to cope with their emotional and behavioral profiles and that may interfere with the expansion of their language, academic, and social skills. Evans (2001) provided several other suggestions for luring children into social interaction and reducing their anxiety, such as fantasy activities, small-group work, opportunities for individual learning, classroom structure and predictability, and organized material. Both in and out of the classroom, use of a more balanced ratio of questions, comments, and phatic acknowledgments when conversing with shy children, and provision of ample time for them to formulate a response (Evans & Bienert, 1992) is advisable for facilitating their initiations within conversations. Scripted speech, choral verbal games, and verbal turn-taking games, such as Fish, may help the shy child participate, feel comfortable speaking, and feel more equal in the exchange. Nonverbal behaviors may also be important, in that when adults smile frequently but do not stare, shy children feel that adults are more trustworthy (Rotenberg et al., 2003), which helps shy children to be more willing to share their thoughts.

Use of a deep vocabulary during conversations and provision of rich shared reading experiences, in which one takes the time to explain the meaning of unfamiliar vocabulary, will likely boost children's semantic knowledge. Specific coaching in social skills, such as asking for help, entering a group, and starting a conversation, may help children to develop pragmatic skills and become more socially confident and assertive. Finally, as previous research (e.g., Hodges, Boivin, Virao, & Bukowski, 1999; Parker & Asher, 1993) has shown, the emotional support of a best friend may be a valuable buffer to help a shy child to be more outgoing with peers.

Providing situations and contexts in which children are likely to experience success academically and socially is also an important principle in working with shy children. Success enhances self-efficacy and may encourage task persistence, motivation, and attempts in the face of uncertainty. Bolstering academic skills may also serve as a protective factor for the child who is less socially skilled. In addition, given that these children are more prone to anxiety, and potentially to test anxiety if they are faring poorly academically, strategies to reduce their anxiety are valuable. These include relaxation techniques, such a deep breathing, progressive muscle relaxation, and calming imagery; test-taking strategies; and good study strategies. While it may appear that encouraging positive self-statements is an effective technique for dealing with anxiety, the effectiveness of positive self-talk is not clear, in that some research has indicated a nonfacilitative or negative relationship between coping statements and task performance (Fox & Houston, 1981), and that self-talk may actually interfere or distract children from the task at hand (Prinz, Groot, & Hanewald, 1994). As such, Kendall (1991) suggested that it is not so much more positive self-talk but less negative self-talk that facilitates performance, underscoring the value of fostering self-esteem in shy children.

FUTURE RESEARCH

Several suggestions that emerged in the course of doing this review are recommended for future researchers. Most language measures have been assessments of vocabulary, and more work needs to address syntactic and pragmatic (e.g., narratives, code switching, discourse) aspects of language in both naturalistic contexts and laboratory settings. Replications of the differential findings with respect to vocabulary and grammar development in shy children would support the notion that the former is more susceptible to socialization and experience, and is less an innate process than the latter. I found very little research on shyness and second language learning in children and adolescents. Gaining facility in a second language—be it additive in learning a second, less dominant language or subtractive in learning the majority language in a culture—may be particularly challenging if shy children are less willing to try out their linguistic knowledge of the new language with peers and in classroom interactions. Studies of academic achievement should differentiate between different subject areas and grade levels rather than presenting composite achievement scores and collapsing results across grade levels given the different demands of mathematics and reading within grade levels, and of language arts in the senior versus the primary grades. More attention should also be given to gender interactions to determine whether the associations with language and academics hold equally for boys and girls. Although the few studies that have reported analyses by sex generally have not observed sex differences, it may be that different mechanisms account for similar results. For example, there may be sex differences in reactivity and passivity in the face of academic difficulties, both of which might interact with inhibition and exert negative effects on academic achievement.

On the methodological front, creativity in setting up test conditions that minimize anxiety when assessing children will also be important in determining whether and, if so, to what extent results may be a function of the conditions and presumed anxiety under which the data are collected. For example, by involving parents as researchers and collecting data in children's homes, further insight may be gained on the language performance–competence debate. Adding observational and noninvasive physiological indices of anxiety in the different testing conditions may also help to clarify this issue. With respect to statistical analyses, studies should examine both linear and curvilinear relations as a way of addressing different relationships at and between the extremes of the distribution from shy to nonshy. It may be the case that the observed linear relationships are to some degree shaped by curvilinear relations, as found most recently by Spere and Evans (2009). Finally, it would be extremely valuable to conduct research that examines the overlap or distinctiveness of the different shyness constructs included in this review, and to facilitate generalizations from the research literature not just in the area of academic and language, but across all domains of shyness inquiry.

ACKNOWLEDGMENTS

Appreciation is extended to Roya Janemi and Kailey Reynolds, who assisted me in locating relevant research and preparation of the reference list.

REFERENCES

American Psychiatric Association. (1994). *Diagnostic and statistical manual of mental disorders* (4th ed.). Washington, DC: Author.

Arbeau, K. A., & Coplan, R. J. (2007). Kindergarten teachers' beliefs and responses to hypothetical prosocial, asocial, and antisocial children. *Merrill–Palmer Quarterly, 53,* 291–318.

Asendorpf, J. B. (1990). Development of inhibition during childhood: Evidence for situational specificity and a two-factor model. *Developmental Psychology, 26,* 721–730.

Asendorpf, J. B. (1994). The malleability of behavior inhibition: A study of individual developmental functions. *Developmental Psychology, 30,* 912–919.

Asendorpf, J. B., & Meier, G. (1993). Personality effects on children's speech in everyday life: Sociability-mediated exposure and shyness-mediated reactivity to social situations. *Journal of Personality and Social Psychology, 64,* 1072–1083.

Birch, S. H., & Ladd, G.W. (1997). The teacher–child relationship and children's early school adjustment. *Journal of School Psychology, 2,* 61–79.

Black, B., & Uhde, T. W. (1995). Psychiatric characteristics of children with selective mutism. *Journal of the American Academy of Child and Adolescent Psychiatry, 34,* 847–856.

Boivin, M., & Hymel, S., (1997). Peer experiences and social self-perceptions: A sequential model. *Developmental Psychology, 33,* 135–145.

Bramlett, R. K., Scott, P., & Rowell, R. K. (2000). A comparison of temperament and social skills in predicting academic performance in first graders. *Special Services in the Schools, 16,* 147–158.

Broberg, A., Hwang, C. P., Lamb, M., & Bookstein, F. L. (1990). Factors related to verbal abilities in Swedish preschoolers. *British Journal of Developmental Psychology, 8,* 335–349.

Broberg, A., Wessels, H., Lamb, M., & Philip, H. (1997). Effects of day care on the development of cognitive abilities in 8-year-olds: A longitudinal study. *Developmental Psychology, 33,* 62–69.

Brophy, J., & McCaslin, M. (1992). Teachers' reports of how they perceive and cope with problem students. *Elementary School Journal, 93,* 3–68.

Bub, K. L., McCartney, K., & Willett, J. B. (2007). Behavior problem trajectories and first grade cognitive ability and achievement skills: A latent growth curve analysis. *Journal of Educational Psychology, 99,* 653–670.

Burgess, K., Rubin, K. H., Cheah, C. S. L., & Nelson, L. J. (2005). Behavioral inhibition, social withdrawal and parenting. In. R. W. Crozier & L. E. Alden (Eds.), *The essential handbook of social anxiety for clinicians* (pp 99–120). New York: Wiley.

Buss, A. H., & Plomin, R. (1984). *Temperament: Early developing personality traits:* Hillsdale, NJ: Erlbaum.

Bzdyra, R., Evans, M. A., & Spooner, A. (2002, August). *The relationship between shyness and self-determination in middle childhood.* Poster presented at the Biennial Meeting of International Society for the Study of Behavioral Development, Ottawa, Canada.

Cazden, C. B. (1972). *Child language and education.* New York: Holt, Rinehart & Winston.

Chang, L. (2003). Variable effects of children's aggression, social withdrawal and prosocial leadership as functions of teacher beliefs and behaviors. *Child Development, 74,* 535–548.

Chen, X., Rubin, K. H., & Li, D. (1997). Relation between academic achievement and social adjustment: Evidence from Chinese children. *Developmental Psychology, 33*, 518–525.

Comadena, M. E., & Comedena, P. M. (1984, May). *Communication apprehension and elementary school achievement: A researcher's note.* Paper presented at the Annual Meeting of the International Communication Association, San Francisco, CA.

Comadena, M. E., & Prusank, D. T. (1988). Communication apprehension and academic achievement among elementary and secondary school students. *Communication Education, 37*, 270–277.

Coplan, R. J., & Arbeau, K. A. (2008). The stresses of a "brave new world": Shyness and social adjustment in kindergarten. *Journal of Research in Childhood Education, 22*, 377–389.

Coplan, R. J., & Armer, M. (2005). Talking yourself out of being shy: Shyness, expressive vocabulary, and socioemotional adjustment in preschool. *Merrill–Palmer Quarterly, 51*, 20–41.

Coplan, R. J., Gavinski-Molina, M. H., Lagacé-Séguin, D. G., & Wichmann, C. (2001) When girls versus boys play alone: Nonsocial play and adjustment in kindergarten. *Developmental Psychology, 37*, 464–474.

Coplan, R. J., Prakash, K., O'Neil, K., & Armer, M. (2004). Do you "want" to play? Distinguishing between conflicted shyness and social disinterest in early childhood. *Developmental Psychology, 40*, 244–258.

Coplan, R. J., & Weeks, M. (2009). Shy and soft-spoken: Shyness, pragmatic language, and socio-emotional adjustment in early childhood [Special issue]. *Infant and Child Development, 18*, 238–254.

Cross, T. G., Nienhuys, T. G., & Kirkman, M. (1983). Parent–child interactions with receptively disabled children: Some determinants of maternal speech style. In K. E. Nelson (Ed.), *Children's language* (Vol. 5, pp. 247–290). New York: Gardner.

Crozier, R., & Badawood, R. (2009). Shyness, vocabulary and children's reticence in Saudi Arabian preschools [Special issue]. *Infant and Child Development, 18*, 255–270.

Crozier, W. R., & Hostettler, K. (2003). The influence of shyness on children's test performance. *British Journal of Educational Psychology, 73*, 317–328.

Crozier, W. R., & Perkins, P. (2002). Shyness as a factor when assessing children. *Educational Psychology in Practice, 18*, 234–244.

Cunningham, C. E., McHolm, A., Boyle, M. H., & Patel, S. (2004). Behavioral and emotional adjustment, family functioning, academic performance, and social relationships in children with selective mutism. *Journal of Child Psychology and Psychiatry, 45*,1363–1372.

Daly, S. (1978). Behavioral correlates of social anxiety. *British Journal of Social and Clinical Psychology, 17*, 117–120.

Daniels, D., & Plomin, R. (1985). Origins of individual differences in infant shyness. *Developmental Psychology, 21*, 118–121.

Davis, G. F., & Scott, M. D. (1978). Communication apprehension, intelligence and achievement among secondary school students. In B. R. Ruben (Ed.), *Communication yearbook* (pp. 458–472). New Brunswick, NJ: Transaction Books.

Dixon, W. E., & Shore, C. (1997). Temperamental predictors of linguistic style during multiword acquisition. *Infant Behavior and Development, 20,* 99–103.

Dixon, W. E., & Smith, P. H. (2000). Links between early temperament and language acquisition. *Merill–Palmer Quarterly, 46,* 417–440.

Dobbs, J., Doctoroff, G. L., Fisher, P. J. H., & Arnold, D. H. (2006). The association between preschool children's socio-emotional functioning and their mathematical skills. *Applied Developmental Psychology, 27,* 97–108.

Dummit, E. S., Klein, R. G., Tancer, N. K., Asche, B., Martin, J., & Fairbanks, J. A. (1997). Systematic assessment of 50 children with selective mutism. *Journal of the American Academy of Child and Adolescent Psychiatry, 36,* 653–660.

Egeland, B., Kalkoske, M., Gottesman, N., & Erickson, M. F. (1990). Preschool behavior problems: Stability and factors accounting for change. *Journal of Child Psychiatry, 31,* 891–909.

Engfer, A. (1993). Antecedents and consequences of shyness in boys and girls: A 6-year longitudinal study. In K. H. Rubin & J. B. Asendorpf (Eds.), *Social withdrawal, inhibition and shyness in childhood* (pp. 49–79). Hillsdale, NJ: Erlbaum.

Evans, M. A. (1987). Discourse characteristics of reticent children. *Applied Psycholinguistics, 8,* 171–184.

Evans, M. A. (1993). Communicative competence as a dimension of shyness. In K. H. Rubin & J. B. Asendorpf (Eds.), *Social withdrawal, inhibition and shyness in childhood* (pp. 189–212). Hillsdale, NJ: Erlbaum.

Evans, M. A. (1996). Reticent primary grade children and their more talkative peers: Verbal, non-verbal, and self-concept characteristics. *Journal of Educational Psychology, 88,* 739–749.

Evans, M. A. (2001). Shyness in the classroom and home. In. W. R Crozier & L. E. Alden (Eds.), *International handbook of social anxiety: Concepts, research and interventions relating to the self and shyness* (pp. 159–183). Chichester, UK: Wiley.

Evans, M. A., & Bienert, H. (1992). Control and paradox in teacher conversations with shy children. *Canadian Journal of Behavioral Science, 24,* 502–516.

Evans, M. A., & Ellis, P. (1992). *Requestive strategies of reticent and verbal children at play.* Paper presented at the Waterloo Conference on Child Development, Waterloo, Canada.

Ford, M. A., Sladeczek, I. E., Carlson, J., & Kratochwill, T. R. (1998). Selective mutism: Phenomenological characteristics. *School Psychology Quarterly, 13,* 192–227.

Fox, J. E., & Houston, B. K. (1981). Efficacy of self-instructional training for reducing children's anxiety in an evaluative situation. *Behaviour Research and Therapy, 19,* 505–509.

Furrer, C., & Skinner, E. (2003). Sense of relatedness as a factor in children's academic engagement and performance. *Journal of Educational Psychology, 95,* 148–162.

Gazelle, H. (2006). Class climate moderates peer relations and emotional adjustment in children with an early history of children with and anxious solitude: A child × environment model. *Developmental Psychology, 42,* 1179–1192.

Gewirtz, J. L. (1948). Studies in word-fluency: II. Its relation to eleven items of child behavior. *Journal of Genetic Psychology, 72,* 177–184.

Gleason, J. B., & Weintraub, S. (1978). The acquisition of routines in child language. *Language in Society, 5,* 129–136.

Gordon, E. M., & Thomas, A. (1967). Children's behavioral style and the teacher's appraisal of their intelligence. *Journal of School Psychology, 5,* 292–300.

Gottlieb, G. (1996). Developmental psychobiological theory. In R. B. Cairns, G. H. Elder, & E. J. Costello (Eds.), *Developmental science: Cambridge studies in social and emotional development* (pp. 63–77). New York: Cambridge University Press.

Green, K. D., Forehand, R., Beck, S., & Vosk, B. (1980). An assessment of the relationship among measures of children's social competence and children's academic achievement. *Child Development, 51,* 1149–1156.

Hadley, N. H. (1994). *Elective mutism: A handbook for educators, counselors, and health care professionals.* Dordrecht, the Netherlands: Kluwer Academic.

Hamre, B. K., & Pianta, R. C. (2001). Early teacher–child relationships and the trajectory of children's school outcomes through eighth grade. *Child Development, 72,* 625–638.

Hodges, V. E., Boivin, B., Virao, F., & Bukowski, W. (1999). The power of friendship: Protection against an escalating cycle of peer victimization. *Developmental Psychology, 35,* 94–101.

Hoff-Ginsberg, E. (1991). Mother–child conversation in different social classes and communicative settings. *Child Development, 62,* 782–796.

HoganBruen, K., Clauss-Ehlers, C., Nelson, D., & Faenza, M. M. (2003). Effective advocacy of school-based mental health programs. In M. D. Wesit, S. W. Evans, & N. A. Lever (Eds.), *Handbook of school mental health: Advancing practice and research* (pp. 45–59). New York: Kluwer Academic/Plenum Press.

Hurt, H. T., & Preiss, R. (1978). Silence isn't necessarily golden: Communication apprehension, desired social choice and academic success among middle school students. *Human Communication Research, 4,* 315–328.

Ialongo, N., Edelsohn, G., Werthamer-Larsson, L., Crockett, L., & Kellam, S. (1995). The significance of self-reported anxious symptoms in first grade children: Prediction of anxious symptoms and adaptive functioning in fifth grade. *Journal of Child Psychology and Psychiatry, 36,* 427–437.

Jones, M. G., & Gerig, T. M. (1994). Silent sixth-grade students: Characteristics, achievement and teacher expectations. *Elementary School Journal, 95,* 169–182.

Kagan, J. (1994). *Galen's prophecy.* New York: Basic Books.

Kagan, J., Resnick, J. S., & Snidman, N. (1986). Temperamental inhibition in early childhood. In R. Plomin & J. Dunn (Eds.), *The study of temperament: Changes, continuities, and challenges* (pp. 53–65). Hillsdale, NJ: Erlbaum.

Kagan, J., Snidman, N., Zentner, M., & Peterson, E. (1999). Infant temperament and anxious symptoms in school-age children. *Development and Psychopathology, 11,* 209–224.

Kashdan, T. B., & Herbert, J. D. (2001). Social anxiety disorder in childhood and adolescence: Current status and future directions. *Clinical Child and Family Psychology Review, 4,* 37–61.

Keogh, B. (2003). *Temperament in the classroom: Understanding individual differences.* Baltimore: Brookes.

Kemple, K. M., David, D. M., & Wang, Y. (1996). Preschoolers' creativity, shyness, and self-esteem. *Creativity Research Journal, 9,* 317–326.

Kendall, P. C. (1991). Guiding theory for therapy with children and adolescents. In P. C. Kendall (Ed.), *Child and adolescent therapy: Cognitive-behavioral procedures* (pp. 3–22). New York: Guilford Press.

Kennedy, W., & Willcutt, H. (1964). Praise and blame as incentives. *Psychological Bulletin, 62,* 323–332.

Kohn, M., & Rosman, B. L. (1972). Relationship of pre-school socio-emotional functioning to later intellectual achievement. *Developmental Psychology, 6,* 445–452.

Kolvin, I., & Fundudis, T. (1981). Elective mute children: Psychological development and background factors. *Journal of Child Psychology and Psychiatry, 22,* 219–232.

Kristensen, H. (2000). Selective mutism and comorbidity with developmental disorder/delay, anxiety disorder, and elimination disorder. *Journal of the American Academy of Child and Adolescent Psychiatry, 39,* 249–256.

Kristensen, H., & Oerbeck, B. (2006). Is selective mutism associated with deficits in memory span and visual memory: An exploratory case–control study. *Depression and Anxiety, 23,* 71–76.

Kristensen, H., & Torgersen, S. (2008). Is social anxiety disorder in childhood associated with developmental deficit/delay? *European Child and Adolescent Psychiatry, 17,* 99–107.

Ladd, G. W., Birch, S. H., & Buhs, E. S. (1999). Children's social and scholastic lives in kindergarten: Related spheres of influence? *Child Development, 70,* 1373–1400.

Landon, S. J., & Sommers, R. K. (1979). Talkativeness and children's linguistic abilities. *Language and Speech, 22,* 269–275.

Lee, K., Chang-Song, Y., & Choi, Y. (2007, April). *The relationship between infants' temperament and early vocabulary acquisition.* Paper presented at the Biennial Meeting of the Society for Research in Child Development, Boston, MA.

Leonard, H., & Topol, D. A. (1993). Elective mutism. *Child and Adolescent Psychiatric Clinics of North America, 2,* 695–707.

Lerner, J. V., Lerner, R., & Zabski, S. ((1985). Temperament and elementary school children's actual and rated academic performance: A test of a goodness-of-fit model. *Journal of Child Psychology and Psychiatry, 26,* 125–136.

Levin, I. P., & Hart, S. (2003). Risk preferences in young children: Early evidence of individual differences in reaction to potential gains and losses. *Journal of Behavioral Decision Making, 16,* 397–413.

Lloyd, B., & Howe, N. (2003). Solitary play and convergent and divergent thinking skills in preschool children. *Early Childhood Research Quarterly, 18,* 22–41.

Ludwig, R. P., & Lazarus, P. J. (1983). Relationship between shyness in children and constricted cognitive control as measured by the Stroop Color–Word Test. *Journal of Clinical and Consulting Psychiatry, 51,* 386–389.

Magnusson, D., & Hakan, S. (1998). Person–context interaction theories. In W.

Damon & R. Lerner (Eds.), *Handbook of child psychology: Vol. 1. Theoretical models of human development* (5th ed., pp. 685–759). Hoboken, NJ: Wiley.

Manassis, K., Tannock, R., Garland, J. E., Minde, K., McInnes, A., & Clark, S. (2007). The sounds of silence: Language, cognition, and anxiety in selective mutism. *Journal of the American Academy of Child and Adolescent Psychiatry, 46*, 1187–1195.

Martin, R. P., & Holbrook, J. (1985). Relationship of temperament characteristics to the academic achievement of first-grade children. *Journal of Psychoeducational Assessment, 3*, 131–140.

Masten, A., Morison, P., & Pellegrini, D. (1985). A Revised Class Play method of peer assessment. *Developmental Psychology, 21*, 523–533.

Maziade, M., Cote, R., Boutin, P., Boudreault, M., & Thivierge, J. (1986). The effect of temperament on longitudinal academic achievement in primary school. *Journal of the American Academy of Child Psychiatry, 25*, 692–696.

McBryde, C., Ziviani, J., & Cuskelly, M. (2004). School readiness and factors that influence decision making. *Occupational Therapy International, 11*, 193–208.

McCarthy, D. (1929). Comparison of children's language in different situations and its relation to personality traits. *Journal of Genetic Psychology, 36*, 583–591.

McCroskey, J. C. (1970). Measures of communication bound anxiety. *Speech Monographs, 37*, 269–277.

McCroskey, J. C., & Daly, J. A. (1976). Teacher expectations of the communication apprehensive child in the elementary school. *Human Communication Research, 3*, 67–72.

McInnes, A., Fung, D., Manassis, K., Fliksenbaum, L., & Tannock, R. (2004). Narrative skills in children with selective mutism: An exploratory study. *American Journal of Speech–Language Pathology, 13*, 304–315.

Nelson, K. E. (1988). Strategies for first language teaching. In M. Rice & R. L. Schiefelbusch (Eds.), *Teachability of language* (pp. 263–310). Baltimore: Brookes.

Nelson, L. J., Rubin, K. H., & Fox, N. A. (2005). Social and nonsocial behaviors and peer acceptance: A longitudinal model of the development of self-perceptions in children ages 4 to 7 years. *Early Education and Development, 20*, 185–200.

Normandeau, S., & Guay, F. (1998). Preschool behavior and first-grade school achievement: The mediational role of cognitive self-control. *Journal of Educational Psychology, 90*, 111–121.

Nowakowski, M. E., Cunningham, C. C., McHolm, A. E., Evans, M.A., Edison, S., St.-Pierre, J. S., et al. (2009). Language and academic abilities in children with selective mutism [Special issue]. *Infant and Child Development, 18*, 271–290.

Nungesser, N. R., & Watkins, R. V. (2005). Preschool teachers' perceptions and reactions to challenging classroom behavior: Implications for speech–language pathologists. *Language, Speech, and Hearing Services in Schools, 36*, 139–151.

Paget, K. D., Nagle, R. J., & Martin, R. P. (1984). Interrelationships between temperament characteristics and first-grade teacher–student interactions. *Journal of Abnormal Child Psychology, 12*, 546–560.

Parker, J. G., & Asher, S. R. (1993). Beyond peer group acceptance: Friendship and friendship quality as distinct dimensions of peer adjustment. In W. H. Jones &

D. Perlman (Eds.), *Advances in personal relationships* (Vol. 4, pp. 261–294). London: Kinsgley Press.

Paulsen, E., Bru, E., & Murberg, T. A. (2006). Passive students in junior high school: The association with shyness, perceived competence and social support. *Social Psychology of Education, 9,* 67–81.

Pianta, R. C., Nimetz, S. L., & Bennett, E. (1997). Mother–child relationships, teacher–child relationships, and school outcomes in preschool and kindergarten. *Early Childhood Research Quarterly, 12,* 263–280.

Prakash, K., & Coplan, R. J. (2007). Socioemotional characteristics and school adjustment of socially withdrawn children in India. *International Journal of Behavioral Development, 31,* 123–132.

Prinz, P., Groot, M., & Hanewald, G. (1994). Cognition in test-anxious children: The role of on-task and coping cognition reconsidered. *Journal of Consulting and Clinical Psychology, 62,* 404–409.

Prior, M., Bavin, E. L., Cini, E., Reilly, S., Bretherton, L., Wake, M., et al. (2008). Influences on communicative development at 24 months of age: Child temperament, behavior problems, and maternal factors. *Infant Behavior and Development, 31,* 270–279.

Prior, M., Smart, D., & Sanson, A. (2000). Does shy-inhibited temperament in childhood lead to anxiety problems in adolescence? *Journal of American Academy of Child and Adolescent Psychiatry, 39,* 461–468.

Rapport, M. D., Denney, C. B., Chung, K. M., & Hustance, K. (2001). Internalizing behavior problems and scholastic achievement in children: Cognitive and behavioral pathways as mediators of outcome. *Journal of Clinical Child Psychology, 30,* 536–551.

Reynolds, K., & Evans, M. A. (2009). Narrative performance and parental scaffolding of shy and non-shy children. *Applied Psycholinguistics, 30,* 1–22.

Rezendes, M., Snidman, N., Kagan, J., & Gibbons, M. J. (1993). Features of speech in inhibited and uninhibited children. In K. H. Rubin & J. B. Asendorpf (Eds.), *Social withdrawal, inhibition and shyness in childhood* (pp. 177–187). Hillsdale, NJ: Erlbaum.

Rimm-Kaufman, S. E., Early, D. M., Cox, M. J., Daluja, G., Pianta, R. C., Bradley, R. H., et al. (2002). Early behavioral attributes and teachers' sensitivity as predictors of competent behavior in the kindergarten classroom. *Applied Developmental Psychology, 23,* 451–470.

Rotenberg, K. J., Eisenberg, N., Cumming, C., Smith, A., Singh, M., & Terlicher, E. (2003). The contribution of adults' nonverbal cues and children's shyness to the development of rapport between adults and preschool children. *International Journal of Behavioral Development, 27,* 21–30.

Rubin, K. H. (1982). Social and social-cognitive characteristics of young isolate, normal, and sociable children. In K. H. Rubin & H. S. Ross (Eds.), *Peer relationships and social skills in childhood* (pp. 353–374). New York: Springer-Verlag.

Rubin, K. H., & Borwick, D. (1984). The communication skills of children who vary with regard to sociability. In H. Sypher & J. Applegate (Eds.), *Social cognition and communication* (pp. 152–170). Hillsdale, NJ: Erlbaum.

Rubin, K. H., Daniels-Beirness, T., & Bream, L. (1982). Social isolation and social problem solving: A longitudinal study. *Journal of Consulting and Clinical Psychology, 52,* 17–25.

Rubin, K. H., & Krasnor, L. R. (1986). Social-cognitive and social behavioral perspectives on problem-solving. In M. Perlmutter (Ed.), *Cognitive perspectives on children's social and behavioral development: The Minnesota symposia on child development* (Vol. 18, pp. 1–68). Hillsdale, NJ: Erlbaum.

Rubin, K. H., & Mills, R. (1988). The many faces of social isolation in childhood. *Journal of Consulting and Clinical Psychology, 56,* 916–924.

Rudasill, K. M., Rimm-Kaufman, S. E., Justice, L. M., & Pence, K. (2006). Temperament and language skills as predictors of teacher–child relationship quality in preschool. *Early Education and Development, 17,* 271–291.

Rydell, A. M., Bohlin, G., & Thorell, L. B. (2005). Representations of attachment to parents and shyness as predictors of children's relationships with teachers and peer competence in preschool. *Attachment and Human Development, 7,* 187–204.

Sameroff, A. J. (1993). Models of development and risk. In C. H. Zeanah, Jr. (Ed.), *Handbook of infant mental health* (pp. 3–13). New York: Guilford Press.

Saranson, I. G. (1972). Experimental approaches to test anxiety: Attention and the uses of information. In C. D. Spielberger (Ed.), *Anxiety: Current trends in theory and research* (Vol. 2, pp. 383–403). New York: Academic Press.

Schoen, M. J., & Nagle, R. J. (1994). Prediction of school readiness from kindergarten temperament scores. *Journal of School Psychology, 32,* 135–147.

Slomkowski, C. L., Nelson, K., Dunn, J., & Plomin, R. (1992). Temperament and language: Relations from toddlerhood to middle childhood. *Developmental Psychology, 28,* 1090–1095.

Snyder-McLean, L. K., & McLean, J. E. (1978). Verbal information gathering strategies: The child's use of language to acquire language. *Journal of Speech and Hearing Disorders, 43,* 306–325.

Spere, K., & Evans, M. A. (2009). Shyness as a continuous dimension and language and literacy scores in young children: Is there a relationship? [Special issue] *Infant and Child Development, 18,* 216–237.

Spere, K. A., Evans, M. A., Hendry, C. A., & Mansell, J. M. (2008). Language skills in shy and non-shy preschoolers and the effects of assessment context. *Journal of Child Language, 35,* 1–19.

Spere, K., Evans, M. A., Mansell, J., & Hendry, C. A. (2007, April). *Are shy children less likely to guess on language and literacy tests?: A look at the response patterns of shy and non-shy children.* Paper presented at the Biennial Meeting of the Society for Research in Child Development, Boston, MA.

Spere, K. A., Schmidt, L. A., Theall-Honey, L. A., & Martin-Chang, S. (2004). Expressive and receptive language skills of temperamentally shy preschoolers. *Infant and Child Development, 13,* 123–133.

Steinhausen, H. C., & Juzi, C. (1996). Elective mutism: An analysis of 100 cases. *American Academy of Child and Adolescent Pychiatry, 35,* 606–614.

Stewart, S. L., & Rubin, K. H. (1995). The social problem solving skills of anxious–withdrawn children. *Development and Psychopathology, 7,* 323–336.

Thijs, J. T., Koomen, H. M. Y., & van der Leij, A. (2006). Teacher's self-reported pedagogical practices toward socially inhibited, hyperactive, and average children. *Psychology in the Schools, 43,* 635–651.

Ting, K. T. (2008). *Shyness, language and children: Can shyness predict children's primary and secondary language ability?* Honor's BA thesis, Chinese University of Hong Kong.

Van Kleeck, A., & Street, R. (1982). Does reticence just mean talking less?: Qualitative differences in the language of talkative and reticent preschoolers. *Journal of Psycholinguistic Research, 11,* 621–641.

Vriniotis, C., & Evans, M. A. (1988). *Children's social communicative competence and its relationship to classroom participation.* Paper presented at the Waterloo Conference on Child Development, Waterloo, Ontario, Canada.

Watson, A. K., & Monroe, E. E. (1990). Academic achievement: A study of relationships of IQ, communication apprehension and teacher perception. *Communication Reports, 3,* 28–36.

Wine, J. (1971). Test anxiety and direction of attention. *Psychological Bulletin, 76,* 311–317.

Wright, H. L. (1968). A clinical study of children who refuse to talk in school. *Journal of the American Academy of Child Psychiatry, 7,* 603–617.

10

Shyness–Inhibition in Childhood and Adolescence
A Cross-Cultural Perspective

XINYIN CHEN

As one of the major socioemotional characteristics, shyness–inhibition plays an important role in social and psychological adjustment in childhood and adolescence (Rubin, Coplan, & Bowker, 2009). It has been found in Western, particularly North American, countries that shyness–inhibition is related to a variety of adjustment problems. Shy–inhibited children are often rejected or isolated by peers and perceived by adults as socially incompetent (e.g., Coplan, Prakash, O'Neil, & Armer, 2004; Gazelle & Ladd, 2003; Rubin, Chen, & Hymel, 1993). Moreover, when they realize their difficulties in social situations, shy–inhibited children may develop negative self-perceptions of their social competence and other psychological problems, such as loneliness, social dissatisfaction, and depression (e.g., Coplan et al., 2004; Crozier, 1995; Prior, Smart, Sanson, & Oberklaid, 2000; Rubin, Chen, McDougall, Bowker, & McKinnon, 1995). Longitudinal research has also indicated that shyness–inhibition in childhood may contribute to later problems, in various areas, such as educational attainment, career stability, and emotional disorder (e.g., Asendorpf, Denissen, & van Aken, 2008; Caspi, Elder, & Bem, 1988; Caspi et al., 2003). Therefore, it has been argued that shyness–inhibition represents a risk factor, if not a symptom, of internalizing problems (Achenbach & Edelbrock, 1981; Rubin et al., 2009).

Nevertheless, shyness–inhibition is a culturally bound phenomenon. Cultural context may affect the exhibition of shy–inhibited behavior through processes of facilitation and suppression. Moreover, cultural norms and values may provide guidance for social evaluations of, and responses to, shy–inhibited behavior and define its meaning (Asendorpf, Chapter 8, this volume; Chen & French, 2008). As a result, shyness–inhibition may develop in different manners across cultures.

In this chapter, I focus on the understanding of children's shyness–inhibition in cultural context. First, I discuss conceptual issues and present a theoretical framework concerning the involvement of cultural norms and values in the development of shyness–inhibition, then discuss methodological issues in conducting cross-cultural research on shyness–inhibition in childhood and adolescence. Next, I review the literature on the prevalence, functional meaning, and developmental pattern of children's shyness–inhibition in different societies. Researchers have recently found that macro-level social, economic, and cultural changes may have a significant impact on children's shyness–inhibition. In the following section, these findings are presented. The chapter concludes with a discussion of future directions in the study of culture and shyness–inhibition.

SHYNESS–INHIBITION
IN CULTURAL CONTEXT:
THEORETICAL ISSUES AND PERSPECTIVES

Research on culture and shyness–inhibition has been conducted from different perspectives with different methods; this has led to some inconsistent findings. Moreover, the lack of clear understanding of shyness–inhibition and related constructs has contributed to the confusion in the field. Thus, it is necessary to discuss the conceptual issues followed by a review of theoretical perspectives.

The Construct of Shyness–Inhibition

Traditionally, researchers who study shyness as a personality trait, especially in adults, focus on feelings of self-consciousness, awkwardness, and anxiety in social interactions (e.g., Cheek & Buss, 1981; Eysenck & Eysenck, 1969). Asendorpf (1990, 1991; Chapter 8, this volume) characterizes shyness as deriving from an internal conflict of approach and avoidance motives in social settings. According to Asendorpf, shy children are interested in social interactions, but this approach motivation is simultaneously hindered by fear and anxiety. In contrast, researchers who study children's temperament and socioemotional functioning are often interested in behavioral inhibition (BI) as a dispositional characteristic of reactivity to social and nonsocial unfamiliar situations (e.g., Fox, Henderson, Marshall,

Nichols, & Ghera, 2005; Kagan, 1997; Rothbart & Bates, 2006). BI is believed to be biologically rooted (e.g., Fox et al., 2005). At the behavioral level, the work of Rubin, Coplan, and their colleagues (Coplan, Rubin, Fox, Calkins, & Stewart, 1994; Rubin, Coplan, Fox, & Calkins, 1995) suggests that inhibition in social situations is indicated largely by the display of reticent behavior in peer group activities. Examples of reticent behavior include watching other children play without joining in (onlooking) and being unoccupied. Based on the converging evidence for conceptual and empirical links between shyness and BI, and their similar behavioral manifestations, Chen and his colleagues (e.g., Chen & French, 2008; Chen, Rubin, & Li, 1995) proposed the concept of "shyness–inhibition," which refers to vigilant, wary, and anxious reactivity to stressful or challenging social situations. Shyness–inhibition may be manifested in different forms in different situations (e.g., social vs. nonsocial) and at different developmental stages (e.g., fearful reactions to social novelty in early childhood vs. social-evaluative anxiety in the later years). This integrative conceptualization allows for an understanding of the phenomenon at multiple levels (e.g., biological, temperamental, behavioral, and sociojudgmental) and provides a framework for research on its developmental origins, processes, and outcomes, with the use of various methods (e.g., observation, self-report, and physiological assessment).

Nevertheless, the construct of shyness–inhibition is different from various types of social withdrawal, such as social disinterest and preference for solitude (e.g., "would rather be alone") (Asendorpf, 1990; Coplan & Armer, 2007; see also Coplan & Weeks, Chapter 4, this volume). According to Asendorpf (1990), social disinterest or unsociability, driven by a low approach motivation, may be manifested by solitary behavior that results from the lack of a desire to interact with others. Social disinterest is evidenced behaviorally through the display of solitary–passive play, including quiet exploration and solitary–constructive activities (Rubin, 1982). Coplan et al. (2004) have argued that socially disinterested or unsociable children may possess object-oriented as opposed to people-oriented personalities; these children may be content to play alone without initiating social contacts.

The distinction between shyness–inhibition and social disinterest is particularly important in cross-cultural research, because cultures may place different values on these sociobehavioral attributes. For example, it has been argued that in North American individualistic societies (Canada, United States), social disinterest or preference for aloneness may not be viewed as maladaptive as shyness–inhibition, because the former is sometimes considered an expression of personal choice and may be conducive to performance on constructive tasks and emotional health (e.g., Burger, 1995; Coplan et al., 2004; Leary, Herbst, & McCrary, 2003). In contrast, in traditional Chinese and some other group-oriented cultures, although shy–inhibited children may be accepted by others, children who prefer solitude and intentionally stay away from the group are often regarded as anticollective and thereby have serious social problems (Casiglia, Lo Coco, & Zappulla, 1998; Chen, 2008; Valdivia, Schneider, Chavez, & Chen, 2005). Therefore, it is critical in cross-cultural research to avoid confounding the meanings of different constructs, such as withdrawn behavior, unsociability, submissiveness, and peer isolation (e.g., Chang et al., 2005; Cheah & Rubin, 2004).

Cultural Values, Social Interaction Processes, and Shyness–Inhibition

Developmental theorists have explored cultural influences on human functioning from different perspectives. Among them, *socioecological theory* (Bronfenbrenner & Morris, 2006; Super & Harkness, 1986) is concerned with how culture affects individual beliefs, attitudes, and behaviors mainly as a part of the socioecological environment. According to socioecological theory, beliefs and practices endorsed within a cultural group may directly affect children's social and cognitive functioning. In addition to its direct effects, culture may play a role in shaping development through organizing various social settings, such as community services, and school and day care arrangements (Bronfenbrenner & Morris, 2006; Super & Harkness, 1986). From a different perspective, *sociocultural theory* (Cole, 1996; Rogoff, 2003; Vygotsky, 1978) focuses on the transmission or internalization of external symbolic systems, such as language, concepts, signs, and symbols, along with their cultural meanings, from the social level to the intrapersonal or psychological level. During development, children master and use these systems as psychological tools to perform various mental processes, such as remembering and recalling. The internalization of external symbolic systems may be facilitated by collaborative or guided learning in which more experienced peers or adults, as skilled tutors and representatives of the culture, assist the child to understand and solve the tasks at hand.

Based on these perspectives, Chen and his colleagues (e.g., Chen & French, 2008; Chen, Wang, & DeSouza, 2006) have recently proposed a contextual–developmental framework concerning cultural values of major socioemotional characteristics and the mediating role of the social interaction process in cultural influence on individual development. According to Chen et al., shy–inhibited behavior is derived from (1) internal anxiety that impedes spontaneous social engagement, leading to a low level of social initiative, and (2) adequate control to constrain behavioral and emotional reactivity toward the self rather than others. Because different values are placed on social initiative and norm-based behavioral control, shy–inhibited behavior may be perceived and evaluated differently across cultures. In Western, self-oriented cultures, where acquiring autonomy and assertive social skills is an important socialization goal, social initiative is viewed as an index of social maturity. As a result, the display of shy–inhibited behavior is considered socially incompetent (Greenfield, Suzuki, & Rothstein-Fisch, 2006). In group-oriented societies, social initiative may not be highly appreciated or valued, because it may not facilitate harmony and cohesiveness in the group. Moreover, to maintain interpersonal and group harmony, individuals need to restrain personal desires and acts in an effort to address the needs and interests of others (Triandis, 1995). Shy–inhibited behavior may be positively valued and encouraged, because it may be conducive to group organization.

The influence of cultural values on shyness–inhibition may occur through the social interaction process (Chen, Chung, & Hsiao, 2009). Specifically, when children display shy–inhibited behavior in social interactions, peers and adults may perceive and evaluate it in manners that are consistent with cultural belief and value systems in the society. Moreover, peers and adults in different cultures may respond differently to this behavior and express different attitudes (e.g., acceptance, rejection) toward the children who display the behavior. Social evaluations and responses, in turn, may regulate children's behavior and, ultimately, its developmental patterns. At the same time, shy–inhibited children may display their reactions (compliance, resistance) to social influence and participate in constructing cultural norms for social evaluations in the peer group (Corsaro & Nelson, 2003). Thus, the social processes are bidirectional and transactional in nature.

METHODOLOGICAL ISSUES IN CROSS-CULTURAL RESEARCH ON CHILDREN'S SHYNESS–INHIBITION

Cross-cultural research relies heavily on comparisons of two or more cultures on the phenomenon of interest. Although this approach may provide valuable information about similarities and differences between samples from different cultures, many methodological obstacles in making valid inferences from the findings may exist in various stages of research, including selection of representative cultural groups, controlling for confounding factors (e.g., socioeconomic status), establishing equivalence in measurement, and making culturally appropriate interpretation of the data (Schneider, French, & Chen, 2006).

Despite the difficulties, however, cross-cultural research on shyness–inhibition and related behaviors has burgeoned in the past 20 years. Among the methods used to assess shyness–inhibition in cross-cultural research are observations; peer evaluations; teacher, parent, and self-reports; qualitative interviews; and, to a lesser extent, physiological assessments. Each of the methods has its strengths and strengths. For example, observational data, either in the controlled laboratory or naturalistic settings, provide objective information about behavioral manifestations of shyness–inhibition in the culture. However, maintaining equivalent conditions in different settings, developing culturally sensitive coding systems, and training coders to code data reliably from different cultures often require significant costs, effort, and time. Peer evaluation (e.g., the *Revised Class Play*; Masten, Morison, & Pellegrini, 1985), another technique used to obtain information about children's social functioning, is particularly useful for cross-cultural research, because it taps the insiders' perspectives of children. However, peer evaluation is used in classrooms, mostly with elementary school children, and does not permit direct cross-cultural comparisons on group mean scores, because peer nomination or rating data often require within-classroom standardization. Parent, teacher, and self-reports are perhaps most commonly used in cross-cultural studies because of relatively low costs for data collection, and advantages in data organization and analysis. However, there are obvious concerns and limitations in self-reports, such as culturally specific response biases; the "reference group" effect; and differences in the understanding of the items and willingness to reveal personal information to others, which can confound the responses of participants (e.g., Peng, Nisbett, & Wong, 1997; Schneider et al., 2006). This is dramatically illustrated by Weisz, Chaiyasit, Weiss, Eastman, and Jackson (1995), who reported that although teachers provided higher behavior problem ratings for Thai than for American students, trained observers found that Thai students displayed fewer behavior problems than their American counterparts. One possible strategy to handle many of the methodological problems noted earlier is to use a multimethod approach, which likely reduces potential biases and errors in data derived from a single source. With data from multiple sources, researchers may focus on general and convergent patterns, rather than specific variables or scores, through integrative analysis.

A major challenge in the cross-cultural study of shyness–inhibition is the understanding of its meaning in cultural context. Consistent with the contextual–developmental perspective (Chen & French, 2008), which emphasizes the role of social interaction in cultural influence on individual behavior, I suggest that researchers examine (1) how shyness–inhibition is associated with social interactions and relationships, particularly in the peer group, and (2) how shyness–inhibition develops (e.g., how it is associated with other culturally relevant variables, and to what developmental outcomes it leads) in the culture. An in-depth examination of shyness–inhibition in the context of social interactions and relationships helps us understand the functional meaning that the culture ascribes to shy–inhibited behavior. Longitudinal research may significantly promote the understanding through tapping into the developmental processes and significance of the behavior.

SHYNESS–INHIBITION IN THE EARLY YEARS: DISPOSITION, SOCIALIZATION, AND CULTURE

Shyness–inhibition in the early years has often been considered a dispositional characteristic (e.g., Fox et al., 2005). However, the manifestation of dispositional influence during development may be constrained by cultural factors. Culture may affect the prevalence of shy–inhibited behavior and the way it contributes to adaptive and maladaptive development.

The Display of Shyness–Inhibition in Early Childhood

One of the primary issues in which cross-cultural researchers are interested is whether children in different societies display different social behaviors (e.g., Parmar, Harkness, & Super, 2004; Whiting & Edwards, 1988). Edwards (2000), for example, reanalyzed the data from the Six Culture Study and found that children in relatively "close" and agricultural communities (e.g., Kenya and India) had significantly lower scores on overall social engagement than children in more open communities (e.g., Okinawa and the United States) where peer interactions were encouraged. Moreover, researchers have found that, compared with their North American counterparts, children in Mayan (Gaskins, 2000), Bedouin Arab (Ariel & Sever, 1980), Kenyan, Mexican, and Indian (Edwards, 2000; Farver & Howes, 1993) cultures tend to be less expressive of their personal styles during peer interactions and engage in few sociodramatic activities that required control of social-evaluative anxiety. These latter results are particularly interesting, because self-expression and assertiveness in social interactions are directly related to shyness–inhibition.

Cross-cultural differences in the display of shyness–inhibition in the early years have been reported mostly between East Asian and North American children (e.g., Farver & Howes, 1988, Kagan, Kearsley, & Zelazo, 1978). In a study of play behavior in Korean preschools in the United States, for example, Farver, Kim, and Lee (1995) found that Korean American children displayed more shy and unoccupied behaviors than did European American children. Moreover, Korean American children's play included less fantastic and self-expressive themes (i.e., extraordinary actions performed by fantasy characters), and these children used fewer self-assertive communicative strategies (Farver & Shin, 1997). The results were consistent with Rubin et al.'s findings (2006) that Korean and Chinese toddlers exhibit more behaviorally inhibited behavior than their Australian, Canadian, and

Italian agemates in a standard BI paradigm (e.g., Kagan, Reznick, & Snidman, 1987). On one of the tasks within the BI paradigm, when the toddler was asked by a female experimenter to touch a potentially scary toy robot, the mean latencies to touch the toy were 18.97 and 13.97 seconds in Korean and Chinese children, but 7.74, 7.70, and 7.74 seconds, respectively, in Australian, Canadian, and Italian children. Moreover, the percentage of children who did not touch the toy during the whole period was 52.2 and 44.4% in Korea and China, respectively, but only 17.3, 23.4, and 28.8% in Australia, Canada, and Italy, respectively.

Chen et al. (1998) conducted a comprehensive analysis of shy–inhibited behavior of Chinese and Canadian children in various free-play and stressful situations. The results indicated that Chinese toddlers were generally more shy, vigilant, and reactive than their Canadian counterparts. Chinese toddlers stayed closer to their mothers and were less likely to explore in mother–child free-play sessions. Moreover, Chinese toddlers displayed more anxious and fearful behaviors when interacting with the stranger, as indicated by their higher scores on the latency to approach the stranger and to touch the toys when they were invited to do so. The percentages of toddlers who made contact with their mothers in the free-play and stressful (stranger with toys) episodes in the Chinese sample (41 and 61%) were almost double those in the Canadian sample (21 and 37%).

It has been found in Western children and adults that serotonin transporter genetic polymorphisms are related to emotional reactivity, vulnerability to stress, and behavioral inhibition (e.g., Fox et al., 2005; Lesch et al., 1996); individuals carrying short alleles of the serotonin transporter (5-HTT)-linked polymorphism (5-HTTLPR) tend to display high reactivity and inhibition. Tsai, Hong, and Cheng (2002) reported that the proportion of people who have 5-HTTLPR short alleles is dramatically higher in Chinese than in Western populations. Tardif (2008) has found that Chinese children show significantly higher cortisol reactivity than American children to a variety of challenging tasks, although they do not differ in nonstressful situations. It should be noted that although these biological/physiological measures are associated with BI in Western children, no research has examined the links in Chinese children. Thus, interpretations of cross-cultural differences in shyness–inhibition from biological perspectives must be made with great caution.

Parent and Peer Attitudes and Responses

There is evidence suggesting that parents in different cultures may respond differently to shy–inhibited behavior (see also Hastings, Nuselovici, Rubin, & Cheah, Chapter 6, this volume). In North America, parents typically react to shy–inhibited behavior with concern, disappointment, rejection, and punishment (Rubin & Burgess, 2002). Chen et al. (1998) found, however, that shy–inhibited behavior in Chinese children was associated with parental acceptance and encouragement. Similarly, Weisz and colleagues (1988) found that Thai parents rated children's shyness and other internalizing behaviors as less serious and worrisome than did American parents.

Peers may also evaluate and respond differently to shy–inhibited behaviors across cultures. Chen, DeSouza, Chen, and Wang (2006) found that, compared with others, shy–inhibited children who made passive and low-power social initiations received fewer positive responses and more rejection from peers in Canada. However, shy–inhibited children who displayed the same behaviors were more likely than others to receive positive responses and support in China. These varying social responses toward shy–inhibited behavior may indicate cultural expectations and values, and, at the same time, constitute social environments within which shy–inhibited children develop.

SHYNESS–INHIBITION FROM CHILDHOOD TO ADOLESCENCE: THE ROLE OF CULTURE IN SHAPING ITS RELATIONS WITH SOCIAL AND PSYCHOLOGICAL ADJUSTMENT

Because cultural beliefs and values serve to guide parental childrearing attitudes and peer evaluations, the experiences of shy–inhibited children are likely to vary in different societies. Therefore, the impact of cultural norms and values may be reflected in the concurrent and predictive relations between shyness–inhibition and social, school, and psychological adjustment.

Shyness–Inhibition and Its Social and Psychological Concomitants

In North America and in Western Europe, shy–inhibited behavior has been found to be associated with the development of social, school, and psychological problems in children and adolescents (e.g., Rubin et al., 2009). In societies where autonomy and assertiveness are not valued or encouraged, shy and restrained behavior is likely to be viewed as less deviant and maladaptive. Although research findings are not highly consistent, existing evidence indicates that relative to what has been found in North America, shyness seems to be less problematic among children in some Asian countries (Eisenberg, Pidada, & Liew, 2001). Eisenberg et al. found that shyness in Indonesian children, as reported by adults, was negatively associated with peer nominations of dislike and behavioral problems, and teacher-rated negative emotionality. Farver et al. (1995) noted that shy and reticent behaviors in Korean American children were consistent with the school expectation of "proper" behavior and cultural values that emphasize group harmony and deemphasize individuality and self-expression.

Cross-cultural variations in the relations between shyness–inhibition and social and psychological adjustment have been found in a series of studies by Chen and his colleagues in Chinese and Canadian children in the early 1990s (e.g., Chen, Chen, & Kaspar, 2001; Chen, Dong, & Zhou, 1997; Chen, Rubin, & Sun, 1992). Specifically, inconsistent with the results from North American samples, shyness was associated with positive peer relationships, school competence, and psychological well-being in China. Shy Chinese children tended to be accepted by peers, to be viewed as competent by teachers, and to perform well in academic areas. These children were also more likely than others to achieve leadership status in the school. Moreover, shy children in China did not feel lonely or depressed, or develop negative perceptions of their competence (Chen et al., 2004). The social and psychological adjustment of Chinese shy children is related to the endorsement of socially restrained behavior. In traditional Chinese culture, shy–inhibited behavior is thought to be associated with virtuous qualities, such as modesty and cautiousness, indicating accomplishment and maturity (e.g., Liang, 1987). The cultural endorsement may help shy children obtain support in social interactions, form social relationships, acquire school achievement, and develop positive views and feelings about self and others.

Chen and Tse (2008) recently found that Chinese children, particularly girls, in Canada (Canadian-born and immigrant) were shyer in the school than children with a European background. The differences were rather robust, based on the evaluations of European Canadian and Chinese Canadian children, as well as children from other cultural backgrounds (e.g., non-Chinese Asian, South American). Interestingly, Chen and Tse found that shyness was associated with social problems, such as peer rejection and victimization, in European Canadian children, but the associations were non-significant or significantly weaker in Chinese Canadian children. The results appear similar to those found in China (e.g., Chen et al., 1992). However, the processes involved in the relations may or may not be the same, because the cultural contexts are different in Canadian and Chinese schools. It is possible that some Chinese cultural practices help children develop skills to cope with adverse outcomes of their shy–inhibited behavior. For example, Chinese children tend to develop relatively advanced regulatory skills in the early years (e.g., Chen et al., 2003; Sabbagh, Xu, Carlson, Moses, & Lee, 2006), which may allow them to express their shyness in a relatively acceptable manner (e.g., engaging in parallel play activities; Asendorpf, 1991) and to minimize the negative consequences of their shy behavior. It is also possible that a stereotypical reputation (e.g., "Chinese are shy") serves to protect shy–inhibited Chinese children in Canada from developing social difficulties in peer interactions and adjustment problems.

DEVELOPMENTAL OUTCOMES OF SHYNESS–INHIBITION

It has been argued that shyness–inhibition represents a risk factor that has "toxic" effects on development (Kagan, 1997; Pennebaker, 1993). Empirically, it has been found in the West that shyness–inhibition is associated with maladaptive developmental outcomes (e.g., Asendorpf et al., 2008; Caspi et al., 2003). Schwartz, Snidman, and Kagan (1999), for example, reported that early inhibition predicted psychopathological symptoms, such as social anxiety, in adolescence. Asendorpf et al. (2008) and Caspi et al. (1988) found that shy–inhibited children, particularly boys, experienced extensive problems in adulthood, including delayed entry into marriage, parenthood, and a stable career. Childhood shyness was also associated with lower occupational achievement and occupational instability in adulthood (see Rubin et al., 2009).

Shyness–inhibition may be related to fewer negative outcomes in less self-oriented and competitive societies. Kerr, Lambert, and Bem (1996) examined the long-term outcomes of shyness in Swedish society, where shy-reserved behavior was viewed more positively than in North America. The researchers followed a sample of children born in a suburb of Stockholm in the mid-1950s to adulthood. The results indicated that although shyness predicted later marriage and parenthood, it did not affect adulthood careers, including occupational stability (as indicated by frequency of job changes), education, or income among Swedish men. According to Kerr et al., the social welfare and support systems that evolved from the egalitarian values in Sweden ensured that people did not need to be assertive or competitive to achieve career success. Interestingly, perhaps because similar social support systems were not yet available for girls during the period in which the study was conducted, shy Swedish girls appeared to attain lower levels of education than did nonshy girls. Kerr et al. expected that shy and nonshy girls would not differ in Sweden today.

Chen, Chen, Li, and Wang (2009) examined relations between shyness–inhibition in toddlerhood, and social and school outcomes in middle childhood in Chinese children. Data on BI were collected through laboratory observations from a sample of 2-year-olds (Chen et al., 1998). The follow-up study was conducted 5 years later, when the children were 7 years of age. Data were collected from multiple sources, including observations of free play, peer interactions, interviews, teacher ratings, and school records. The results indicated that inhibition in toddlerhood was positively associated with later cooperative behavior, peer liking, perceived social integration, positive school attitudes, and school competence. Behavioral inhibition was negatively associated with later learning problems. Further extreme group analyses (extremely inhibited and uninhibited groups identified with the criteria at the top and bottom [15 or 8%] of the distribution) showed that the associations were mainly due to the differences between highly inhibited children and other children; children who were shy–inhibited in toddlerhood were more competent and successful in social and school performance, and had fewer behavioral and learning problems in middle childhood than did "average" and uninhibited children.

The positive contributions of shyness–inhibition to later social, school, and psychological adjustment have also been found in a longitudinal study from middle childhood to adolescence in China (Chen, Rubin, Li, & Li, 1999). In this study, children's shyness was assessed by peer evaluations when the children were 8 and 10 years old. In the follow-up study conducted 4 years later, children were administered a sociometric nomination measure and completed measures of self-perceptions of competence. Teachers and parents rated children's school-related competence and behavioral problems. Data on children's leadership, distinguished studentship, and academic achievement were obtained from the school records. Chen et al. found that shyness was not associated with later adjustment problems, either externalizing or internalizing. Moreover, shyness was positively predictive of adolescent adjustment, including teacher-assessed competence, leadership, academic achievement, and self-perceptions of competence. Thus, shy–inhibited Chinese children continue to be well adjusted to social and school environments in adolescence.

Taken together, the findings from various projects suggest that shyness–inhibition in some cultures, such as China and Sweden, does not necessarily predict maladaptive development, as has been found in North America. In these cultures, shy–inhibited children may not experience evident obstacles in getting involved in social interactions. Moreover, these children are likely to receive social support and encouragement from others that help them develop confidence and ability to establish relationships. The engagement in activities with peers, in turn, may provide the opportunity for shy–inhibited children to learn norms and skills to behave appropriately in social situations. At the same time, social relationships that shy–inhibited children establish in school may be beneficial to the development of positive attitudes toward the school and motivation to achieve success in education and career.

The Impact of Social and Cultural Changes on Relations between Shyness–Inhibition and Adjustment

Human lives carry the imprint of particular social worlds that are themselves subject to historical change (e.g., Bronfenbrenner & Morris, 2006; Elder, 1998). Examining the implications of macro-level social and cultural changes for children's socioemotional functioning helps us better understand the role of context in human development. The impact of social and cultural changes on socialization, children's and adolescents' attitudes and behaviors, and social relationships has been demonstrated by the effects of the Great Depression in the 1930s on family organization and child functioning (Elder, 1974), the effects of urbanization of Turkish society in the past 30 years on parental socialization and parent–child relationships (Kagitcibasi & Ataca, 2005), and the effects of dramatic societal change in Eastern European nations after the fall of the Berlin Wall on children and adolescents' value systems, life course, and interactional styles (Flanagan, 2000; Little, Brendgen, Wanner, & Krappmann, 1999; Silbereisen, 2000).

Chen and colleagues (Chen, Cen, Li, & He, 2005; Chen & Chen, in press) have explored how the ongoing social transformation in China is altering parenting beliefs and practices, and children's socioemotional functioning. A major aspect of the project was to examine the significance of shyness–inhibition for adjustment in children at different periods of the societal transition and in different regions of country. China has changed dramatically since the early 1980s, particularly in the past 15 years, toward a market-oriented society. Along with social and economic reforms, Western individualistic values and ideologies have been gradually appreciated and accepted in the country (Zhang, 2000). For example, many schools in China have changed their education goals, policies, and practices to facilitate the development of social skills. A variety of strategies has been used to help children learn these skills (e.g., encouraging students to engage in public debate, and to propose and implement their own plans about extracurricular activities). Relative to some other aspects of socioemotional functioning, shyness–inhibition may be particularly susceptible to the influence of the macro-level changes (Chen, Wang, et al., 2006). Shy, anxious, and wary behavior that impedes exploration and self-expression in stressful situations is incompatible with the requirements of a competitive society. As a result, shyness may no longer be regarded as adaptive and competent in social and psychological adjustment in the new environment. Shy–inhibited children may be at a disadvantage in obtaining social approval, and may experience adjustment difficulties (Hart et al., 2000; Xu, Farver, Chang, Zhang, & Yu, 2007).

Chen et al. (2005) examined the relations between shyness and social, school, and psychological adjustment in urban China in three cohorts (1990, 1998, and 2002) of elementary school children. Whereas children in the 1990 cohort experienced relatively limited influence of the comprehensive reform, and children in the 2002 cohort were socialized in an increasingly self-oriented cultural context, the 1998 cohort represented an intermediate phase, in which children might have mixed socialization experiences in the family and the peer group. The analysis revealed significant cross-cohort differences in the relations between shyness and adjustment variables. Whereas shyness was positively associated with peer acceptance, leadership, and academic achievement in the 1990 cohort, it was negatively associated with peer acceptance and teacher-rated social competence, and positively associated with peer rejection and depression in the 2002 cohort. The patterns of the relations between shyness and peer relationships and adjustment variables were nonsignificant or mixed in the 1998 cohort. The results indicated that by the early part of the 21st century, as the country became more deeply immersed in a market economy, shy–sensitive children, unlike their counterparts in the early 1990s, were perceived as incompetent and problematic by teachers and were rejected by peers, displayed school problems, and reported high levels of depression.

An interesting finding of Chen et al.'s study (2005) is that shyness was positively associated with both peer acceptance and peer rejection in the 1998 cohort. The analysis of the sociometric classification revealed that shy children in this cohort were controversial; they were liked and disliked by peers at the same time. These results indicate mixed attitudes of peers toward shy–inhibited children, which, to some extent, may reflect the cultural conflict between the new values of initiative and traditional Chinese values of self-control. Another interesting finding in that, in the 2002 cohort, shyness was associated with negative peer, teacher, and self-attitudes and evaluations, but not with school performance, such as distinguished studentship and academic achievement. Thus, the impact of the social and historical changes on different aspects of socioemotional functioning and adjustment may be an ongoing process that occurs gradually and cumulatively. The findings also support the argument that social attitudes and relationships serve as major mediators of contextual influence on individual development (Chen & French, 2008; Chen, French, & Schneider, 2006).

There are substantial regional, particularly urban–rural, differences in social and economic development. The massive social and economic reform, such as the opening of stock markets in China, has been largely limited to urban centers and cities. Families in rural China have lived mostly agricultural lives, and rural children do not have as much exposure as urban children to the influence of the market economy (Cui, 2003). In many rural areas, traditional Chinese values, such as self-control, are still highly emphasized (Fuligni & Zhang, 2004; Shen, 2006). Several studies have examined urban–rural differences in children's social attitudes and socioemotional functioning in China. Guo, Yao, and Yang (2005), for example, found that, based on teacher evaluations and self-reports, relative to urban children, rural children were more group-oriented, displayed greater social responsibility, and were less likely to pursue individual interests. Chen, Wang, and Wang (2009) in a recent study in Beijing, found that shyness was associated with social and school problems and depression in urban children, similar to the results in Chen et al.'s study (2005) with urban children in Shanghai. However, shyness was generally associated with indices of adjustment, such as leadership, teacher-rated competence, and academic achievement, in rural children in migrant children's schools. Similar results were found in a rural sample in the countryside of Henan province in China in 2006 (Chen & Chen, in press). Thus, like their urban counterparts in the early 1990s, shy rural children are not yet regarded as problematic; these children still obtain approval from peers and adults, and achieve success in social and academic areas. It is important to note that many rural regions of China are currently undergoing rapid changes. Urban and Western values increasingly influence socialization beliefs and practices, and socioemotional development in rural children. It will be interesting to investigate how rural children adapt to the changing environment.

CONCLUSIONS AND FUTURE DIRECTIONS

Children in most societies display shy–inhibited behavior in the early years. The early characteristic constitutes a major dispositional basis for the development of socioemotional functioning. Through socialization and social interaction processes, however, cultural norms and values determine, in part, the exhibition and functional significance of shyness–inhibition. Consequently, the prevalence of shyness–inhibition and its relations with social and psychological adjustment may vary across cultures. As social and cultural contexts change, the significance and developmental patterns of shyness–inhibition may change accordingly.

Research on culture and shyness–inhibition has focused on direct or indirect cross-cultural comparisons. Although cross-cultural similarities and differences are interesting in demonstrating the role of cultural context, this approach provides little information about the processes in which cultural beliefs and values affect children's shy–inhibited behavior. It will be important to investigate how cultural values guide social interactions and organize social relationships, which in turn regulate children's shy–inhibited behavior and development (Chen & French, 2008).

In this chapter, I have focused on shyness–inhibition, without tapping social disinterest, preference for solitude, and other types of social withdrawal. Researchers have conducted a number of studies involving mixed aspects of social withdrawal among children in different countries, such as China, Cuba, India, and Italy (Attili, Vermigli, & Schneider, 1997; Chang et al., 2005; Chen, 2008; Prakash & Coplan, 2007; Valdivia et al., 2005). In general, the results indicate that, across cultures, when the components of social disinterest or preference for solitude are included in measures, socially withdrawn or constrained behavior is associated with problems in peer relationships and psychological adjustment, similar to what has been found in North America. Little cultural variation in the linkage between withdrawn behavior and adjustment variables seems to suggest that the lack of tendency to approach the social situation is a universal antecedent of maladaptive social and psychological functioning. Nevertheless, further investigation is needed to examine more specific types of social withdrawal. Chen (2008), for example, has argued that preference for solitude may be related to different reactions in different cultures. If preference for solitude is based on the personal "choice" (Coplan et al., 2004), it represents an autonomous action of the individual. As such, it does not necessarily indicate "failure" or incompetence in Western individualistic cultures that endorse personal decision making and self-direction, but it may be considered anticollective or selfish in group-oriented cultures that emphasize social affiliation. In Western culture, shyness–inhibition and unsociability tend to merge in school-age children (Asendorpf, 1991). There is also a similar trend of amalgamation in urban Chinese children as shyness becomes increasingly maladaptive in the competitive environment (Chen et al., 2005). It will be interesting to examine how shyness–inhibition is associated with unsociability, and how they jointly contribute to socioemotional development in different societies.

Coplan and his colleagues have recently studied children's knowledge of shyness and other social behaviors (e.g., Coplan, Girardi, Findlay, & Frohlick, 2007). For example, they analyzed the content of children's self-generated descriptions of their classmates' fearful or self-conscious shyness, active isolation, and social disinterest, and found that children at different ages provided different reasons why children are shy or play alone. Moreover, children displayed different attitudes and responses to shyness and social disinterest in hypothetical vignettes. To what extent children's perspectives on shyness and social withdrawal are similar or different across cultures, and how cultural beliefs and values affect children's understanding and reaction will be important questions to address.

Finally, like China and Eastern European nations, many countries are currently undergoing rapid changes during globalization. The political, economic, and cultural exchanges and interactions across nations may lead to the merger and coexistence of diverse value systems (Kagitcibasi, 2005; Tamis-LeMonda et al., 2008). Moreover, within-culture variations are likely to increase remarkably during this process. Researchers should investigate how shy–inhibited children integrate diverse values in their adaptation to the changing global community.

REFERENCES

Achenbach, T. M., & Edelbrock, C. (1981). Behavioural problems and competencies reported by parents of normal and disturbed children aged four through sixteen. *Monographs of the Society for Research in Child Development, 46* (Serial No. 188).

Ariel, S., & Sever, I. (1980). Play in the desert and play in the town: On play activities of Bedouin Arab children. In H. B. Schwartzman (Ed.), *Play and culture* (pp. 164–175). West Point, NY: Leisure Press.

Asendorpf, J. (1990). Beyond social withdrawal: Shyness, unsociability and peer avoidance. *Human Development, 33,* 250–259.

Asendorpf, J. B. (1991). Development of inhibited children's coping with unfamiliarity. *Child Development, 62,* 1460–1474.

Asendorpf, J. B., Denissen, J. J. A., & van Aken, M. A. G. (2008). Inhibited and aggressive preschool children at 23 years of age: Personality and social transition into adulthood. *Developmental Psychology, 44,* 997–1011.

Attili, G., Vermigli, P., & Schneider, B. H. (1997). Peer acceptance and friendship patterns among Italian schoolchildren within a cross-cultural perspective. *International Journal of Behavioral Development, 21,* 277–288.

Bronfenbrenner, U., & Morris, P. A. (2006). The bioecological model of human development. In W. Damon (Series Ed.) & R. M. Lerner (Vol. Ed.), *Handbook of child psychology: Vol 1. Theoretical models of human development* (pp. 793–828). New York: Wiley.

Burger, J. M. (1995). Individual difference in preference for solitude. *Journal of Research in Personality, 29,* 85–108.

Casiglia, A. C., Lo Coco, A., & Zappulla, C. (1998). Aspects of social reputation and peer relationships in Italian children: A cross-cultural perspective. *Developmental Psychology, 34,* 723–730.

Caspi, A., Elder, G. H., Jr., & Bem, D. J. (1988). Moving away from the world: Life-course patterns of shy children. *Developmental Psychology, 24,* 824–831.

Caspi, A., Harrington, H., Milne, B., Amell, J. W., Theodore, R. F., & Moffitt, T. E. (2003). Children's behavioral styles at age 3 are linked to their adult personality traits at age 26. *Journal of Personality, 71,* 495–513.

Chang, L., Lei, L., Li, K. K., Liu, H., Guo, B., Wang, Y., et al. (2005). Peer acceptance and self-perceptions of verbal and behavioural aggression and withdrawal. *International Journal of Behavioral Development, 29,* 49–57.

Cheah, C. L., & Rubin, K. H. (2004). European American and Mainland Chinese mothers' responses to aggression and social withdrawal in preschoolers. *International Journal of Behavioral Development, 28,* 83–94.

Cheek, J. M., & Buss, A. H. (1981). Shyness and sociability. *Journal of Personality and Social Psychology, 41,* 330–339.

Chen, X. (2008). Shyness and unsociability in cultural context. In A. S. Lo Coco, K. H. Rubin, & C. Zappulla (Eds.), *L'isolamento sociale durante l'infanzia* [Social withdrawal in childhood] (pp. 143–160). Milan: Unicopli.

Chen, X., Cen, G., Li, D., & He, Y. (2005). Social functioning and adjustment in Chinese children: The imprint of historical time. *Child Development, 76,* 182–195.

Chen, X., & Chen, H. (in press). Children's social functioning and adjustment in the changing Chinese society. In R. K. Silbereisen & X. Chen (Eds.), *Social change and human development: Concepts and results.* London: Sage.

Chen, X., Chen, H., & Kaspar, V. (2001). Group social functioning and individual socio-emotional and school adjustment in Chinese children. *Merrill–Palmer Quarterly, 47,* 264–299.

Chen, X., Chen, H., Li, D., & Wang, L. (2009). Early childhood inhibition and social and school adjustment in Chinese children: A five-year longitudinal study. *Child Development, 80,* 1692–1704.

Chen, X., Chung, J., & Hsiao, C. (2009). Peer interactions, relationships and groups from a cross-cultural perspective. In K. H. Rubin, W. Bukowski, & B. Laursen (Eds.), *Handbook of peer interactions, relationships, and groups* (pp. 432–451). New York: Guilford Press.

Chen, X., DeSouza, A., Chen, H., & Wang, L. (2006). Reticent behavior and experiences in peer interactions in Canadian and Chinese children. *Developmental Psychology, 42,* 656–665.

Chen, X., Dong, Q., & Zhou, H. (1997). Authoritative and authoritarian parenting practices and social and school adjustment. *International Journal of Behavioral Development, 20,* 855–873.

Chen, X., & French, D. (2008). Children's social competence in cultural context. *Annual Review of Psychology, 59,* 591–616.

Chen, X., French, D., & Schneider, B. (2006). Culture and peer relationships. In X. Chen, D. French, & B. Schneider (Eds.), *Peer relationships in cultural context* (pp. 123–147). New York: Cambridge University Press.

Chen, X., Hastings, P., Rubin, K. H., Chen, H., Cen, G., & Stewart, S. L. (1998). Childrearing attitudes and behavioral inhibition in Chinese and Canadian toddlers: A cross-cultural study. *Developmental Psychology, 34,* 677–686.

Chen, X., He, Y., De Oliveira, A. M., Lo Coco, A., Zappulla, C., Kaspar, V., et al.. (2004). Loneliness and social adaptation in Brazilian, Canadian, Chinese and Italian children. *Journal of Child Psychology and Psychiatry, 45,* 1373–1384.

Chen, X., Rubin, K. H., Li, B., & Li, Z. (1999). Adolescent outcomes of social functioning in Chinese children. *International Journal of Behavioural Development, 23,* 199–223.

Chen, X., Rubin, K. H., & Li, Z. (1995). Social functioning and adjustment in Chinese children: A longitudinal study. *Developmental Psychology, 31,* 531–539.

Chen, X., Rubin, K. H., Liu, M., Chen, H., Wang, L., Li, D., et al. (2003). Compliance in Chinese and Canadian toddlers. *International Journal of Behavioral Development, 27,* 428–436.

Chen, X., Rubin, K. H., & Sun, Y. (1992). Social reputation and peer relationships in Chinese and Canadian children: A cross-cultural study. *Child Development, 63,* 1336–1343.

Chen, X., & Tse, H. C. (2008). Social functioning and adjustment in Canadian-born children with Chinese and European backgrounds. *Developmental Psychology, 44*,1184–1189.

Chen, X., Wang, L., & DeSouza, A. (2006). Temperament and socio-emotional functioning in Chinese and North American children. In X. Chen, D. French, & B. Schneider (Eds.), *Peer relationships in cultural context* (pp. 123–147). New York: Cambridge University Press.

Chen, X., Wang, L., & Wang, Z. (2009). Shyness–sensitivity and social, school, and psychological adjustment in rural migrant and urban children in China. *Child Development, 80*, 1499–1513.

Cole, M. (1996). *Cultural psychology.* Cambridge, MA: Harvard University Press.

Coplan, R. J., & Armer, M. (2007). A "multitude" of solitude: A closer look at social withdrawal and nonsocial play in early childhood. *Child Development Perspectives, 1*, 26–32.

Coplan, R. J., Girardi, A., Findlay, L. C., & Frohlick, S. L. (2007). Understanding solitude: Young children's attitudes and responses towards hypothetical socially-withdrawn peers. *Social Development, 16*, 390–409.

Coplan, R. J., Prakash, K., O'Neil, K., & Armer, M. (2004). Do you "want" to play?: Distinguishing between conflicted-shyness and social disinterest in early childhood. *Developmental Psychology, 40*, 244–258.

Coplan, R. J., Rubin, K. H., Fox, N. A., Calkins, S. D., & Stewart, S. L. (1994). Being alone, playing alone, and acting alone: Distinguishing among reticence and passive and active solitude in young children. *Child Development, 65*, 129–137.

Corsaro, W. A., & Nelson, E. (2003). Children's collective activities and peer culture in early literacy in American and Italian preschools. *Sociology of Education, 76*, 209–227.

Crozier, W. R. (1995). Shyness and self-esteem in middle childhood. *British Journal of Educational Psychology, 65*, 85–95.

Cui, C. (2003). Adapting to the city and adjusting rural-urban relations: A study of migrant children's school and live circumstances in Beijing. In B. Li (Ed.), *The peasant worker: An analysis of social and economic status of Chinese rural-to-urban migrants* (pp. 161–171). Beijing: Social Sciences and Documentation Publishing House.

Edwards, C. P. (2000). Children's play in cross-cultural perspective: A new look at the Six Cultures Study. *Cross-Cultural Research, 34*, 318–338.

Eisenberg, N., Pidada, S., & Liew, J. (2001). The relations of regulation and negative emotionality to Indonesian children's social functioning. *Child Development, 72*, 1747–1763.

Elder, G. H., Jr. (1974). *Children of the Great Depression.* Chicago: University of Chicago Press.

Elder, G. H., Jr. (1998). The life course and human development. In W. Damon (Series Ed.) & R. M. Lerner (Vol. Ed.), *Handbook of child psychology: Vol 1. Theoretical models of human development* (pp. 939–991). New York: Wiley.

Eysenck, H. J., & Eysenck, S. B. G. (1969). *Personality structure and measurement.* London: Routledge & Kegan Paul.

Farver, J. M., & Howes, C. (1988). Cultural differences in social interaction: A comparison of American and Indonesian children. *Journal of Cross-Cultural Psychology, 19,* 203–315.

Farver, J. M., & Howes, C. (1993). Cultural differences in American and Mexican mother–child pretend play. *Merrill–Palmer Quarterly, 39,* 344–358.

Farver, J. M., Kim, Y. K., & Lee, Y. (1995). Cultural differences in Korean- and Anglo-American preschoolers' social interaction and play behaviors. *Child Development, 66,* 1088–1099.

Farver, J. M., & Shin, Y. L. (1997). Social pretend play in Korean- and Anglo-American preschoolers. *Child Development, 68,* 544–556.

Flanagan, C. A. (2000). Social change and the "social contract" in adolescent development. In L. J. Crockett & R. K. Silbereisen (Eds.), *Negotiating adolescence in times of social change* (pp. 191–198). New York: Cambridge University Press.

Fox, H. A., Henderson, H. A., Marshall, P. J., Nichols, K. E., & Ghera, M. M. (2005). Behavioral inhibition: Linking biology and behavior within a developmental framework. *Annual Review of Psychology, 56,* 235–262.

Fuligni, A. J., & Zhang, W. X. (2004). Attitudes toward family obligation among adolescents in contemporary urban and rural China. *Child Development, 74,* 180–192.

Gaskins, S. (2000). Children's daily activities in a Mayan village: A culturally grounded description. *Cross-Cultural Research, 34,* 375–389.

Gazelle, H., & Ladd, G. W. (2003). Anxious solitude and peer exclusion: A diathesis–stress model of internalizing trajectories in childhood. *Child Development, 74,* 257–278.

Greenfield, P. M., Suzuki, L. K., & Rothstein-Fisch, C. (2006). Cultural pathways through human development. In K. A. Renninger & I. E. Sigel (Eds.), *Handbook of child psychology: Vol. 4. Child psychology in practice* (pp. 655–699). New York: Wiley.

Guo, L., Yao, Y., & Yang, B. (2005). Adaptation of migrant children to the city: A case study at a migrant children school in Beijing. *Youth Study, 3,* 22–31.

Hart, C. H., Yang, C., Nelson, L. J., Robinson, C. C., Olson, J. A., Nelson, D. A., et al. (2000). Peer acceptance in early childhood and subtypes of socially withdrawn behaviour in China, Russia and the United States. *International Journal of Behavioral Development, 24,* 73–81.

Kagan, J. (1997). Temperament and the reactions to unfamiliarity. *Child Development, 68,* 139–143.

Kagan, J., Kearsley, R. B., & Zelazo, P. R. (1978). *Infancy: Its place in human development.* Cambridge, MA: Harvard University Press.

Kagan J., Reznick, J. S., & Snidman, N. (1987). The physiology and psychology of behavioral inhibition in children. *Child Development, 58,* 1459–1473.

Kagitcibasi, C. (2005). Autonomy and relatedness in cultural context: Implications for self and family. *Journal of Cross-Cultural Psychology, 36,* 403–422.

Kagitcibasi, C., & Ataca, B. (2005). Value of children and family change: A three-decade portrait from Turkey. *Applied Psychology: An International Review, 54,* 317–337.

Kerr, M., Lambert, W. W., & Bem, D. J. (1996). Life course sequelae of childhood shyness in Sweden: Comparison with the United States. *Developmental Psychology, 32,* 1100–1105.

Leary, M. R., Herbst, K. C., & McCrary, F. (2003). Finding pleasure in solitary activities: Desire for aloneness or disinterest in social contact? *Personality and Individual Differences, 35,* 59–68.

Lesch, K. P., Bengel, D., Heils, A., Sabol, S. Z., Greenberg, B. D., Petri, S., et al. (1996). Association of anxiety-related traits with a polymorphism in the serotonin transporter gene regulatory region. *Science, 274,* 1527–1531.

Liang, S. (1987). *The outline of Chinese culture.* Shanghai: Xue Lin.

Little, T. D., Brendgen, M., Wanner, B., & Krappmann, L. (1999). Children's reciprocal perceptions of friendship quality in the sociocultural contexts of East and West Berlin. *International Journal of Behavioral Development, 23,* 63–89.

Masten, A., Morison, P., & Pellegrini, D. (1985). A Revised Class Play method of peer assessment. *Developmental Psychology, 21,* 523–533.

Parmar, P., Harkness, S., & Super, C. M. (2004). Asian and Euro-American parents' ethnotheories of play and learning: Effects on preschool children's home routine and school behaviour. *International Journal of Behavioral Development, 28,* 97–104.

Peng, K., Nisbett, R. E., & Wong, N. Y. (1997). Validity problems comparing values across cultures and possible solutions. *Psychological Methods, 2,* 329–344.

Pennebaker, J. W. (1993). Overcoming inhibition: Rethinking the roles of personality, cognition, and social behaviors. In H. C. Traue & J. W. Pennebaker (Eds.), *Emotion, inhibition and health* (pp. 100–115). Kirkland, WA: Hogrefe & Huber.

Prakash, K., & Coplan, R. J. (2007). Socioemotional characteristics and school adjustment of socially withdrawn children in India. *International Journal of Behavioral Development, 31,* 123–132.

Prior, M., Smart, D., Sanson, A., & Oberklaid, F. (2000). Does shy–inhibited temperament in childhood lead to anxiety problems in adolescence? *Journal of the American Academy of Child and Adolescent Psychiatry, 39,* 461–468.

Rogoff, B. (2003). *The cultural nature of human development.* New York: Oxford University Press.

Rothbart, M. K., & Bates, J. E. (2006). Temperament. In N. Eisenberg (Ed.), *Handbook of child psychology: Vol. 3. Social, emotional, and personality development* (pp. 99–166). New York: Wiley.

Rubin, K. H. (1982). Non-social play in preschoolers: Necessarily evil? *Child Development, 53,* 651–657.

Rubin, K. H., & Burgess, K. (2002). Parents of aggressive and withdrawn children. In M. Bornstein (Ed.), *Handbook of parenting* (2nd Ed., Vol. 1, pp. 383–418). Hillsdale, NJ: Erlbaum.

Rubin, K. H., Chen, X., & Hymel, S. (1993). Socio-emotional characteristics of aggressive and withdrawn children. *Merrill–Palmer Quarterly, 39,* 518–534.

Rubin, K. H., Chen, X., McDougall, P., Bowker, A., & McKinnon, J. (1995). The Waterloo Longitudinal Project: Predicting adolescent internalizing and externalizing problems from early and mid-childhood. *Development and Psychopathology, 7,* 751–764.

Rubin, K. H., Coplan, R. J., & Bowker, J. C. (2009). Social withdrawal and shyness in childhood and adolescence. *Annual Review of Psychology, 60,* 141–171.

Rubin, K. H., Coplan, R. J., Fox, N. A., & Calkins, S. (1995). Emotionality, emotion regulation, and preschoolers' social adaptation. *Development and Psychopathology, 7,* 49–62.

Rubin, K. H., Hemphill, S. A., Chen, X., Hastings, P., Sanson, A., Lo Coco, A., et al. (2006). A cross-cultural study of behavioral inhibition in toddlers: East–west–north–south. *International Journal of Behavioral Development, 30,* 219–226.

Sabbagh, M. A., Xu, F., Carlson, S. M., Moses, L. J., & Lee, K. (2006). The development of executive functioning and theory of mind: A comparison of Chinese and U.S. preschoolers. *Psychological Science, 17,* 74–81.

Schneider, B., French, D., & Chen, X. (2006). Peer relationships in cultural perspective: Methodological reflections. In X. Chen, D. French, & B. Schneider (Eds.), *Peer relationships in cultural context* (pp. 489–500). New York: Cambridge University Press.

Schwartz, C. E., Snidman, N., & Kagan, J. (1999). Adolescent social anxiety as an outcome of inhibited temperament in childhood. *Journal of the American Academy of Child and Adolescent Psychiatry, 38,* 1008–1015.

Shen, R. (2006). Problems and solutions for child education for migrant rural worker families. *Journal of China Agricultural University (Social Science Edition), 64,* 96–100.

Silbereisen, R. K. (2000). German unification and adolescents' developmental timetables: Continuities and discontinuities. In L. A. Crockett, & R. K. Silbereisen (Eds.), *Negotiating adolescence in times of social change* (pp. 104–122). Cambridge, UK: Cambridge University Press.

Super, C. M., & Harkness, S. (1986). The developmental niche: A conceptualization at the interface of child and culture. *International Journal of Behavioral Development, 9,* 545–569.

Tamis-LeMonda, C. S., Way, N., Hughes, D., Yoshikawa, H., Kalman, R. K., & Niwa, E. (2008). Parents' goals for children: The dynamic co-existence of collectivism and individualism in cultures and individuals. *Social Development, 17,* 183–209.

Tardif, T. (2008, March). *Physiological reactions of Chinese and American children in daily activities.* Paper presented at the Joint Meeting on Culture and Child Development, Ann Arbor, MI.

Triandis, H. C. (1995). *Individualism and collectivism.* Boulder, CO: Westview Press.

Tsai, S. J., Hong, C. J., & Cheng, C. Y. (2002). Serotonin transporter genetic polymorphisms and harm avoidance in the Chinese. *Psychiatric Genetics 12,* 165–168.

Valdivia, I. A., Schneider, B. H., Chavez, K. L., & Chen, X. (2005). Social withdrawal and maladjustment in a very group-oriented society. *International Journal of Behavioral Development, 29,* 219–228.

Vygotsky, L. S. (1978). *Mind in society: The development of higher psychological processes.* Cambridge, MA: Harvard University Press.

Weisz, J. R., Chaiyasit, W., Weiss, B., Eastman, K. L., & Jackson, E. E. (1995). A multimethod study of problem behavior among Thai and American children in school: Teacher reports versus direct observations. *Child Development, 66,* 402–415.

Weisz, J. R., Suwanlert, S., Chaiyasit, W., Weiss, B., Walter, B. R., & Anderson, W. W. (1988). Thai and American perspectives on over-and undercontrolled child behavior problems: Exploring the threshold model among parents, teachers, and psychologists. *Journal of Consulting and Clinical Psychology, 56,* 601–609.

Whiting, B. B., & Edwards, C. P. (1988). *Children of different worlds.* Cambridge, MA: Harvard University Press.

Xu, Y., Farver, J. M., Chang, L., Zhang, Z., & Yu, L. (2007). Moving away or fitting in?: Understanding shyness in Chinese children. *Merrill–Palmer Quarterly, 53,* 527–556.

Zhang, W. W. (2000). *Transforming China: Economic reform and its political implications.* New York: St. Martin's Press.

11

Electronic Communication

Escape Mechanism or Relationship-Building Tool for Shy, Withdrawn Children and Adolescents?

BARRY H. SCHNEIDER
YAIR AMICHAI-HAMBURGER

Early adolescence is a developmental stage at which friendship emerges as a crucial element in psychosocial adjustment (Sullivan, 1953). At that stage, socially withdrawn and socially anxious individuals experience increased rejection by their peers, loneliness, and depression (Rubin & Coplan, 2004). Despite the appearance of a few influential studies in recent years, little is known about the role of electronic communication as both a tool that could facilitate individuals' social contacts and/or an escape mechanism that helps to perpetuate their relationship difficulties. This chapter begins with consideration of the features of electronic communication as a relationship-building tool, together with some theoretically based conjectures with regard to specific use by socially withdrawn children and adolescents. We then examine the empirical basis for the theoretically driven arguments. In doing so, we borrow at times from the literature on Internet use by the general population given the paucity of specific data on socially withdrawn young people.

Mentioned in this chapter are studies with participants identified as "socially withdrawn," "socially anxious," "socially phobic," "shy," and "lonely." There are both commonalities and important distinctions among these terms. Rubin and Burgess (2001) describe "social withdrawal" as

avoiding other people and choosing solitude to escape the trials of forming and maintaining social relationships. They note that isolating oneself
is not necessarily problematic. Social withdrawal is not a clinical disorder
but is associated with several clinical disorders, including depression, psy-
chosis, and anxiety disorder. Some children withdraw from interacting with
peers because they are essentially "loners," who simply prefer to be on their
own. Others, however, withdraw because they are wary and anxious of
what would happen if they approached their peers, including being rebuffed
or evaluated negatively. Rubin and Burgess describe the relation between
social withdrawal and anxiety as "dialectical and cyclical" (p. 411). They
note that anxiety may be "marked by frequent withdrawal from, and avoidance of, peer interaction" (p. 411), and that anxiety can be the cause of
social withdrawal. Social withdrawal may also deprive children of needed
opportunities to develop normal social skills, causing or exacerbating social
anxiety.

The temperamental construct of shyness is used in both developmental
psychology and clinical psychology literatures. Rapee and Heimberg (1997)
contend that "shyness" is a term that can characterize social anxiety problems that are relatively mild and that are likely not to correspond to the full
diagnostic criteria for social phobia. In contrast, developmental researchers
Rubin and Asendorpf (1993), in their groundbreaking volume on social
withdrawal in childhood, referred to "shyness" as inhibited responses to
novel social situations.

Anxiety is the central feature of social phobia. According to an influential review by Rapee and Heimberg (1997), individuals with social phobia
live in fear of being evaluated negatively by others. Their anxiety about the
negative evaluation by others is manifest in their beliefs about themselves
and others, and in selective, disproportionate attention to cues they interpret as indicating that others are likely to view them negatively. Rapee and
Heimberg note that there is not a one-to-one correspondence between social
anxiety and actual performance in social situations. Nevertheless, children
diagnosed with social phobia or social anxiety have been found to be uncom-
municative, unresponsive, and generally passive in their peer interactions
(Alfano, Biedel, & Turner, 2006; Spence, Donovan, & Brechman-Toussaint,
1999). Social anxiety has been found to correlate with loneliness, especially
among girls (Hymel, Franke, & Freigang, 1985; Inderbitzen-Pisaruk, Clark,
& Solano, 1992).

ACCESS TO ELECTRONIC COMMUNICATION

Electronic communication is by now available to the vast majority of children and adolescents in most developed countries. It is also increasingly

accessible in developing nations. In the United States, the number of children between the ages of 12 and 17 going online reached 87% in July 2005; 51% of teenagers say that they go online at least once a day. Much of Internet time involves social interaction: After homework, e-mail and electronic messaging are adolescents' most common activities on the Internet; 85% of online teens use electronic messaging and e-mails to communicate (Lenhart, Rainie, & Lewis, 2001). Working in two Greek cities, Vekiri and Chronaki (2008) found that 91% of elementary school pupils indicated in a survey that they used computers outside of school. Although only 47% reported regular access to the Internet at home, 90% said that they used the Internet outside of school, logging on either at friends' or relatives' homes or in Internet cafés, if necessary. Internet cafés have mushroomed in much of the developing world, even though relatively few people in those countries have connections at home. For example, Ybarra, Kiwanuka, Emenyonu, and Bangsberg (2006) found that 48% of the adolescents surveyed in the town of Mbarara, Uganda, accessed the Internet regularly; these researchers believe that Internet access in towns like Mbarara is greater than in smaller villages, but not as common as in large Ugandan cities.

Although the digital gap still exists in certain societies, the advent of near-universal access to electronic communication in many countries means, quite obviously, that this technology is probably available to most shy, withdrawn children and adolescents who choose to use it. Accessibility also means that certain individual differences, evident only a few years ago, may have disappeared: Individuals with particularly strong needs to use the Internet, which might include shy, withdrawn children and adults, may not necessarily use the Internet any more than most of their neighbors or make any greater economic sacrifice to access the Net.

SPECIFIC IMPLICATIONS OF RECENT TRENDS FOR SOCIALLY WITHDRAWN INDIVIDUALS

In understanding the implications of electronic communication for socially withdrawn individuals, it is important to take into account the trends already discussed about access to electronic communication in general. Some socially withdrawn individuals live in communities or societies where the Internet is available to people who want it, but not so available as to be present in almost every home, school, and major street. In this situation, the socially withdrawn person may be drawn to the Internet because of his or her difficulties in face-to-face (FtF) relational communication. Substituting the electronic medium may either help or hinder the individual's interpersonal relationships depending on how he or she uses the technology. One option, widely discussed in the popular press a few years ago, is to replace social action of any kind with nonsocial use of the Internet, such as seeking information, playing games, and so forth. In this case, the Internet may be the culprit that many people feel it is, one that exacerbates social withdrawal. On the other hand, the socially withdrawn person might use the Internet to find friends, perhaps in chat rooms. If used in this way, the electronic medium might actually enhance relationships, to the extent, of course, that the individuals befriended in the chat rooms are genuine and not there to exploit in some way the people they meet. It is also conceivable that the socially withdrawn person may be able to use e-mail to extend and enhance his or her limited network of acquaintances, perhaps helping these relationships develop into true friendships. This beneficial effect might occur, for example, if an individual knows what to say to a friend but feels anxious doing so FtF.

On the other hand, a socially withdrawn person might live in a place where Internet access and electronic communication have become almost universal. In this situation, being able to use electronic communication to extend and enhance relationships initiated FtF is a general expectation and a vital social skill. Socially withdrawn individuals might be at a disadvantage in this situation if they are not skilled in using electronic communication for the types of relationship communication that the socially competent members of their social circles practice. Unfortunately, little is known at this point about the extent to which individuals lacking in FtF social skills are also deficient in the analogous skills in electronic communication. In an innovative study conducted with university undergraduates, Brunet and Schmidt (2007) paired university undergraduates with other participants with whom they were not acquainted. The dyads exchanged conversation for 10 minutes in two conditions: with and without a live webcam. Participants who rated themselves as shy engaged in little self-disclosure when the webcam was in use; there were no significant differences between shy participants and others during free chat without the webcam. These results suggest that shyness is context-dependent, and that the specific features of electronic communication may help or hinder interpersonal communication by shy people.

Of course, the socially withdrawn person still has the option of "withdrawing" into nonsocial uses of the Internet, such as online games, sites providing information about some subject of interest, and so forth. In any case, the implications of electronic communication for the social lives of shy, withdrawn people might elude any research study in which the different applications of the Internet are not separated.

INDIVIDUAL DiFFERENCES AS PREDICTORS OF RELATIONSHIP FORMATION ONLINE

Individual differences in disposition and self-efficacy beliefs may determine reasons for Internet usage and its effects (LaRose, Eastin, & Gregg, 2001).

The "rich get richer" hypothesis (Kraut et al., 1998) predicts that the Internet is used primarily by extraverts to expand their network of contacts. In contrast, the "social compensation" hypothesis (e.g., Hamburger & Ben-Artzi, 2000) maintains that introverts, lonely, depressed, and socially anxious people are drawn to the Internet to compensate for their anxieties during offline social interaction. In turn, their preference for virtual communication may exacerbate their personal problems (research useful in evaluating these contradictory positions is discussed later). People who are socially anxious report that they find forging and maintaining relationships with others easier online than in person (McKenna & Bargh, 2000). The anonymity of online relationships, especially in their early stages, may reduce inhibition, because online communicators may feel that they are shielded from the consequences of disclosing personal information (McKenna & Bargh, 2000). This anonymity allows individuals to manipulate their self-presentations with ease, often to the point of online identity "experimentation" (e.g., Valkenburg, Schouten, & Peter, 2005), which is discussed in greater detail later. The shy adolescents interviewed by Henderson, Zimbardo, Smith, and Buell (2000) indicated that they preferred to talk about personal and emotional issues online to a greater degree than do nonshy students. Maczewski (2002) proposed that ineffectual, powerless youth can use the Internet to their benefit to assume a more powerful stance in their interpersonal interactions. Thus, electronic communication can make it easy to avoid intimacy, if that is what one wants to do. However, if one's goal is to pursue a relationship to a stage of heightened intimacy, the Internet can permit the necessary relational communication even if geography and circumstances make FtF contact difficult.

THE PSYCHOLOGICAL FEATURES
OF ELECTRONIC COMMUNICATION

The Internet creates a unique psychological environment for its users. McKenna, Green, and Gleason (2002) suggested four major factors that differentiate between Internet and FtF interactions: (1) greater anonymity; (2) decreased importance of physical appearance; (3) greater control; and (4) capacity to find similar others.

Greater Anonymity

Many websites allow surfers to move around freely, without disclosing any personal information. In fact, even when people do divulge personal information on the Net, they still subjectively feel relatively anonymous (McKenna & Bargh, 2000; McKenna et al., 2002). The "online disinhibition effect" results in a sense of anonymity that frees people from social norms in their physical environment and reduces personal inhibitions (Joinson, 2007; Suler, 2004a). On the Internet, surfers frequently share personal information with one another, including individuals totally unknown to them, whom they are unlikely to come across again. This has been compared to the "strangers on a train phenomenon" (Z. Rubin, 1975), in which people share personal information with fellow travelers, strangers whom they have no likelihood of seeing again (Barak & Gluck-Ofri, 2007; Bargh, McKenna, & Fitzsimmons, 2002; Joinson, 2007). The relative anonymity of the Internet may reduce the inhibitions of socially anxious, shy users. Socially anxious children are known to believe that others regard them disapprovingly and will probably rebuff their bids for social interchange (e.g., Banerjee & Henderson, 2001). This maladaptive belief may have less effect on social overtures if the person contacted has little knowledge of the individual initiating the contact.

Decreased Importance of Physical Appearance

Physical appearance significantly influences the ways a person is perceived and judged by others. One factor in their judgment is as a result of the "*halo effect*" (Asch, 1946), a phenomenon whereby one positive characteristic of a person leads observers to believe that other positive characteristics are present (e.g., an attractive person may be perceived as possessing superior personality traits), whereas people who are physically unappealing are frequently judged unfavorably on unrelated issues. Online social interactions are typically text-based; consequently, participants' physical characteristics remain unknown. This may appeal to people with unattractive physical characteristics or visible disabilities, who are likely to suffer from prejudice and discrimination in FtF interactions. Because socially anxious people may be prone to poor body image, as has been demonstrated in at least one study with university students (Izgic, Akyuz, Dogan, & Kugu, 2004), the unimportance of physical appearance may attract socially anxious children and adolescents to electronic communication. Online, they have an opportunity to present themselves in any way they choose (Suler, 2004b). In some cases, this may lead to deception.

Greater Control

One of the unique features of Internet communication is that participants can explore the world and meet exotic strangers from the safety and comfort of their own homes. Internet users feel that they are in greater control of their social interactions, because they can easily escape from an interaction, remain unidentified, and experience a subjective sense of privacy (Madell &

Muncer, 2007). Perceived lack of control has been shown to relate to social anxiety, at least in adults (Rapee, 1997).

Capacity to Find Similar Others

The need to "belong" is one of the significant needs in Maslow's (1971) hierarchy. For individuals, being a member of a group that shares goals and interests is likely to enhance self-esteem (Tajfel & Turner, 1986), which in turn is an important factor in overall well-being (Branden, 1969). The Internet is an extremely effective tool for discovering like-minded others due to the vast numbers of people online and the efficient search facilities. This is particularly relevant to people who belong to stigmatized or minority groups, since they frequently experience difficulties both in locating similar others offline and finding opportunities to interact with them FtF. Both of these challenges are made easier in cyberspace. Indeed, as McKenna et al. (2002) pointed out, once one finds similar others, group identification frequently develops faster online than offline. Perhaps the Internet helps shy, withdrawn individuals connect with each other, share, and overcome their difficulties in interacting with others.

Together, these different features form a highly protected environment for the Net surfer. The security that comes from this anonymity is likely to encourage Internet users to express themselves more freely online than in their offline interactions. In other words, they may well feel freed from their usual, undeviating offline persona and be able to express aspects of themselves online that they are unable to articulate in FtF interactions. This may result in their displaying a huge variety of behaviors on the net. For example, an individual may produce social skills that he or she was unable or possibly too shy to engage in offline, or may even exhibit extremely uninhibited, aggressive behavior both within the protected Net environment.

CONNECTING INDIVIDUALS' ONLINE AND OFFLINE WORLDS

Kraut et al. (1998) expressed many people's greatest fear regarding the Internet, when they argued that the Internet is an isolated environment that has a negative impact on our "real world." Despite this negative outlook, there appear to be increasing instances when the reverse is true, when skills acquired in cyberspace may impact the offline world in a positive way. Below we discuss two major examples of the process of transformation from the Internet to the offline environment. In the first, individuals discover and shape their identity online before bringing it offline. In the second, people meet and form a relationship in cyberspace and later move it offline. Making the transition between the two may be particularly important for socially withdrawn users. Electronic communication may be very helpful to them in establishing social contacts. However, and despite the fact that online-only relationships do exist, it has yet to be demonstrated that a relationship that remains limited to electronic media is as rewarding as an FtF friendship.

Identity Construction

The Internet's secure environment may help young people to find an answer to the all-pervasive question "Who am I?" Erikson (1968) suggested that this is the most important question with which adolescents deal. He believed that identity may be effectively constructed through the use of games. Turkle (1995) argued that Internet identity games help to bring about psychological maturity. This maturity is achieved by being able to discover different aspects of the self and experiencing flexible transitions between the different identities.

There has been one recent empirical study of the possible consequences of Internet identity games for socially anxious young people. Valkenburg and Peter (2008), working with a large sample of 10- to 17-year-olds in the Netherlands, found that socially anxious participants were slightly (but not significantly) more likely than others to engage in identity experiments. Loneliness was, however, a significant predictor of identity experimentation. Contrary to common impressions, these researchers found that the use of identity experiments to communicate with a wide range of different people was linked with *greater* social competence in general.

Turkle (1995) believes that the Internet supplies an individual with space, warmth, safety, and understanding. This is, in fact, a similar setting to that provided by psychotherapy, so that both the Internet and the psychotherapy room may create a safe environment in which to rework elements from the past and try out different alternatives for the present and the future. In addition, the Internet supplies an environment that helps to create a "time-out" for the individual, so it can serve as a moratorium, as was recommended by Erickson for adolescents in our society (Turkle, 2004).

One of unique components in Jung's (1939) personality theory is the understanding that the personality comprises opposites that together can create a significant whole. The concept of opposites is common in Eastern philosophy as, for example, demonstrated in the Taoist symbols of yin and yang, which stand for a complex of inexorable opposites. According to Jung, opposites produce a tension, creating the psychic energy that enables life to exist. Jung believed the danger that lies in one side expresses itself so strongly that the opposing side is prevented from expressing itself in a satisfactory way.

Amichai-Hamburger (2005a) suggested that the Internet environment, because of the protection it provides, may be the place where many people feel comfortable to express their less dominant sides. He focused mainly on introverts as an example of the types of person who may use the Internet to express their opposite, in this case, extraverted, side. Maldonado, Mora, Garcia, and Edipo (2001) evaluated computer-mediated messages and found that introverted subjects send messages with an extraverted tone. Their messages contained more information than those sent by extraverted subjects. It seems that on the Net, introverts do not act in accordance with their usual behavior patterns, instead, due to the secure environment, conducting themselves in ways associated with extraverts in offline relationships (see also Amichai-Hamburger, Wainapel, & Fox, 2002).

The anonymity of the Net, and the feelings of safety it brings, provide opportunities for people to discuss topics that may be awkward or even taboo offline. Magid (1998) found that older children are much more likely than younger children to use chat rooms and online forums to discuss relationships and sexual activity. Stern (2002) believes that the Internet provides a forum for teenage girls to express themselves as they undergo social and sexual changes in their lives. As well as providing a place for such discussions, the Internet was also found to be a place where teenagers sought advice, information, and support around socially taboo topics (Subrahmanyam, Greenfield, & Tynes, 2004; Suzuki & Calzo, 2004; Gray, Klein, Noyce, Sessellberg, & Cantrill, 2005).

When someone identifies with a group that is negatively perceived by the surrounding society, this may seriously impact the person's self-esteem (Tajfel & Turner, 1986). This may be particularly true in the case of hidden or stigmatized groups in which people's group identity is not obvious. In such cases, group members may not only experience difficulties in locating other like-minded people but may also be exposed to hearing others, for example, work colleagues, expressing negative stereotypes against their group, unaware that they work with someone from this stigmatized group. This too adds to their low self-esteem (Frable, 1993). The Internet can be a very helpful tool for such people. Finding the similar others is straightforward on the Net and can be done without embarrassment or exposure. Moreover, researchers claim that the support and positive reinforcement experienced online by such group members may actually encourage them to "come out" in the offline world (McKenna & Bargh, 1998).

For the members of Generation X (i.e., people born during the "baby bust" in North America from the 1960s to the 1980s), the Internet was initially presented as a futuristic and mysterious concept, whereby communication between two or more computers was possible through a phone line. Initially, people's online behavior was generally similar to their offline activities, for example, writing e-mails instead of sending letters. However, for Web-savvy children growing up in the era of the Internet, a distinct virtual existence is very possible. Their borders between online and offline worlds can appear blurred at times. Livingstone and Bovill (2001) argue that the online activity of young people (ages 9–19) cannot be separated from their offline lives, both because they construct and experiment with their identities, and because of otherwise separate offline activities, such as talking to friends on the same day using instant messages, the phone, FtF, and Facebook. Valentine and Holloway (2002) concur that children (ages 5–16) use the Internet to construct private and public identities, just as they do in the offline environment.

FORMING FRIENDSHIPS ONLINE

For many people, the Internet is an excellent medium through which to meet people and in some cases start romantic relationships that may eventually become FtF meetings. Friendships and intimate relationships evolve through the development of disclosure and mutual trust (Jourard, 1971). Offline, this gradual revelation may develop over a long period, the exception being those who meet as strangers, with no intention of forming a relationship or even meeting again, "the strangers on a train phenomenon" (Z. Rubin, 1975). As discussed later in this chapter, forming and maintaining rewarding friendships with socially competent peers is an important challenge for socially withdrawn children and youth, one at which they often do not succeed.

The process of meeting in cyberspace may be seen as much more akin to "the strangers on a train phenomenon" than the usual gradual emergence of intimacy seen in the FtF world. This is due to the cyberspace environment, with its opportunities to "disappear off the train" into oblivion, coupled with protection that allows for anonymity. This results in speedier self-disclosure than is found in the offline world (McKenna et al., 2002; Ben-Ze'ev, 2005). Indeed, accelerated and increased self-disclosure is typical in virtual interpersonal relationships (e.g., Joinson & Paine, 2007). This self-disclosure tends to be reciprocated (Barak & Gluck-Ofri, 2007).

In many situations in the offline world, physical impressions are crucial (e.g., Fiske & Taylor, 1991). This puts individuals who belong to stigmatized social groups (e.g., those with physical disabilities) at a major disadvantage. Such people may find it easier to meet others in an environment where they can control how they wish to be portrayed. The Internet provides such an environment where interaction is text-based, physical cues are limited, and individuals are free to choose whom they wish to interact with and when (e.g. Ben-Ze'ev, 2005; McKenna et al., 2002).

Simulation experiments have been used successfully to understand the differences between online and offline communication by adults; we are aware of no similar studies with children or adolescents. McKenna et al. (2002, Study 3) assigned undergraduates randomly in cross-sex pairs. The pairs were to meet initially either FtF or in an Internet chat room. After the meeting, those who had met in online chat rooms more often reported feeling that they knew the other person better and liked him or her more than did participants who had met FtF. This effect was retained when participants met their original dating partner on two further separate occasions, over the Internet and FtF. It is important to add that participants were unaware that they were meeting with the same partner FtF and online.

McKenna et al. (2002) describe online dating sites as a "relatively non-threatening environment" in which people who experience shyness, social anxiety, or a lack of social skills can feel free to meet others without the fear of instant rejection. Internet dating has been found to improve individuals' well-being by reducing feelings of loneliness and depression, and also providing social support and encouraging openness among users (Valkenburg et al., 2006; Valkenburg & Peter, 2007a, 2007b).

There are some individuals who, because of their social inhibitions, experience major anxieties and in some cases feel unable to communicate with a potential partner FtF. Amichai-Hamburger and Furnham (2007) proposed a four-stage process to help such people gradually combat their social anxiety in the FtF interactions. The stages include (1) text-based interaction only, (2) text and video (via live webcam), (3) audio and video, and (4) FtF interaction. Amichai-Hamburger, McKenna, and Azran (2008) argue that this process illustrates the power of the Internet, for not only can people learn new social skills and use them to interact online, they can also utilize their new proficiency in FtF interactions. This theoretical model currently awaits application in intervention studies.

Peter, Valkenburg, and Schouten (2006) proposed a model to explain how introverted people, presumably including shy, withdrawn children and adolescents, form friendships online. Included in the model are several links established in previous research: Introverted people self-disclose online more than others and use electronic communication more than others. Introverts are also motivated to turn to online communication to compensate for social communication deficits they encounter in FtF interactions. This social compensation motive also leads to greater online self-disclosure, regardless of one's introversion. Peter et al. found empirical support for the path model in a study with 600 Dutch participants ages 9–18 years. Their data also confirmed that girls self-disclose more than boys online. Older adolescents communicated more online than the younger participants in the study, but younger participants formed more friendships online. Unfortunately, in this one-wave, cross-sectional study, the brief questionnaires provided little specificity about the modalities of online communication used by the participants.

What might be the quality and stability of online friends? Schneider, Coplan, Amichai-Hamburger, Tessier, Vitoroulis, Miller, Koszycki, Flament, Baiocco, Laghi, d'Alessio, Lohan, Hudson, and Rapee are currently conducting a large-scale longitudinal study with early adolescents in Canada, Italy, and Australia to compare both the stability and quality of online and offline friendships. Their study will also provide data about the reasons for the termination of the friendships and the predictors of long-term survival of relationships conducted on- and offline. This is important, because many of the studies to date (and those discussed in this chapter) have considered only relationship quality, not relationship stability. Mesch and Talmud (2007), in an interview study of Israeli adolescents, found that the respondents felt less close to their online friendships. Their data did not elucidate the reasons for this. It is possible that online relationships do not weather the "test of time" very well; if there is a conflict, the relationship can be easily "turned off." Furthermore, the physical indicators of closeness are, of course, not available online at moments of difficulty in the relationship.

None of the studies noted thus far considered the similarity of the friends contacted online in terms of physical features or psychological makeup. This is an important consideration, especially in the study of the friendships of socially withdrawn children and adolescents. Although these children and youth do indeed have friendships that are not totally devoid of rewarding qualities, many of their friends are themselves socially withdrawn to a certain degree (Rubin, Wojslawowicz, Rose-Krasnor, Booth-LaForce, & Burgess, 2006; Schneider, 1999). This is not surprising given the well-known homophily process in friendships: People of all ages tend to select others who are similar to themselves as friends. Although it is heartening that socially withdrawn children and youth do have some friends, they may not have friends who can help them practice age-appropriate social skills or integrate into the larger social groups that surround the friendship dyads.

There is reason to believe that homophily is less important for friendships formed online than for those formed FtF, especially in schools. The greater willingness to befriend peers who are somewhat dissimilar may stem from the absence of cues online that would indicate many aspects of similarity. In their study featuring home interviews with almost 1,000 Israeli adolescents, Mesch and Talmud (2007) found that homophily was far less evident in online than in offline relationships. Thus, electronic communication may be helpful to socially anxious, withdrawn children and youth in two dissimilar ways: forming friends with other socially anxious children and youth (due to the facilitation of contact with similar others, discussed earlier), and forming friends with others who are more socially competent (due to the decreased importance of physical indicators of homophily).

EXISTING STUDIES WITH SOCIALLY
WITHDRAWN CHILDREN AND YOUTH

As discussed earlier, most research to date consists of "one-shot" correlational studies that cannot elucidate authoritatively the long-run costs and
benefits of Internet use. Many of these studies have included data on social
anxiety, social withdrawal, and depression or loneliness. Despite their limitations, these studies are useful as a starting point.

According to the Youth Internet Safety Survey (Wolak, Mitchell, &
Finkelhor, 2006), conducted by telephone in the United States, youth who
reported depressive symptoms use the Internet more frequently than others and use the Internet more extensively to disclose personal information
and feelings. In a study by Gross, Juvonen, and Gable (2002) with seventh
graders in California, lonely and socially anxious participants were found
to use the Internet more often for relational communication than others. In
contrast with other studies, Gross (2004), who studied logs of instant messages sent by California high school students over a 4-day period, found no
significant correlations between Internet use and measures of psychological
adjustment (depression, loneliness, social anxiety). Many of the participants
had developed online friends. Gross concluded that Internet use is becoming
so normative that differences between online and offline social communication are starting to disappear. Similarly, Amichai-Hamberger (2005b) predicted that many individual differences in Internet use and its consequences
will disappear as use extends to the majority of the populace in many societies. Thus, data collected even a few years ago may already be outdated.
Furthermore, it is very possible that with time, young people will change
their relative frequencies of use of the different applications of the medium
(for gaming, information gathering, meeting new people, communicating
with people already known, etc.).

In one of the most important studies published to date on the implications of electronic communication for the friendships of young people,
Valkenburg and Peter (2007a) considered the possible effects of social anxiety. Their analysis of data obtained from 794 Dutch participants ages 10–16
years revealed that social anxiety predicted electronic relational communication. Importantly, online communication predicted closeness to friends.
Socially anxious participants tend to communicate online, which, in turn,
leads to closeness in relationships with friends. These findings illustrate the
potential benefit of electronic relational communication for socially withdrawn, anxious children and adolescents, and may dispel some common
fears about the potential harm of this technology. Importantly, the benefits
were only evident for participants who used electronic communication with
friends they already had rather than with strangers. It should be noted that

chat room and messaging were not differentiated, and that the design was cross-sectional rather than longitudinal.

A more specific study with adolescents in the Netherlands yields a somewhat different picture of the possible effects (and antecedents) of electronic communication. Importantly, though, this study did not include measures of social anxiety or loneliness, making the results applicable only to the general population. Working with 663 young people ages 12–15 years old, van den Eijnden, Meerkerk, Vermulst, Spijkerman, and Engels (2008) used questionnaires that differentiated among the major electronic communication media—instant messaging, e-mail, and chat rooms. They employed a two-wave longitudinal design and found that instant messenger use predicted depressive feelings 6 months later. Structural equation modeling suggested that instant messenger use more likely caused the depressive feelings than vice versa. However, loneliness was linked to *reduced* instant messenger use at Time 2, perhaps because lonely young people develop a maladaptive, avoidant interpersonal style. The use of e-mail and participation in chat rooms were unrelated to either loneliness or depressive feelings.

In a longitudinal study in Toronto, Canada, Blais, Craig, Pepler, and Connolly (2008) explored the relationship implications of Internet use by 884 adolescents ages 14–18 years. Instant messaging was correlated positively with the quality of both best-friend and romantic relationships. However, visiting chat rooms and participating in online games were negative predictors of friendship qualities. Again, participant characteristics, such as social withdrawal or social anxiety, were not considered in this study. Interestingly, friendship quality was studied both in this Canadian research and in the Dutch study by Valkenberg and Peter (2007b); in both cases, some forms of electronic communication emerged as positive correlates of friendship quality. Nevertheless, this conclusion can only be considered very tentative until far more data become available. Clearly, it is much too early to conclude that electronic communication is good or bad for relationships or adjustment, either for socially withdrawn individuals or for the general population.

Space permits us to mention only these recent, influential studies. However, previous research has yielded similar discrepancies, perhaps due to variations in the independent and dependent measures. Thus, despite the contributions of the studies to date, many glaring gaps remain. The studies we have discussed include use of data about social anxiety, loneliness, and introversion among the variables to discover the predictors of electronic relational communication and/or its consequences. Useful as this may be, these correlational analyses of population data would be complemented quite usefully by a more specific focus on the extreme group of participants known to be experiencing difficulty because of social withdrawal. To remedy this, an anxiety clinic sample is included in the ongoing international longitudinal study of electronic communication, friendship formation, friendship dissolution, and friendship quality by Schneider and colleagues cited earlier. That study also includes a longitudinal follow-up of the friendships in which participants are involved. This is important, because many of the benefits children and adolescents derive from their friendships may depend on friendship bonds that endure long enough for intimacy and social support to crystallize.

ELECTRONIC VICTIMIZATION OF SOCIALLY WITHDRAWN CHILDREN

Sadly, it is very possible that the electronic communication experience of many socially withdrawn children and adolescents may include being victimized by cyberbullies. About one-third of the teenagers interviewed as part of the Pew Internet and American Life Project in 2007 reported being bullied on line, with unwanted disclosure of private information being the most common form of cyberbullying. Although there appears to be no research on the cyberbullying of socially withdrawn children or adolescents specifically, it has been found that individual roles in online bullying are often the same as those in bullying behavior in person (Raskauskas & Stoltz, 2007). Thus, because socially withdrawn children and adolescents are known to be frequent victims of *in vivo* bullies at school (e.g., Schwartz, 2000), they may well be among the typical victims of cyberbullies. Empirical confirmation that depressed adolescents tend to be singled out as victims by cyberbullies (Ybarra, 2004) provides some findings in a separate but not unrelated area of psychological symptomatology.

There has also been some concern that electronic communication may make socially withdrawn adolescents more prone to victimization by people they do not know. Gross et al. (2002) found that introverted adolescents are more likely than others to communicate with strangers over the Internet; this was not replicated by Peter, Valkenburg, and Schouten (2006).

FUTURE DIRECTIONS

Antecedents of Online Relating

In many existing studies, online relational communication is studied as an isolated phenomenon. In many others, personality characteristics such as introversion–extraversion have been considered as determinants of relationship behavior online. Researchers are only beginning to study the "real-world" processes that may determine how people relate online. In a groundbreaking study, Ledbetter (2009) discovered that young adults from families in which conversation is warm and lively, and young people are encouraged to participate, have the closest friendships. Both online and FtF relational communication were found to mediate the link between home life and friendship quality. Some research has established that dimensions of parenting such as parental warmth, control, and encouragement are linked to social withdrawal in childhood (e.g., Coplan, Arbeau, & Armer, 2008). Therefore, studies with children and adolescent participants that parallel Ledbetter's may be very revealing.

Gender and Cultural Differences

The limited data available at this stage do very little to elucidate the specific possibilities the Internet offers to shy, withdrawn people of different genders and cultures. Electronic communication must be understood in light of broader gender and cultural differences. Suler (2004a) argues that women, in particular, benefit from being able to reframe their identities and self-definition online, especially in patriarchal societies, where they would have difficulty doing so using other media. Boneva, Kraut, and Frohlich (2001) observed that men and women in Western societies tend to use the Internet in different ways. Women and girls express emotions more extensively online and generally use e-mail more often. Men and boys, however, use electronic communication in more instrumental ways, such as setting times for contacts with friends and associates or gathering information related to recreational pursuits. In many cultures with strong gender role distinctions, parents and peers may provide greater support to boys than to girls in learning to use technology. Vekiri and Chronaki (2008) found that female elementary school pupils perceived less parental and peer support than did boys for becoming proficient with electronic technology.

Electronic communication also provides unique opportunities for self-expression in societies where direct expression of emotion is discouraged. Kamibeppu and Suguira (2005) conducted a questionnaire study with Japanese early adolescents. Socially effective students used the Internet or cell phones to expand and consolidate existing relationships with others in close proximity. This phenomenon may apply more strongly in Japan than elsewhere (the "rich get richer" hypothesis is discussed later in this chapter). Kamibeppu and Suguira describe many cases of pathological Internet addiction among Japanese youth. They also describe the use of electronic communication as a criterion for inclusion in the circle of popular peers: Groups of popular children exclude potential group members who do not have cell phones or access to the Internet.

Ishii and Ogasahara (2007) compared the functions of online communities in Korea and Japan in a survey study with adults. In Korea, most online communities are made up of people who know each other in real life. Unique virtual communities are prevalent in Japan. Ishii and Ogasahara interpret the results as indicating cultural differences between Japan and Korea, with Japanese adults avoiding the expression of emotion FtF. Parallel findings have been reported for Internet use in various ethnic communities in the United States. For example, Matei and Ball-Rokeach (2003) found evidence of cultural differences in their study of adults in Los Angeles who were members of seven diverse ethnic communities. Participants of Korean and Japanese origin were far more likely than others to have close relationships maintained exclusively online.

Many other cultural differences in the relationship implications of electronic communication remain to be explored. It is not unimaginable that electronic communication may actually have some effect on the core features of some societies. For example, in cultures with little tolerance for diversity, the Internet may become a vehicle for members of minority groups to contact each other and achieve greater social success and satisfaction. As is known by totalitarian regimes that block access to certain Internet sites, the Internet has the potential to make exercise of absolute authority more difficult for authority figures. This could change the nature of societies in which authority figures are highly revered (known as cultures high in "power distance" in Hofstede's [1983] schema). Finally, since children and adolescents may acquire electronic communication skills faster than do adults, electronic communication may promote the development of more distinct children's or adolescents' cultures in societies where the extended family has been the most important social unit.

Moving beyond Self-Report and Other Methodological Improvements

Researchers studying electronic communication are beginning to tackle the methodological problems they share with colleagues in any field where self-report data predominate. Questionnaire and survey methods, whether completed on paper or, less often, online have become the mainstay of research in this area. Self-reporting in this area of inquiry is a logical method: The respondent knows best about his or her online communication. However, the problems inherent in questionnaire research are the same as those in paper-and-pencil methods to study any other relationship phenomenon. First of all, the respondent may wish to convey to the researcher impressions that are socially desirable. Second, study participants who complete a questionnaire at a single point of time may not accurately remember or accurately portray the events occurring over a longer period of time. Their responses may be affected by their mood at the moment; this may be particularly troublesome in probes of participants' loneliness or anxiety.

In the vast majority of studies to date, the questionnaire responses are used in correlational analyses of data obtained at a single point in time. There are many problems with this strategy, although it is by no means easy for researchers to improve on it. The newspaper headlines in 1998 that proclaimed to the world the Internet was causing people to be lonely were based on a one-shot correlational study by Kraut et al. (1998). Even the journalists who commented on that contention a few days later were aware that, as is made clear in any basic textbook on research methods, correlations cannot indicate the direction of causation: Any correlation between Internet use and loneliness, for example, may indicate that either Internet use causes loneliness or that people who are lonely already start to use the Internet more than others (see Amichai-Hamburger & Ben-Artzi, 2003). Furthermore, it is possible that some other variable might explain the connection, if any, between loneliness and Internet use. Along these lines, with supporting data obtained from university students, Caplan (2007) argued that the correlation between Internet use and loneliness is spurious, because social anxiety probably explains both loneliness and Internet use. Thus, even if the current dependence on self-report measures continues, studies featuring more than one time point and more comprehensive measurement of "outcome" will hopefully increase.

Another important consideration is the researcher's selection of the applications of electronic communication to be measured. Many of the early studies were based on the amount of time the study participants spent online. That variable, of course, obscures the many possible uses of the Net. Many more recent studies focus on participants' use of the many tools available online. In gauging the effects of electronic communication on socially withdrawn individuals, it makes an enormous difference, of course, whether a participant spends time avoiding relationships by gathering information about his or her favorite performer or sports hero, or uses chat rooms to meet potential friends. Thus, researchers from now on should be looking at how and why shy, withdrawn children and adolescent use the Internet, not how much they log on. In one of the most-quoted lines in this literature, McKenna and Bargh (2000, p. 1) remarked that "the Internet by itself is not a main effect cause of anything."

Synthesizing the Database

Although the scope of this chapter does not permit complete cataloguing of studies on the purported benefits and dangers of electronic communication, we did find and report many contradictions among the results of studies that superficially appear quite similar. As the database evolves and expands, it will become more possible and surely more profitable to review data judiciously using the most sophisticated techniques in data synthesis, such as statistical meta-analysis. In this way, systematic patterns in the data may emerge, resolving some of the contradictions and replication failures.

Diverse Technologies

The scope of the technology studied by a researcher may also affect the conclusions. At the moment this chapter was written, the Internet tends to be used for different relationship-building and relationship-maintaining functions from the cellular phone. Kim, Kim, Park, and Rice (2007), in a study with Korean adults, showed that cell phone short message services are used to expand and consolidate existing relationships; e-mail is used to establish and develop new contacts and to deepen relationships. This may change, however, as more communication functions, including e-mail, are incorporated into cellular phones. The iPhone, introduced in 2008, combines the functions of the Internet and the cell phone in a package that appeals widely to young people.

Developmental Differences

Finally, it is important to remember that developmental issues are essentially ignored by researchers studying the relationship implications of electronic communication. As time goes on, electronic communication is being used by younger children and adolescents. A U.S. Census Bureau Population survey in 2001 (*www.census.gov/prod/2001pubs/p23-207.pdf*) indicated that 24% of 5-year-olds used the Internet regularly, with the proportion of Internet users exceeding 50%, starting at age 9; the percentages have probably increased since the date of that report. The visual appearance of webpages is increasingly being adapted to the tastes of younger users. It is commonly perceived that children and adolescents use electronic communication far more extensively than do adults to form and maintain relationships. This is not an illogical contention, because electronic communication has been available to today's younger generation during the developmental phases in which people learn to relate with others. Nevertheless, there has been little speculation or research about possible age differences in the extent or ways that electronic communication is used to relate. Much more data are available about electronic communication by adults than by children or adolescents. As in any other area of inquiry, there are many problems in extrapolating the results of research with adults to form conclusions about the social behavior of children and adolescents. Therefore, more research must be designed to compare the implications of electronic communication for different age groups, including younger children who are increasingly relating to others online.

CONCLUSION

The current literature contains a number of useful correlational studies suggesting that the Internet harms, helps, and has no effect on the social relationships, adjustment, and feelings of belonging of children and adolescents. Some, but not all, of the more recent and comprehensive studies tend to indicate a correlation between Internet use and greater involvement in relationships. Therefore, in contrast with earlier impressions in the popular press, current research and theory tend not to confirm that the Internet is damaging the current younger generation in any way. Nevertheless, the correlational data are difficult to interpret. The prevailing opinion seems to be that electronic communication tends to be used by individuals who are already socially competent to expand and deepen their social relationships. Electronic communication, then, is used now the way written letters and messages were used in the past, and the way landline telephones are still used. This, of course, would mean that socially withdrawn children and adolescents are left out regardless of the modality of contact. This has yet to be confirmed in a specific study targeting this group. Such targeted studies should become an important priority for research.

Nevertheless, even more focused descriptive studies cannot demonstrate that the full potential of electronic communication in helping withdrawn, anxious children and youth has been realized. To do that, scholars will have to move beyond studying how children and adolescents tend to use electronic communication. They will have to introduce and evaluate interventions in which the participants are taught how to communicate optimally online to form satisfying relationships in a safe context that may sometimes be continued in person. There is no reason why that social skill cannot be taught and learned like any other.

REFERENCES

Alfano, C. A., Beidel, D. C., & Turner, S. M. (2006). Cognitive correlates of social phobia among children and adolescents. *Journal of Abnormal Child Psychology, 34,* 189–201.

Amichai-Hamburger, Y. (2005). Personality and the Internet. In Y. Amichai-Hamburger (Ed.), *The social net: Human behavior in cyberspace* (pp. 27–55). New York: Oxford University Press.

Amichai-Hamburger, Y. (2005a). Internet minimal group paradigm. *Cyberpsychology and Behavior, 8,* 140–142.

Amichai-Hamburger, Y. (Ed.). (2005b). *The social net: Human behaviour in cyberspace.* New York: Oxford University Press.

Amichai-Hamburger, Y., & Ben-Artzi, E. (2003). Loneliness and Internet use. *Computers in Human Behavior, 19,* 71–80.

Amichai-Hamburger, Y., & Furnham, A. (2007). The positive Net. *Computers in Human Behavior, 23,* 1033–1045.

Amichai-Hamburger, Y., McKenna, K. Y. A., & Azran, T. (2008). Internet empowerment. *Computers in Human Behavior, 24,* 1776–1789.

Amichai-Hamburger, Y., Wainapel, G., & Fox, S. (2002). "On the Internet no one knows I'm an introvert": Extroversion, neuroticism and Internet interaction. *CyberPsychology and Behavior, 5,* 25–28.

Asch, S. (1946). Forming impressions of personality. *Journal of Abnormal and Social Psychology, 41,* 258–290.

Banerjee, R., & Henderson, L. (2001). Social-cognitive factors in child social anxiety: A preliminary investigation. *Social Development, 10,* 558–571.

Barak, A., & Gluck-Ofri, O. (2007). Degree and reciprocity of self-disclosure in online forums. *CyberPsychology and Behavior, 10,* 407–417.

Bargh, J. A., McKenna, K. Y. A., & Fitzsimons, G. M. (2002). Can you see the real me?: Activation and expression of the "true self" on the Internet. *Journal of Social Issues, 58,* 33–48.

Ben-Ze'ev, A. (2005). "Deattachment": The unique nature of online romantic relationships. In Y. Amichai-Hamburger (Ed.), *The social net: The social psychology of the internet* (pp. 115–138). New York: Oxford University Press.

Blais, J., Craig, W. M., Pepler, D. J., & Connolly, J. (2008). Adolescents online: The importance of Internet activity choices to salient relationship. *Journal of Youth and Adolescence, 37,* 49–58.

Branden, N. (1969). *The psychology of self-esteem.* New York: Bantam.

Boneva, B., Kraut, R., & Frohlich, D. (2001). Using e-mail for personal relationships: The difference gender makes. *American Behavioral Scientist, 45,* 530–549.

Brown, M., King, E., & Barraclough, B. (1995). Nine suicide pacts: A clinical study of a consecutive series 1974–1993. *British Journal of Psychiatry, 167,* 448–451.

Brunet, P. M., & Schmidt, L. A. (2007). Is shyness context specific?: Relation between shyness and online self-disclosure with and without a webcam in young adults. *Journal of Research in Personality, 41,* 938–945.

Caplan, S. E. (2007). Relations among loneliness, social anxiety, and problematic Internet use. *CyberPsychology and Behavior, 10,* 234–241.

Coplan, R. J., Arbeau, K. A., & Armer, M. (2008). Don't fret, be supportive!: Maternal characteristics linking child shyness to psychosocial and school adjustment in kindergarten. *Journal of Abnormal Child Psychology, 36,* 359–371.

Doring, N. (2002). Personal homepages on the Web: A review of research. *Journal of Computer Mediated Communication, 7*(3). Retrieved October 2004 from *www.ascusc.org/jcmc/vol7/issue3/doering.html.*

Enochsson, A. B. (2001). *Meningen med webben: en studie om internetsokning utifranerfarenheter I en fjardeklass.* Linkopings: Institutionen for utbildnings-vetenskap.

Erikson, E. H. (1968). *Identity: Youth and crisis.* New York: Norton.

Fiske, S. T., & Taylor, S. E. (1991). *Social cognition.* New York: McGraw-Hill.

Fogel, J. S. M., Albert, F., Schnabel, B. A., Ditkoff, A., & Neugut, I. (2002). Use of the Internet by women with breast cancer. *Journal of Medical Internet Research, 4,* e9.

Frable, D. E. S. (1993). Being and feeling unique: Statistical deviance and psychological marginality. *Journal of Personality, 61,* 85–110.

Gray, N. J., Klein, J. D., Noyce, P. R., Sessellberg, T. S., & Cantrill, J. A. (2005). Health information-seeking behaviour in adolescence: The place of the Internet. *Social Science and Medicine, 60,* 1467–1478.

Greenfield, P. M. (2004). Developmental considerations for determining appropriate Internet use guidelines for children and adolescents. *Journal of Applied Developmental Psychology, 25,* 751–762.

Gross, E. F. (2004). Adolescent Internet use: What we expect, what teens report. *Applied Developmental Psychology, 25,* 633–649.

Gross, E. F., Juvonen, J., & Gable, S. L. (2002). Internet use and well-being in adolescence. *Journal of Social Issues, 58,* 75–90.

Hamburger, Y. A., & Ben-Artzi, E. (2000). The relationship between extraversion and neuroticism and the different uses of the Internet. *Computers in Human Behavior, 16,* 441–449.

Henderson, L., Zimbardo, P., Smith, C., & Buell, S. (2000). Shyness and technology use in high school students. Retrieved from *www.shyness.com.*

Hofstede, G. (1983). Dimensions of national cultures in fifty countries and three regions. In J. Deregowski, S. Dzuirawiec, & R. Annis (Eds.), *Explications in cross-cultural psychology* (pp. 335–355). Lisse, the Netherlands: Swets & Zeitlinger.

Hymel, S., Franke, S., & Freigang, R. (1985). Peer relationships and their dysfunction: Considering the child's perspective. *Journal of Social and Clinical Psychology, 3,* 405–415.

Inderbitzen-Pisaruk, H., Clark, M. L., & Solano, C. H. (1992). Correlates of loneliness in midadolescence. *Journal of Youth and Adolescence, 21,* 151–167.

Ishii, K., & Ogasahara, M. (2007). Links between real and virtual networks: A comparative study of online communities in Japan and Korea. *CyberPsychology and Behavior, 10,* 252–257.

Izgic, F., Akyuz, G., Dogan, O., & Kugu, N. (2004). Social phobia among university students and its relation to self-esteem and body image. *Canadian Journal of Psychiatry, 49,* 630–634.

Joinson, A. N. (2007). Disinhibition and the Internet. In J. Gackenbach (Ed.), *Psychology and the Internet: Intrapersonal, interpersonal and transpersonal implications* (2nd ed., pp. 76–92). San Diego: Elsevier Academic Press.

Joinson, A. N., & Paine, C. B. (2007). Self-disclosure, privacy and the Internet. In A. N. Joinson, K. Y. A. McKenna, T. Postmes, & U.-D. Reips (Eds.), *Oxford handbook of Internet psychology* (pp. 237–252). Oxford, UK: Oxford University Press.

Jourard, S. M. (1971). *Self-disclosure: An experimental analysis of the transparent self.* New York: Wiley.

Jung, C. G. (1939). *The integration of the personality.* New York: Farrar & Rinehart.

Kamibeppu, K., & Sugiura, H. (2005). Impact of the mobile phone on junior high-school students' friendships in the Tokyo metropolitan area. *CyberPsychology and Behavior, 8,* 121–130.

Kim, H., Kim, G. J., Park, H. W., & Rice, R. E. (2007). Configurations of relation-ships in different media: FtF, email, instant messenger, mobile phone, and SMS. *Journal of Computer-Mediated Communication, 12*(4), article 3. Retrieved February 2nd, 2009, from *jcmc.indiana.edu/vol12/issue4/kim.html.*

Kraut, R., Kiesler, S., Bonever, B., Cummings, J., Helgeson, V., & Crawford, A. (2002). Internet paradox revisited. *Journal of Social Issues, 58,* 49–74.

Kraut, R., Lundmark, V., Patterson, M., Kiesler, S., Mukopadhyay, T., & Scherlis, W. (1998). Internet paradox: A social technology that reduces social involve-ment and psychological well-being. *American Psychologist, 53,* 1017–1031.

LaRose, R., Eastin, M., & Gregg, J. (2001). Reformulating the Internet paradox: Social cognitive explanations of Internet use and depression. *Journal of Online Behavior, 1*(2). Available from *www.behavior.net/job/v1n2/paradox.html.*

Ledbetter, A. M. (2009). Family communication patterns and relational mainte-nance and behaviour: Direct and mediated associations with friendship close-ness. *Human Communication Research, 35,* 130–147.

Lenhart, A., Rainie, L., & Lewis, O. (2001). *Teenage life online: The rise of the instant-message generation and the internet's impact on friendships and fam-ily relationships.* Washington, DC: Pew Internet & American Life Project. Retrieved September 8, 2009 from *www.pewinternet.org/Reports/2001/Teen-age-Life-Online.aspx.*

Livingstone, S., & Bovill, M. (2001). *Children and their changing media environ-ment: A European comparative study.* London: Erlbaum.

Livingstone, S., & Bober, M. (2003). *UK children go online: Listening to young people's experiences.* London School of Economics, Department of Media and Communication. Retrieved URL October, 2003 from *www.children-goonline. net.*

Maczewski, M. (2002). Exploring identities through the Internet: Youth experiences online. *Child and Youth Care Forum, 31,* 111–129.

Madell, D. E., & Muncer, S. J. (2007). Control over social interactions: An impor-tant reason for young people's use of the Internet and mobile phones for com-munication. *CyberPsychology and Behavior, 10,* 137–140.

Magid, L. J. (1998). *Child safety on the information highway.* National Center for Missing and Exploited Children. Retrieved from *www.safekids.com/child_ safety.htm.*

Maldonado, G. J., Mora, M., Garcia, S., & Edipo, P. (2001). Personality, sex and computer comunication mediated through the Internet. *Anuario de Psicologia, 32,* 51–62.

Maslow, A. (1971). *The farther reaches of human nature.* New York: Viking Press.

Matei, S., & Ball-Rokeach, S. (2003). The Internet in the communication infrastructure of urban residential communities: Macro- or mesolinkage? *Journal of Communication, 53*, 642–657.

McKenna, K. Y. A., & Bargh, J. A. (1998). Coming out in the age of the internet: Identity "demarginalization" through virtual group participation. *Journal of Personality and Social Psychology, 75*, 681–694.

McKenna, K. Y. A., & Bargh, J. A. (2000). Plan 9 from Cyberspace: The implications of the Internet for personality and social psychology. *Personality and Social Psychology Review, 4*(1), 57–75.

McKenna, K. Y. A., Green, A. S., & Gleason, M. J. (2002). Relationship formation on the Internet: What's the big attraction? *Journal of Social Issues, 58*, 9–32.

Mesch, G. S., & Talmud, I. (2007). Similarity and the quality of online and offline social relationships among adolescents in Israel. *Journal of Research in Adolescence, 17*, 455–466.

Peter, J., Valkenburg, P. M., & Schouten, A. P. (2006). Characteristics and motives of adolescents talking with strangers on the Internet. *CyberPsychology and Behavior, 9*, 526–530.

Rapee, R. M. (1997). Perceived threat and perceived control as predictors of the degree of fear in physical and social situations. *Journal of Anxiety Disorders, 11*, 455–461.

Rapee, R. M., & Heimberg, R. G. (1997). A cognitive-behavioral model of anxiety in social phobia. *Behaviour Research and Therapy, 35*, 741–756.

Raskauskas, J., & Stoltz, A. D. (2007). Involvement in traditional and electronic bullying among adolescents. *Developmental Psychology, 43*, 564–575.

Rice, R. E. (2001). Primary issues in Internet use: Access, civic and community involvement, and social interaction and expression. In L. A. Lievrouw & S. Livingstone (Eds.), *The handbook of new media* (pp. 105–129). London: Sage.

Rubin, K. H., & Asendorpf, J. (Eds.) (1993). *Social withdrawal, inhibition and shyness in childhood*. Hillsdale, NJ: Erlbaum.

Rubin, K., & Burgess, K. B. (2001). Social withdrawal and anxiety. In M. W. Vasey & M. R. Dodds (Eds.), *The developmental psychopathology of anxiety* (pp. 407–434). Oxford, UK: Oxford University Press.

Rubin, K. H., & Coplan, R. J. (2004). Paying attention to and not neglecting social withdrawal and social isolation. *Merrill–Palmer Quarterly, 50*, 506–534.

Rubin, K. H., Wojslawowicz, J. C., Rose-Krasnor, L., Booth-LaForce, C., & Burgess, K. B. (2006). The best friendships of shy/withdrawn children: Prevalence, stability, and relationship quality. *Journal of Abnormal Child Psychology, 34*, 143–157.

Rubin, Z. (1975). Disclosing oneself to a stranger: Reciprocity and its limits. *Journal of Experimental Social Psychology, 11*, 233–260.

Schneider, B. H. (1999). A multimethod exploration of the friendships of children considered socially withdrawn by their school peers. *Journal of Abnormal Child Psychology, 27*, 115–123.

Schwartz, D. (2000). Subtypes of victims and aggressors in children's peer groups. *Journal of Abnormal Child Psychology, 28*, 181–192.

Spence, S. H., Donovan, C., & Toussaint, M. (1999). Social skills, social outcomes, and cognitive features of childhood social phobia, *Journal of Abnormal Psychology, 108,* 211–221.

Stern, S. (2002). Sexual selves on the World Wide Web: Adolescent girls' home pages assites for sexual self-expression. In J. D. Brown, J. E. Steele, & K. Walsh-Childers (Eds.), *Sexual teens, sexual media: Investigating media's influence on adolescent sexuality* (pp. 265–285). Mahwah, NJ: Erlbaum.

Subrahmanyam, K., Greenfield, P. M., & Tynes, B. (2004). Constructing sexuality and identity in an online teen chat room. *Journal of Applied Developmental Psychology, 25,* 651–666.

Suler, J. (2004a). The online disinhibition effect. *CyberPsychology and Behavior, 7,* 321–326.

Suler, J. (2004b). The psychology of text relationships. In R. Kraus, J. Zack, & G. Stricker (Eds.), *Online counseling: A handbook for mental health professionals* (pp. 19–50). San Diego: Elsevier Academic Press.

Sullivan, H. S. (1953). *Conceptions of modern psychiatry.* New York: W. W. Norton.

Suzuki, L. K., & Calzo, J. P. (2004). The search for peer advice in cyberspace: An examination of online teen bulletin boards about health and sexuality. *Journal of Applied Developmental Psychology, 25,* 658–698.

Tajfel, H., & Turner, J. C. (1986). The social identity theory of inter-group behavior. In S. Worchel & L. W. Austin (Eds.), *Psychology of intergroup relations* (pp. 7–24). Chicago: Nelson-Hall.

Turkle, S. (1995). *Life on the screen: Identity in the age of the Internet.* New York: Simon & Schuster.

Turkle, S. (2004). Whither psychoanalysis in computer culture? *Psychoanalytic Psychology, 21,* 16–30.

Valentine, G., & Holloway, S. L. (2002). Cyberkids?: Exploring childen's identities and social networks in online and offline worlds. *Annals of the Association of American Geographers, 92*(2), 302–319.

Valkenburg, P. M., & Peter, J. (2007a). Preadolescents' and adolescents' online communication and their closeness to friends. *Developmental Psychology, 43,* 267–277.

Valkenburg, P. M., & Peter, J. (2007b). Online communication and adolescent well-being: Testing the stimulation versus the displacement hypothesis. *Journal of Computer-Mediated Communication, 12,* 1169–1182.

Valkenburg, P. M., & Peter, J. (2008). Adolescents' identity experiments on the Internet: Consequences for social competence and self-concept unity. *Communication Research, 35,* 208–231.

Valkenburg, P. M., Peter, J., & Schouten, A. P. (2006). Friend networking sites and their relationship to adolescents' well-being and social self-esteem. *Cyberpsychology and Behavior, 9,* 584–590.

Valkenburg, P. M., Schouten, A. P., & Peter, J. (2005). Adolescents' identity experiments on the internet. In *New Media and Society, 7,* 383–402.

van den Eijnden, R. J. J. M., Meerkerk, G.-J., Vermulst, A. A., Spijkerman, R., & Engels, R. C. M. E. (2008). Online communication, compulsive Internet use, and psychosocial well-being among adolescents: A longitudinal study. *Developmental Psychology, 44,* 655–665.

Vekiri, I., & Chronaki, A. (2008). Gender issues in technology use: Perceived social support, computer self-efficacy and value beliefs, and computer use beyond school. *Computers and Education, 51,* 1392–1404.

Wolak, J., Mitchell, K., & Finkelhor, D. (2006). *Online victimization of youth: Five years later.* Alexandria, VA: National Center for Missing and Exploited Children.

Ybarra, M. L. (2004). Linkages between depressive symptomatology and Internet harassment among young regular Internet users. *CyberPsychology and Behavior, 7,* 247–257

Ybarra, M. L., Kiwanuka, J., Emenyonu, N., & Bangsberg, D. R. (2006). Internet use among Ugandan adolescents: Implications for HIV intervention. *PLoS Medicine, 3,* 2104–2112.

12

"Once Upon a Time There Were a Blushful Hippo and a Meek Mouse"

A Content Analysis of Shy Characters in Young Children's Storybooks

ROBERT J. COPLAN
KATHLEEN HUGHES
HILARY CLAIRE ROWSELL

"Shyness" is typically described as wariness in the face of social novelty and perceived social evaluation (Rubin, Coplan, & Bowker, 2009). Although shy children may desire social interaction, this social approach motivation is simultaneously inhibited by social fear and anxiety (Coplan, Prakash, O'Neil, & Armer, 2004). Shyness has been historically "understudied," particularly in comparison to constructs such as aggression and other externalizing problems (Rubin & Asendorpf, 1993; Rubin & Coplan, 2004). However, as evidenced by this very volume, recent years have witnessed a steep increase in the study of childhood shyness.

This steady swell in research attention has also likely contributed to an accompanying "rise in awareness" about shyness in parents, teachers, and the media. For example, 25 years ago, it was argued that shyness in early childhood was largely ignored in the classroom by teachers, who, if anything, might encourage such behaviors as a means of maintaining order in the classroom (e.g., Rubin, 1982). More recently, results from a number of studies have indicated that teachers spend increased time with shy children at school, view shyness as having negative consequences, and are just as likely to intervene to assist shy versus aggressive children (Arbeau

& Coplan, 2007; Coplan & Arbeau, 2008). In addition, parents (Rubin & Mills, 1992) and even young children (Coplan, Girardi, Findlay, & Frohlick, 2007) now seem to perceive shyness as a problem.

Recent years have also witnessed overall increased efforts by social scientists to engage in "knowledge translation," which involves the communication of relevant empirical research results to relevant stakeholders (e.g., parents, teachers, politicians). Notwithstanding, "nonacademic" sources, such as the media, remain major forces for the communication of ideas to parents and children (e.g., Anderson et al., 2003).

In this chapter, we explore how the construct of *shyness* has been portrayed in a form of media that is readily available for young children—picture storybooks. We proceeded under the assumption that parents of young, shy children might seek out age-appropriate storybooks with shy central characters. Our goal was to examine the overall *message* that parents and children might be receiving about shyness when they sit down together to read such a storybook together.

INFLUENCE OF CHILDREN'S STORYBOOKS

For decades, storybook reading has been a favorite pastime of parents and young children (Clark, Guilmain, Saucier, & Tavarex, 2003). Along with enhancing the intellectual development of young children (e.g., Senechal, Pagan, Lever, & Ouellette, 2008), storybooks provide a context for children to learn about social roles, expectations, and values, including desirable emotions, appropriate social-communicative skills, and the importance of emotional self-regulation (Cooper, 2007; Tsai, Louie, Chen, & Uchida, 2007).

Content analyses of children's books can be found on a wide range of topics, from the depiction of gender (Clark et al., 2003) and race (Mullen, 2004) to the challenges of starting school (Dockett, Perry, & Whitton, 2006) and the loss of a pet (Corr, 2003). Researchers have also begun to focus on the portrayal of themes related to children's "socioemotional functioning," including autism (Dyches, Prater, & Cramer, 2001), stuttering (Bushey & Martin, 1988), and bullying (Gregory & Vessey, 2004). For example, in their study of the descriptions of bullying in children's books, Oliver, Young, and LaSalle (1994) reported that violence was the most common reaction depicted in response to bullying, followed by avoidance. In contrast, positive resolution was found to be an infrequent response.

However, our review of the literature did not reveal any previous studies that provided a qualitative description of the portrayal of shy storybook characters. The manner in which shy characters are depicted in storybooks can be viewed as a conduit for transmitting information about shyness to parents and young children. We were particularly interested in information that might influence parents' understanding and beliefs about the origins and nature of shyness (e.g., trait vs. state) and how shyness is generally manifested (e.g., emotions, behaviors). We also sought to explore the implicit and explicit portrayal of attitudes and responses toward shyness (e.g., others' reactions to shyness; shyness as a problem). Finally, we examined representations of interventions and outcomes (e.g., changes in the shy character; antecedents of such changes). For each of these categories, we evaluated the "accuracy" of each of these storybook representations of shyness through comparison with relevant theory and data from extant published psychological literature.

METHODOLOGY

Selection of Books

Our inclusion criteria for book selection were as follows: (1) a storybook with a narrative; (2) a central character described as "shy" (or a related term); (3) appropriate for preschool-age children (ages 4–6 years); and (4) accessible via local libraries, children's bookstores, or common book-selling websites (e.g., Amazon). After an extensive search, we were able to obtain books ($N = 20$) that met these criteria. This sample size is comparable to other, recent content analysis studies of children's storybooks (e.g., Clark & Fink, 2004).

Not surprisingly, the distribution of publication years was heavily weighted with books from the last 20 years, primarily due to many older books being out of print (thus, not available). Of the 20 books included, 12 (60%) were published between 2000 and 2008, 5 (25%) between 1990 and 1999, 2 (10%) from 1980 to 1989, and 1 (5%) in 1946. In addition to differences in publication dates, the books varied in terms of length (from 8 to 40 pages) and format (e.g., hard vs. soft cover, paper vs. board pages). A complete listing of the books can be found in Appendix 12.1.

Coding the Data

We developed a coding scheme for the content of the storybooks using an iterative process that included multiple coders. This protocol was based upon earlier procedures for developing coding schemes to analyze the content of children's literature (e.g., LaDow, 1976; Weitzman, Eifer, Holeada, & Ross, 1972).

The first set of coding categories assessed the *depictions* of shyness. This included the demographic characteristics of the shy character (e.g., animal vs. person, gender), descriptions of the origins of shyness (e.g., stable trait vs. changeable state), types of situations that provoke shyness, as well as the behaviors and feelings of shy characters. We were also interested in how the *implications* of shyness were implicitly and explicitly portrayed. Accordingly, we coded the quality (positive, neutral, negative) of words used to describe shy characters, how shy characters felt about their own shyness, how others (i.e., parents, teachers, peers) responded to shy characters, and whether shyness was presented as causing social difficulties. The final category assessed *outcomes and changes* in shyness. In this regard, we coded whether shy characters changed at all (i.e., became less shy) and the presented "causes" of this change. A complete copy of the coding scheme is available from the authors.[1]

RESULTS OF CONTENT ANALYSES

In terms of the presentation of results, we focused primarily on descriptive statistics and frequencies. Where appropriate, we also conducted chi-square analyses and Cochran's Q tests (used to compare the frequency distribution of related variables).

Depictions of Shyness

In 45% of the books, the shy character was a person; in remaining books, the shy character was an animal. The gender distribution of the characters was relatively even, with 60% of the shy characters being male. We noted that this representation was consistent with previous empirical results demonstrating a *lack* of sex differences in the prevalence or frequency of shyness and related constructs (Rubin et al., 2009).

In 11 books that specifically addressed this issue, shyness was significantly more likely to be described as a stable personality *trait*, with origins in early childhood. For example, shy characters were described as "born that way," being shy "as long as she can remember," or in the case of Buster (a shy dog), as "shy ever since he was a puppy." In comparison, in only one book, was shyness presented as a later emerging response to a specific situation (e.g., "He used to talk to the neighbor but won't anymore").

In terms of stability across *situations*, almost two-thirds of the storybooks depicted the main character as being shy in more than one social context (e.g., at home and at school). It was most common for the characters to be shy in *novel* social settings (e.g., meeting a new person) and in situations where they felt they were being socially *evaluated* (e.g., answering questions in class, performing in front of others). Other contexts that elicited shy responses included instances of social difficulty (e.g., being teased), as well as a number of nonspecific (but typically familiar) social contexts (e.g., going shopping; playing with other children that he or she knows).

Social withdrawal (e.g., "running away" or "hiding" from social situations) was the most frequently described shy *behavior*. About half of the books also depicted other shy behaviors, including physiological responses (e.g., blushing, heart pounding), gaze aversion (e.g., looking down at shoes), speech reticence (e.g., not speaking in class), and automanipulatives (e.g., finger biting; hair twirling). In terms of emotional response, shy characters were also almost equally characterized as displaying either fear/anxiety (e.g., "felt scared to play with others") or self-consciousness/embarrassment (e.g., "afraid that everyone would watch and laugh at her"). In a few cases, the shy character was also described (or portrayed in a picture) as feeling physically sick (e.g., nauseous).

These findings suggest that parents and children are presented with a mostly "accurate" depiction of the nature of shyness in these storybooks. For example, shyness was generally presented as a characteristic that appears early in childhood and is stable across time (Kagan, Snidman, Kahn, & Towsley, 2007) and situations (Coplan, DeBow, Schneider, & Graham, in press). Consistency across time and contexts is often cited as a defining quality of a personality trait (Asendorpf & van Aken, 1991). Moreover, these books also portrayed the (somewhat complex) notion that there are both stable individual differences in shyness and specific contexts that evoke shy behavior—including unfamiliar situations and situations that require one to be the center of attention (Buss, 1986).

Consistent with the psychological literature, shy children were also described as tending to withdraw from social situations (e.g., Coplan et al., 2004) but when faced with social contact, to respond by blushing, avoiding eye contact, refraining from speaking, and appearing anxious (e.g., Crozier, 2001; Evans, 1987). As well, the portrayal of shyness as evoking both fearful and self-conscious emotions is consistent with the two most common "forms" of shyness discussed by researchers and theorists (i.e., fearful vs. self-conscious shyness; Buss, 1986). Thus, overall, we viewed these storybooks as presenting a fairly complex and nuanced portrayal of shyness that is quite consistent with the extant psychological literature.

Implications of Shyness

Shy characters were described using terms coded as carrying a *neutral* (e.g., shy, quiet) or *negative* valence (e.g., "shrinking," "cowardly") in all books except one. This remaining book contained the only instances of using *positive* words (e.g., "hopeful," "mindful," and "thoughtful") to describe the shy. This ambivalent-to-negative evaluation of shyness was also mirrored in the *self-perceptions* and attitudes of the shy characters themselves. In the

14 books in which this issue was explicitly addressed, shy characters were significantly more likely to be portrayed as unhappy with and wanting to change their shyness (e.g., "wished that she wasn't so shy"; "wanted to be more like his more outgoing friend") than as accepting or talking positively about their shyness (e.g., "accepts that he is shy"). In addition, in 80% of the books, the shy character explicitly experienced problems with social relationships. This occurred significantly, most often as difficulties in peer relations (e.g., teased at school), followed by problems with parents (e.g., "fights with his mom, disappoints his dad") then with teachers (e.g., "does not answer the teacher").

Particularly when considered within the context of a storybook for young children, these results represent quite a negative portrayal of shyness. Such a depiction provides further support for the well-established notion that shyness is not positively valued in Western societies (Rubin et al., 2009). Moreover, the storybook depictions refer to the most frequently described socioemotional difficulties associated with shyness in the psychological literature. For example, shy characters were generally portrayed as being unhappy with themselves, supporting empirical research linking shyness with negative self-regard (e.g., Coplan, Findlay, & Nelson, 2004; Crozier, 1995). Shy young children are also at an increased risk for experiencing peer rejection, exclusion, and even victimization in their peer relationships (Gazelle & Ladd, 2003; Perren & Alsaker, 2006), as well as less positive relationships with teachers (Arbeau, Coplan, & Weeks, in press; Rydell, Bohlin, & Thorell, 2005). In addition, parents tend to respond negatively to and are more often angry or embarrassed by their children's shyness (Coplan, Prakash, et al., 2004; Rubin & Mills, 1992).

There is growing evidence to suggest that shyness is a greater risk factor for boys than for girls during childhood and adolescence. For example, shy boys are more likely than shy girls to be excluded and rejected by peers (e.g., Coplan, Prakash, et al., 2004). As well, mothers tend to respond more negatively to shy behaviors in boys than in girls (e.g., Stevenson-Hinde, 1989). It has been argued that these findings arise from shyness being viewed as more socially acceptable in girls and less tolerable in boys in Western cultures (Rubin & Coplan, 2004). With this in mind, we sought to determine whether a similar gender "bias" might be reflected in the portrayal of shy male versus female characters in the storybooks. Accordingly, we computed a variable representing the *severity* of the social difficulties that the shy characters experienced. Results from a comparison between genders indicated that shy *male* characters were depicted to experience significantly more pervasive social adjustment difficulties than were shy *female* characters.

We can only speculate about the "intentionality" of the storybook authors in these gendered depictions. We concede that it is possible that authors were aware of the growing number of psychological studies suggesting this gender difference (Rubin et al., 2009) and sought to accurately represent these events in the texts. However, we would suggest that this differential pattern of responses to shy boys and girls emerged less intentionally and was instead reflective of the authors own "real-world" experiences with such children.

A similar notion was forwarded by Arcus (1989), who reported that shy cartoon characters in Disney films were more likely than their more outgoing counterparts to be rendered with blue eyes. Although the nature of this association is not well understood, shy white children are more likely to have blue eyes than brown eyes (Coplan, Coleman, & Rubin, 1998; Rosenberg & Kagan, 1987; Rubin & Both, 1989). Arcus (1989) postulated that the illustrators of these characters may have been (subconsciously) influenced by their own personal experiences with blue-eyed shy children.

Outcomes and Change

By the end of the storybooks, almost all of the shy characters (90%) had undergone a notable *change*. Most frequently, this change came in the form of becoming less shy (e.g., "became more comfortable," "stopped blushing," "became brave enough," "finds the courage to talk"). In three other cases, the shy child became more accepted by friends and family members (e.g., "Other kids liked him and thought it was cool"; "His friend lets him know he's got lots of other positive characteristics besides being shy").

Finally, we examined the *reasons* (i.e., circumstances, experiences, people) why story characters became less shy. Various agents of change were described. However, in 85% of the books, either parents (e.g., support and encouragement) and/or peers (e.g., the formation of new friendships) were depicted as contributing toward this change. The experience of a positive social event (e.g., going to a party and everyone was nice) and overcoming a challenge (e.g., helping another peer in distress) were also presented as putative reasons for children becoming less shy.

These "happy endings" represent a stark contrast when considered against the backdrop of the storybook portrayals of shyness as a stable trait associated with a wide range of socioemotional difficulties. It should not come as a surprise that authors would create positive endings to storybooks intended for young children. Yet these ending suggest to parents (and their preschoolers) that shyness is readily "changeable." The implications of such a conclusion are varied. On the one hand, results from research related to implicit theories of personality suggest that individuals with "incremental" self-theories of personality (i.e., not stable, subject to change) are more likely to pursue such change actively with regard to undesirable characteristics they possess (e.g., Erdley, Cain, Loomis, Dumas-Hines, & Dweck, 1997; Molden & Dweck, 2006). However, the notable changes in shyness portrayed in storybooks may also foster unrealistic expectations in children and parents in terms of how easily and quickly shyness might be altered.

Notwithstanding, the storybooks did portray a representative account of *how* shy individuals may be influenced to change. Both parents and peers have been implicated as factors that may lead to changes in the stability and outcomes of childhood shyness (Rubin et al., 2009). As well, despite the limited research related to early intervention and prevention techniques in this area (Greco & Morris, 2001), some success has been noted in the use of both parents (e.g., Rapee, Kennedy, Ingram, Edwards, & Sweeney, 2005) and peers (Coplan, Schneider, DeBow, & Graham, 2009) as promoters of positive outcomes for extremely shy children.

SOME CLOSING THOUGHTS

Our goal in this chapter was to explore how shyness is generally portrayed in young children's storybooks. We were particularly interested in the messages that parents and their children may receive after reading preschoolers' books about shy characters. After completing a content analysis of the depiction of these shy characters, the overriding message for parents and children can be summarized as follows:

1. Shyness is a personality trait with origins in early childhood that is stable across time and contexts. Shyness is most often displayed in response to social novelty and in situations of perceived social evaluation.
2. Shy children tend to withdraw from social situations. However, when they are unable to avoid social contact, shy children tend to blush, avoid eye contact, refrain from speaking, and are more likely to feel fearful, worried, and embarrassed.
3. Shy children feel less positive about themselves and tend to experience difficulties in their social relationships with family, friends, and teachers. Moreover, it is particularly problematic to be a shy boy.
4. Almost all shy children can change in a relatively short period of time. The best way to elicit this change is to seek help and support from parents and friends.

We noted two particularly striking aspects of this overall portrayal of shyness. To begin with, storybook authors are providing a complex and nuanced portrayal of shyness that is remarkably consistent with the current state of theoretical and empirical knowledge in the psychological sciences (Rubin et al., 2009). However, the one aspect of this depiction that varies from the extant empirical literature is that shyness is relatively easy to change. As described earlier, this latter representation regarding change may suggest both positive and negative messages for readers. However, it must be acknowledged that the nature of the change depicted in these books was far from uniform. Indeed, no two books depicted change in shy children identically, and the changes described could be characterized as being of greater (e.g., becoming outgoing at school) or smaller magnitude (speaking to one other character).

Some potentially intriguing possibilities for future research arise from our findings. For example, children's storybooks represent only one type of media that may depict shy characters. Researchers may also consider an exploration of the portrayal of shyness in other media, such as movies, television, novels of fiction, and the Internet.

It is also currently unknown whether portrayals of shyness in children's literature (or other forms of media) directly affect child and parental attitudes toward shyness. Researchers could examine such attitudes and beliefs both before and after exposure to storybooks (which could themselves be modified to project differing messages about the nature and implications of shyness). Indeed, the use of such storybooks could become integrated into early intervention and prevention programs, which may help to create even more "happy endings" for shy children.

REFERENCES

Anderson, C. A., Berkowitz, L., Donnerstein, E., Huesmann, L. R., Johnson, J. D. & Linz, D. (2003). The influence of media violence on youth. *Psychological Science in the Public Interest, 4,* 81–110.

Arbeau, K. A., & Coplan, R. J. (2007). Kindergarten teachers' beliefs and responses to hypothetical prosocial, asocial, and antisocial children. *Merrill–Palmer Quarterly, 53,* 291–318.

Arbeau, K. A., Coplan, R. J., & Weeks, M. (in press). Shyness, teacher–child relationships, and socio-emotional adjustment in grade 1. *International Journal of Behavioural Development.*

Arcus, D. (1989). Vulnerability and eye color in Disney cartoon characters. In J. S. Reznick (Ed.), *Perspectives on behavioral inhibition* (pp. 291–297). Chicago: University of Chicago Press.

Asendorpf, J. B., & van Aken, M. A. (1991). Correlates of the temporal consistency of personality patterns in childhood. *Journal of Personality, 59,* 689–703.

Bushey, T., & Martin, R. (1988). Stuttering in children's literature. *Language, Speech, and Hearing Services in Schools, 19,* 235–250.

Buss, A. H. (1986). A theory of shyness. In W. H. Jones, J. M. Cheek, & S. R. Briggs (Eds.), *Shyness: Perspectives on research and treatment* (pp. 39–46). New York: Plenum Press.

Clark, R., & Fink, H. (2004). A multicultural feminist analysis of picture books for children. *Youth and Society, 36,* 102–126.

Clark, R., Guilmain, J., Saucier, P. K., & Tavarex, J. (2003). Two steps forward, one step back: The presence of female characters and gender stereotyping in award winning picture books between the 1930s, and the 1960s. *Sex Roles, 49,* 439–449.

Cooper, P. M. (2007). Teaching young children self-regulation through children's books. *Early Childhood Education Journal, 34,* 315–322.

Coplan, R. J., & Arbeau, K. A. (2008). The stresses of a brave new world: Shyness and adjustment in kindergarten. *Journal of Research in Childhood Education, 22,* 377–389.

Coplan, R. J., Coleman, B., & Rubin, K. H. (1998). Shyness and Little Boy Blue: Iris pigmentation, gender, and social wariness in preschoolers. *Developmental Psychology, 32,* 37–44.

Coplan, R. J., DeBow, A., Schneider, B. H., & Graham, A. (in press). The social behaviors of extremely inhibited children in and out of preschool. *British Journal of Developmental Psychology.*

Coplan, R. J., Findlay, L. C., & Nelson, L. J. (2004). Characteristics of preschoolers with lower perceived competence. *Journal of Abnormal Child Psychology, 32,* 399–408.

Coplan, R. J., Girardi, A., Findlay, L. C., & Frohlick, S. L. (2007). Understanding solitude: Young children's attitudes and responses towards hypothetical socially withdrawn peers. *Social Development, 16,* 390–409.

Coplan, R. J., Prakash, K., O'Neil, K., & Armer, M. (2004). Do you "want" to play?: Distinguishing between conflicted-shyness and social disinterest in early childhood. *Developmental Psychology, 40,* 244–258.

Coplan, R. J., DeBow, A., Schneider, B. H., & Graham, A. (2009). *"Play skills" for shy children: Preliminary effectiveness of a social skills-facilitated play intervention program for extremely inhibited preschoolers.* Manuscript currently under review.

Corr, C. A. (2003). Pet loss in death related literature for children. *Omega: Journal of Death and Dying, 48,* 389–414.

Crozier, W. R. (1995). Shyness and self-esteem in middle childhood. *British Journal of Educational Psychology, 65,* 85–95.

Crozier, W. R. (2001). Blushing and the exposed self: Darwin revisited. *Journal of the Theory of Social Behaviour, 31,* 61–72.

Dockett, S., Perry, B., & Whitton, D. (2006). Picture storybooks and starting school. *Early Child Development and Care, 176,* 835–848.

Dyches, T. T., Prater, M. A., & Cramer, S. F. (2001). Characterization of mental retardation and autism in children's books. *Education and Training in Mental Retardation and Developmental Disabilities, 36,* 230–243.

Erdley, C. A., Cain, K. M., Loomis, C. C., Dumas-Hines, F., & Dweck, C. S. (1997). Relations among children's social goals, implicit personality theories, and responses to social failure. *Developmental Psychology, 33,* 263–272.

Evans, M. A. (1987). Discourse characteristics of reticent children. *Applied Psycholinguistics, 8,* 171–184.

Gazelle, H., & Ladd, G. W. (2003). Anxious solitude and peer exclusion: A diathesis–stress model of internalizing trajectories in childhood. *Child Development, 74,* 257–278.

Greco, L. A., & Morris, T. L. (2001). Treating childhood shyness and related behavior: Empirically evaluated approaches to promote positive social interactions. *Clinical Child and Family Psychology Review, 4,* 299–318.

Gregory, K. E., & Vessey, J. A. (2004). Bibliotherapy: A strategy to help students with bullying. *Journal of School Nursing, 20,* 127–133.

Kagan, J., Snidman, N., Kahn, V., & Towsley, S. (2007). The preservation of two infant temperaments into adolescnce. *Monographs of the Society for Research in Children Development, 72,* 76–91.

LaDow, M. (1976). *A content analysis of selection picture books examining the portrayal of sex roles and representation of males and females.* East Lansing, MI: National Center for Research on Teacher Learning.

Molden, D. C., & Dweck, C. S. (2006). Finding "meaning" in psychology: A lay theories approach to self-regulation, social perception, and social development. *American Psychologist, 61,* 192–203.

Mullen, B. (2004). Sticks and stones can break my bones, but ethnophaulisms can alter the portrayal of immigrants to children. *Personality and Social Psychology Bulletin, 30,* 250–262.

Oliver, R., Young, T. A., & LaSalle, S. M. (1994). Early lessons in bullying and victimization: The help and hindrance of children's literature. *The School Counselor, 42,* 137–146.

Perren, S., & Alsaker, F. D. (2006). Social behavior and peer relationships of victims, bully-victims, and bullies in kindergarten. *Journal of Child Psychology and Psychiatry, 47,* 45–57.

Rapee, R., Kennedy, S., Ingram, M., Edwards, S., & Sweeney, L. (2005). Prevention and early intervention of anxiety disorders inhibited preschool children. *Journal of Consulting Clinical Psychology, 73,* 488–497.

Rosenberg, A., & Kagan, J. (1987). Iris pigmentation and behavioral inhibition. *Developmental Psychobiology, 20,* 377–392.

Rubin, K. H. (1982). Nonsocial play in preschoolers: Necessarily evil? *Child Development, 533,* 651–657.

Rubin, K. H., & Asendorpf, J. B. (1993). *Social withdrawal, inhibition and shyness in childhood.* Hillsdale, NJ: Erlbaum.

Rubin, K. H., & Both, L. (1989). Iris pigmentation and sociability in childhood: A re-examination. *Developmental Psychobiology, 22,* 1–9.

Rubin, K. H., & Coplan, R. J. (2004). Paying attention to and not neglecting social withdrawal and social isolation. *Merrill–Palmer Quarterly, 50,* 506–534.

Rubin, K. H., Coplan, R. J., & Bowker, J. (2009). Social withdrawal in childhood. *Annual Review of Psychology, 60,* 11.1–11.31.

Rubin, K. H., & Mills, R. S. L. (1992). Parents' ideas about the development of aggression and withdrawal. In I. Sigel, J. Goodnow, & A. McGillicuddy-deLisi (Eds.), *Parental belief systems* (pp. 41–68). Hillsdale, NJ: Erlbaum.

Rydell, A. M., Bohlin, G., & Thorell, L. B. (2005). Representations of attachment to parents and shyness as predictors of children's relationships with teachers and peer competence in preschool. *Attachment and Human Development, 7,* 187–204.

Senechal, M., Pagan, S., Lever, R., & Ouellette, G. P. (2008). Relations among the frequency of shared reading and 4-year-old children's vocabulary, morphological and syntax comprehension, and narrative skills [Special issue: Parent–Child Interaction and Early Literacy Development]. *Early Education and Development, 19,* 27–44.

Stevenson-Hinde, J. (1989). Behavioral inhibition: Issues of context. In J. S. Reznick (Ed.), *Perspectives on behavioral inhibition* (pp. 125–138). Chicago: University of Chicago Press.

Tsai, J. L., Louie, J. Y., Chen, E. E., & Uchida, Y. (2007). Learning what feelings to desire: Socialization of ideal affect through children's storybooks. *Personality and Social Psychology, 33,* 17–30.

Weitzman, L., Eifer, D., Holcada, E., & Ross, C. (1972). Sex-roles socialization in picture books for preschool children. *American Journal of Sociology, 77,* 1125–1150.

---

[1]Interrater reliability was initially established between two raters based on coding of half the books in the sample. Overall, interrater agreement was 86%. The two researchers then independently coded the remaining books in the sample. Interrater reliability for the second half of the books was 89%.

APPENDIX 12.1. LIST OF CHILDREN'S STORYBOOKS INCLUDED IN THE STUDY

1. Baguley, E. & Pedler, C. (2008). *Little Pip and the rainbow wish.* Intercourse, PA: Good Books. (24 pp)
2. Bechtold, L. (1999). *Buster: The very shy dog.* Boston: Houghton Mifflin. (15 pp)
3. Best, C. (2001). *Shrinking Violet.* New York: Farrar, Straus & Giroux. (24 pp)
4. Broyles, A. (2000). *Shy mama's Halloween.* Gardiner, ME: Tilbury House. (37 pp)
5. Cain, B. (1999). *I don't' know why ... I guess I'm shy.* Washington, DC: Magination Press. (29 pp)
6. Dierssen, A. (2003). *Timid Timmy.* New York: North–South Books. (24 pp)
7. Goldsmith, H. (1998). *Shy little turtle.* New York: McGraw-Hill. (30 pp)
8. Hargreaves, R. (1981). *Little Miss Shy.* New York: Price Stern Sloan. (31 pp)
9. Hood, S. (2000). *Tyler is shy.* Montreal: Reader's Digest Children's Books. (31 pp)
10. Lawrence, E. (2002). *Shy little moth.* Hauppauge, NY: Barron's Educational Series. (8 pp)
11. Mack, D. (2007). *The shy creatures.* New York: A Feiwel and Friends Books. (33 pp)
12. Maier, I. (2005). *When Lizzy was afraid of trying new things.* Washington, DC: Magination Press. (30 pp)
13. Morrison, V. (2004). *So shy.* New York: North–South Books. (20 pp)
14. Nascimbeni, B. (2002). *Shy Edward.* London: Campbell Books. (10 pp)

15. Raschka, C. (1996). *The blushful hippopotamus.* New York: Orchard Books. (27 pp)

16. Schaefer, C. E. (1992). *Cat's got your tongue: A story for children afraid to speak.* Washington, DC: Magination Press. (28 pp)

17. Schurr, C. (1946). *The shy little kitten.* New York: Golden Books Publishing. (24 pp)

18. Sheehan, I. (2001). *Mitsie the meekest mouse.* Red Reef. (40 pp)

19. Tibo, G. (2002). *Shy guy.* New York: North–South Books. (22 pp)

20. Wells, R. (1992). *Shy Charles.* Toronto: Puffin Books. (28 pp)

PART V

CLINICAL RESEARCH, PRACTICE, AND TREATMENT

13

Temperament and the Etiology of Social Phobia

RONALD M. RAPEE

The purpose of this chapter is to review the role of temperament in the etiology of social phobia. A number of very similar temperamental types or constructs of relevance to the development of social phobia have been described in the literature. Some of the terms used include "inhibition," "sociability," "negative emotionality," "approach," "withdrawal," and "shyness." Although each may have slightly different properties and features, and some of these terms overlap more than others, for the purpose of this review I focus on the similarities between these temperamental constructs. For ease of discussion, I restrict myself to two main terms. I use the term "inhibition" to refer to a style characterized by behavioral restraint, cautiousness, timidity, and low rates of approach, particularly in response to novel and unfamiliar situations or situations involving potential threat. I use the term "shyness" to refer to a subset of inhibition that occurs specifically in response to social cues or settings. In contrast, I use "social phobia" to refer to a clinical syndrome as described in the fourth edition of the *Diagnostic and Statistical Manual of Mental Disorders* (American Psychiatric Association, 1994). The key features of social phobia include (1) marked and excessive fear of social interactions or performance in which the person is exposed to potential scrutiny, (2) fear of being evaluated negatively, (3) extensive avoidance of social situations, and (4) life interference as a result of these features.

SOCIAL ANXIETY DISORDER AND SHYNESS

Central to any discussion of the role of shyness in the etiology of social phobia must be consideration of the relation between these constructs. There has been commentary that the demarcation between "normal" social reticence and "abnormal" social fearfulness is somewhat arbitrary (e.g., Rettew, 2000). As a result, several authors have described a continuum of social reticence along which shyness and social phobia (and even avoidant personality disorder) differ in degree (Hofmann, Heinrichs, & Moscovitch, 2004; McNeil, 2001; Rapee, 1995).

Surprisingly, empirical examination of the relation between shyness and social phobia has been very limited. Few differences on the quality and degree of symptoms and behaviors have been shown between a population selected on the basis of extreme shyness and a clinical population meeting diagnostic criteria for social phobia (Turner, Beidel, & Townsley, 1990). However, standard, clinically derived measures of social phobia share only approximately 20% of their variance with personality-focused measures of shyness, and among highly shy individuals, severity of shyness explains only around 20% of the variance in social phobia (Heiser, Turner, & Beidel, 2003). Put another way, although groups that score at the upper extreme on measures of shyness are more likely to meet criteria for social phobia, a sizable proportion of these groups do not meet clinical criteria, and a proportion of people scoring at moderate levels on shyness nevertheless demonstrate the clinical disorder (Chavira, Stein, & Malcarne, 2002). Hence, the limited evidence suggests that although shyness and social phobia are positively related, they are most likely not part of a single, common construct.

Despite this conclusion, determining the differences between these constructs has not been easy and, once again, empirical evidence is lacking. Possibly the key demonstrated difference reflects the impact or life interference associated with the symptoms (Chavira et al., 2002; Heiser et al., 2003). People meeting diagnostic criteria for social phobia appear to report higher levels of avoidance compared with equally shy people not meeting diagnostic criteria (Turner et al., 1990). As a result, they report higher levels of life impairment, especially with respect to career and social functioning (Chavira et al., 2002). Those with the clinical disorder also appear to have a broader focus, pointing to the possible importance of other factors in its development. Specifically, compared to highly shy individuals without social phobia, those with social phobia report higher levels of neuroticism, introversion, and diagnostic comorbidity (Chavira et al., 2002; Heiser et al., 2003).

One final issue that needs to be considered is the existence of and relations between possible subtypes of social phobia. Whether social phobia itself is a single entity that differs along a continuum, or whether there exist qualitatively distinct subtypes is an issue that has a long and complicated history (Hofmann et al., 2004). There is not space in this chapter to consider this issue in detail, and the reader is referred to previous reviews (Heimberg, Holt, Schneier, Spitzer, & Leibowitz, 1993; Hofmann et al., 2004; Hook & Valentiner, 2002). However, there currently exists some indication that specific fears surrounding public speaking may represent a somewhat distinct form of social phobia (Stein & Deutsch, 2003). For this reason, this chapter focuses primarily on the etiology of what might better be referred to as "generalized" or "noncircumscribed" social phobia.

Of key importance to this chapter, the limited knowledge at this stage suggests that temperament or personality dimensions, such as inhibition and shyness, are related to and overlap with the clinical diagnostic entity of social phobia, but they are not synonymous. As has been argued previously (Chavira et al., 2002; Rapee & Spence, 2004), I assume, in this chapter, that one of the key differences between these constructs is to be found in the interference and life impact associated with the clinical disorder. Etiological factors that infer risk for shyness mostly also infer risk for (noncircumscribed) social phobia. But additional factors that may infer risk for social phobia may not be relevant to shyness.

TEMPERAMENT

There is abundant evidence that several temperamental and personality constructs are related to social phobia. The most common relations have been with temperamental styles that reflect inhibition and shyness. Cross-sectionally, people with social phobia score high on measures of neuroticism or negative affectivity, and low on measures of extraversion or positive affectivity (van Velzen, Emmelkamp, & Scholing, 2000; Weinstock & Whisman, 2006). In fact, the combination of high-negative and low-positive affect appears to be a relatively specific profile that distinguishes social phobia from other anxiety disorders, although this profile is also shared with depression (Brown, Chorpita, & Barlow, 1998).

More importantly, several longitudinal studies have demonstrated that children who rate high on measures of inhibited temperament early in life are at increased risk for social phobia during later childhood, adolescence, and into adulthood (e.g., Hayward, Killen, Kraemer, & Taylor, 1998; Schwartz, Snidman, & Kagan, 1999). The specificity of this effect, however, is limited. One long-term study demonstrated that children who were inhibited at 3 years of age were at increased risk for a broad range of psychopathology in adulthood (Caspi, Moffitt, Newman, & Silva, 1996). Similarly, follow-up studies have shown inhibited young children to be at increased risk for a variety of anxiety disorders several years later (Prior, Smart, Sanson, &

Oberklaid, 2000). Nevertheless, social phobia appears to show the strongest associations with prior inhibition, suggesting that an inhibited temperament provides greater risk for social phobia than for other clinical disorders. One confound that may help to explain some of the overlap is the way in which inhibition is assessed. Current measures of inhibited temperament typically include components tapping both social and physical inhibition (Neal, Edelmann, & Glachan, 2002; Rubin, Hastings, Stewart, Henderson, & Chen, 1997). Research has suggested that it is inhibition toward social stimuli (referred to here as "shyness") that confers the greatest and most specific risk for social phobia, whereas inhibition toward physical stimuli appears to confer a more general risk for later anxiety (Neal et al., 2002). Consistent with the personality links between social phobia and depression described earlier, there is some evidence that inhibition toward social stimuli also confers risk for later depression (Gladstone & Parker, 2006).

Importantly, shyness appears to be one of the more stable temperaments, especially after the toddler years (Pedlow, Sanson, Prior, & Oberklaid, 1993). Similarly, social phobia appears to be one of the most stable mental disorders (Massion et al., 2002). Social phobia in adulthood is most commonly preceded by adolescent social phobia (Pine, Cohen, Gurley, Brook, & Ma, 1998). In adulthood, remission over 8 years has been estimated at only 35%, with the majority of remission occurring in the first 1–2 years (Yonkers, Dyck, & Keller, 2001). Therefore, it seems that a subgroup of people with social phobia may remit relatively quickly, whereas the majority shows a chronic and persistent course. This more consistent course seems to occur less frequently in the presence of comorbid personality disorders, especially avoidant personality disorder (Massion et al., 2002), suggesting that stability of social phobia is greater at higher levels of shyness (Rapee & Spence, 2004). In addition, where changes do occur, they are more likely to constitute small moves along a gradient of social anxiousness rather than large dramatic shifts in functioning (Merikangas, Avenevoli, Acharyya, Zhang, & Angst, 2002).

A different possible description of the relation between temperament and social phobia is that social phobia may be preceded by a combination of temperaments rather than just one. There has been recent interest in the adult literature on the importance of poor emotion regulation in the expression of anxiety disorders. It is argued that people with anxiety disorders not only experience greater amounts of emotion but also have fewer coping resources and more difficulty in managing and controlling their negative emotions than do people without anxiety disorders (Rodebaugh & Heimberg, 2008). A parallel suggestion has been made in the temperament field. Fox, Henderson, Marshall, Nichols, and Ghera (2005) have argued that risk for anxiety disorders is increased in children who score high on inhibition and show difficulty with effortful control. In particular it is suggested that an aspect of effortful control that involves voluntary attentional regulation is vital for the management of excess emotion and thereby central to the development of anxiety disorders. Empirical evidence has demonstrated that effortful and attentional control explain variance in symptoms of anxiety that is independent of neuroticism, and that the combination of high neuroticism and low attentional control provides the greatest risk (Muris, Meesters, & Blijlevens, 2007; Muris, Meesters, & Rompelberg, 2007).

The assumption that shyness and social phobia are distinct constructs is supported by evidence that high levels of inhibition are insufficient to lead to social phobia. Most theories of the development of anxiety disorders rate inhibition as a key risk for the development of disorder through its influence on the effects of other risk factors (e.g., Chorpita & Barlow, 1998; Manassis & Bradley, 1994; Rapee & Spence, 2004). As I describe later in this chapter, consistent evidence suggests that temperament interacts with other risks to better predict social anxiety (or anxiety more generally).

GENETIC FACTORS

There is abundant evidence that anxiety disorders, including social phobia, have a marked and significant genetic component (Gregory & Eley, 2007; Hettema, Neale, & Kendler, 2001). Considered together, the empirical literature suggests that approximately 30–50% of the variance in anxiety disorders and/or symptoms of anxiety is heritable. For example, Kendler, Neale, Kessler, Heath, and Eaves (1992) reported a genetic contribution to social phobia of .31 in 2,163 female twin pairs. This research group subsequently reexamined the genetic influence on social phobia, taking into account the reliability of measurement across an 8-year interval. The heritability estimate increased to around .50 (Kendler, Karkowski, & Prescott, 1999). Similar results were reported in a twin study of children and adolescents in which trait anxiety was shown to have a markedly stronger heritability than state anxiety (Lau, Eley, & Stevenson, 2006). These data suggest that it may be the persistence and stability of social phobia that is especially strongly under genetic influence.

It is widely assumed that the genes responsible for social phobia are mostly broad, general ones that are common across the anxiety and mood disorders (Andrews, 1996; Eley, 1999). For example, a common genetic component has been found to influence social phobia, depression, and alcohol abuse to varying degrees, with a disorder-specific contribution being evident for only alcohol abuse (Nelson et al., 2000). Interestingly, several studies have demonstrated that a smaller but significant proportion of the variance in symptoms of social phobia can be attributed to genetic factors that are unique to the disorder. For example, Kendler, Myers, Prescott, and

Neale (2001) found that as much as 13% of the variance in social fears was accounted for by genetic factors unique to this type of fear. Another twin study examined genetic and environmental influences across four fear dimensions: situational, illness–injury, social, and fear of small animals (Sundet, Skre, Okkenhaug, & Tambs, 2003). In addition to the common genetic and environmental influences, significant fear-specific genetic and environmental factors were demonstrated. More recent research has shown that social phobia appears to share only modest genetic overlap with several other anxiety disorders (Hettema, Prescott, Myers, Neale, & Kendler, 2005) and appears to share substantial genetic commonality with both extraversion and neuroticism (Bienvenu, Hettema, Neale, Prescott, & Kendler, 2007).

It is often assumed that temperament represents a more fundamental and basic phenotype that has a significantly heavier genetic loading compared with clinical disorders (Clark, 2005; Thomas & Chess, 1977). However, twin studies of shyness and inhibition indicate a similar level of heritability to that shown for the clinical disorder of social phobia (Robinson, Kagan, Reznick, & Corley, 1992; Stein, Jang, & Livesley, 2002), although one study has shown a somewhat stronger heritability for shyness in 4-year-old children (Eley et al., 2003). Similar effects have been shown for adult personality factors such as extraversion and neuroticism (e.g., Bienvenu et al., 2007). Thus, the expressions of shyness and inhibition are themselves likely to be strongly influenced by nongenetic risks.

ENVIRONMENTAL RISK FACTORS

Consistent with the data described earlier, several studies have demonstrated that social phobia runs in families (Lieb et al., 2000; Stein et al., 1998). Interestingly, these studies have shown somewhat greater diagnostic specificity than have the twin studies described in the previous section (Hettema et al., 2001). For example, a large study of familial transmission of phobic disorders indicated that first-degree relatives of individuals with social phobia were at specifically increased risk for social phobia (Fyer, Mannuzza, Chapman, Martin, & Klein, 1995). Combining these effects would appear to suggest that the emergence of specific symptom patterns (as opposed to broad, general emotional difficulties) may be more an effect of factors shared across a family.

Studies comparing pairs of twins allow researchers not only to determine the genetic contribution to disorders but also to examine the variance in a behavior contributed by environmental factors. These studies have generally indicated that a major proportion of the variance in social anxiety (and indeed in all anxiety disorders) is accounted for by nonshared environmental factors (i.e., environmental factors that occur differently to each twin; Kendler et al., 1999; Nelson et al., 2000). In contrast, estimates of the contribution of shared environmental factors (environmental factors that affect both twins more comparably) have been more variable. In general, studies of anxiety in adult twins have tended to indicate little or no contribution from the shared environment (Hettema et al., 2001), while studies of anxiety in child twins have shown some, or even substantial, shared environmental contributions (Gregory & Eley, 2007). Interestingly, social phobia is one of the few disorders where shared environmental effects have been demonstrated in adult twins (Hettema et al., 2005; Kendler et al., 2001). Therefore, social phobia may be influenced by not only environmental factors, such as individual life events or differential parent treatment, but also by factors such as parent attitudes or socioeconomic factors.

DEMOGRAPHIC FACTORS

One of the most consistent risk factors for social phobia is female gender. Epidemiological studies in adults indicate a female to male ratio of around 1.5 to 2:1 (e.g., Kessler, Chiu, Demler, & Walters, 2005). This gender difference appears to also be present in younger populations that meet diagnostic criteria for social phobia (Essau, Conradt, & Peterman, 1999). Studies of gender differences in shyness and other forms of inhibited temperament have not been as consistent. While some studies have reported higher levels of shyness and inhibition in females than in males (La Greca & Lopez, 1998), others have reported relatively similar gender ratios (Coplan, Gavinski-Molina, Lagacé-Séguin, & Wichmann, 2001; Hirshfeld-Becker et al., 2004). It is likely, however, that some of this confusion may be a result of confounding with age. There appears to be a slow shift in the association of gender with anxiety across development, with little difference before 5 years of age and a gradual increase in preponderance for females across childhood and adolescence (Roza, Hofstra, van der Ende, & Verhulst, 2003). Given that studies of temperament often involve very young children, it may appear that inhibition is more evenly displayed in both genders than is social phobia, but this difference may disappear once groups are matched on age.

The apparent shift in gender displays of shyness across age may reflect an important cultural influence on the expression of social fears. Several authors have suggested that many cultures view shy, withdrawn behaviors more negatively in males than in females (Rapee & Spence, 2004; Rubin, Coplan, & Bowker, 2009). Subsequently, some research has indicated that parents respond more positively to shyness in girls than in boys (Simpson & Stevenson-Hinde, 1985). As a result, in Western countries, shyness in boys appears to be associated with more associated problems and life interference (Caspi, Elder, & Bem, 1988; Coplan et al., 2001; Stevenson-Hinde &

Glover, 1996). In some countries, where shyness is not associated with the same negativity, longer-term effects are not especially negative (see Chen, Chapter 10, this volume).

Age of onset of social phobia is one of the more complicated issues to determine. Unlike many forms of psychopathology, there does not appear to be an abrupt onset or sudden shift in functioning in people with social phobia, and their reports of onset are generally broad and nonspecific. Therefore, determining a clear age of onset is extremely difficult. Nevertheless, retrospective studies in adults typically point to onset during early to midadolescence (Kessler, Berglund, Demler, Jin, & Walters, 2005), with a slightly earlier onset reported by those with greater severity of disorder (Tran & Chambless, 1995). In contrast, shyness and other forms of inhibited temperament are reported very early in life. There is little doubt that social phobia can also be diagnosed early in life. However, the retrospective data noted earlier suggest that diagnosis is more likely with development and should reach a peak in midadolescence. Perhaps surprisingly, epidemiological studies have provided mixed evidence on whether the prevalence of social phobia increases across childhood (Canino et al., 2004; Ford, Goodman, & Meltzer, 2003); however, the issue has not received extensive investigation. From a theoretical perspective, it might be expected that shy behaviors produce increasing life interference across development, and that maximum interference should occur during the adolescent years, when autonomy from family and interactions with peers take on greatest importance (Rapee & Spence, 2004).

PARENT–CHILD RELATIONSHIPS

An extensive literature has documented associations between anxiety disorders and parenting styles reflecting excessively controlling or overprotective parenting, excessively harsh or critical parenting, and their interaction (Bögels & Brechman-Toussaint, 2006; McLeod, Wood, & Weisz, 2007; Rapee, 1997; Wood, McLeod, Sigman, Hwang, & Chu, 2003). Although there are some hints that social phobia may show particularly strong associations with these parenting styles, the associations appear to be relatively consistent across the anxiety disorders and are also shown with other disorders (Rapee, 1997). Of the styles of parenting associated with anxiety, the largest effect sizes and most consistent findings have been with an overly controlling and protective style of parenting (McLeod et al., 2007). Theoretically, it has been argued more specifically that parenting that excessively protects the child from potential threat, and in this way fits in with his or her natural tendency to avoid, may provide the most critical risk for social phobia and other anxiety disorders (Edwards, Rapee, & Kennedy, in press).

Overprotective parenting has also been associated with shyness and related temperament in younger children (Rubin & Burgess, 2002). Therefore, overprotection appears to be a common risk that may influence expression of the more basic phenotype. Whether overprotection plays a causal role in the development of social phobia is a difficult issue to address; there has been very little research on this question. Theoretically, it is generally assumed that anxiety and parental overprotection interact in a cyclical fashion, thereby representing a temperament–environment correlation (Rubin et al., 2009). In other words, the anticipation of threat, distress, and avoidance that characterize the shy child is likely to elicit protective behaviors from the parent, which in turn reinforce and exacerbate the child's shyness. It is further predicted that higher levels of parental anxiety will lead to greater overprotection (Hudson & Rapee, 2004).

As noted, empirical support for these causal relations has been limited. Evidence for the elicitation of parental protection by shyness in children, but not the reverse, was demonstrated in a longitudinal study of preschool children (Rubin, Nelson, Hastings, & Asendorpf, 1999). Child shyness at age 2 predicted parent protection at age 4, but the reverse relationship was nonsignificant. In contrast, a recent longitudinal study demonstrated that maternal overprotection at age 4 predicted child anxiety 12 months later and the child's anxiety at age 4 predicted maternal overprotection 12 months later (Edwards et al., in press). Furthermore, mothers' own anxiety cross-sectionally predicted their degree of overprotection. Slightly different results were demonstrated in a longitudinal study in which an interaction between inhibited behavior in 2-year-old children and their mothers' degree of intrusiveness predicted child shyness 2 years later (Rubin, Burgess, & Hastings, 2002). Similarly, evidence for the importance of an interaction between temperament and maternal behavior in predicting symptoms of anxiety was demonstrated in a longitudinal study of 228 boys assessed across ages 2–10 (Feng, Shaw, & Silk, 2008). Child shyness at age 2 was associated with higher levels of anxiety across the time frame, while a combination of maternal negativity and intrusiveness predicted the exacerbation of anxiety in those who were shy (see also Hane, Cheah, Rubin, & Fox, 2008, for similar findings).

A somewhat different but related construct, parent–child attachment, has also been linked with anxiety disorders (Chorpita & Barlow, 1998; Manassis & Bradley, 1994; see Hastings, Nuselovici, Rubin, & Cheah, Chapter 6, this volume, for a review). Some research has indicated that insecure attachment predicts anxiety disorders in preschool children independently of their level of inhibition (Shamir-Essakow, Ungerer, & Rapee, 2005). In an especially long-term study, insecure–ambivalent attachment style assessed at 1 year of age significantly predicted anxiety disorders in adolescents when they were 17 years old (Warren, Huston, Egeland, &

Sroufe, 1997). Again, this effect was independent of infant temperament, as well as maternal anxiety. In contrast, insecure attachment was not shown to predict anxiety symptoms in the longitudinal study of 2- to 10-year-old boys (Feng et al., 2008).

To date, there have been almost no attempts to evaluate the importance of parent–child interactions for anxiety through experimental manipulation. In one pilot study, mothers were asked to assist their unselected children in preparation of a speech and were randomly allocated to act in either an overintrusive and overprotective manner, or a minimally involved but supportive manner (de Wilde & Rapee, 2008). On a subsequent speech, children whose mothers had previously acted in an overprotective manner displayed greater levels of overt anxiety.

PEER RELATIONSHIPS

One of the key aspects of shyness and inhibition in young children is their association with social withdrawal and impaired peer relationships. Shy children have fewer friends and are often less popular than nonshy children (Gazelle & Ladd, 2003; Inderbitzen, Walters, & Bukowski, 1997; Rubin, Wojslawowicz, Rose-Krasnor, Booth-LaForce, & Burgess, 2006). Similar poverty of social relationships has been shown in clinically diagnosed children and adults with social phobia (Alden & Taylor, 2004). By adulthood, social phobia interferes with social relationships; adults with social phobia are less likely to have close friends and confidants (Whisman, Sheldon, & Goering, 2000), and to be married or in a significant romantic relationship (Lampe, Slade, Issakidis, & Andrews, 2003; Magee, Eaton, Wittchen, McGonagle, & Kessler, 1996). Finally, the relationships of adults and children with shyness and social phobia are characterized by less intimacy and support (La Greca & Moore, 2005; Whisman et al., 2000).

Along similar lines, there is evidence that social anxiety is strongly related to teasing and bullying during the childhood years (e.g., Hawker & Boulton, 2000; Storch & Masia-Warner, 2004). Adults with social phobia have also reported greater frequency of being bullied as a child than have adults with other anxiety disorders (McCabe, Antony, Summerfelt, Liss, & Swinson, 2003).

It is possible that the poverty of social relationships is in part due to decrements in social performance and interactions. By adulthood, it appears that adults with social phobia do not lack social skills and knowledge. However, they do appear to demonstrate poorer social performance than do nonanxious adults (Beidel, Turner, & Jacob, 1989). It seems that the anxiety elicited by social interactions may interfere with their ability to produce competent social skills (Thompson & Rapee, 2002). Research indicates that shy children lack social skills (e.g., Simonian, Beidel, Turner, Berkes, & Long, 2001; Spence, Donovan, & Brechman-Toussaint, 1999; Stewart & Rubin, 1995). Regardless, data suggest that interaction partners have less desire to interact with shy adults and children (Spence et al., 1999). Importantly, some research suggests that children's lack of skills mediates between shyness and peer rejection (Greco & Morris, 2005).

Although poor social relationships are clearly one effect of being shy, it is possible that this lack of relationships in turn contributes to the maintenance and exacerbation of shyness and social phobia. In one longitudinal examination, shy kindergarten children who were excluded by their peers were much more likely to maintain and slightly increase their levels of shyness over the following 4 years than were shy children who were not excluded by peers (Gazelle & Ladd, 2003). Similarly, in a longitudinal study of peer victimization, it was shown that experiences of bullying by early adolescents led to increases in anxiety 12 months later (Bond, Carlin, Thomas, Rubin, & Patton, 2001).

LEARNING/MODELING

Following theories described earlier on the role of parent–child interactions in the development of social phobia, some models have also suggested that observation by young children of their parents' behaviors and attitudes may play a similar role in the disorder (Chorpita & Barlow, 1998; Hudson & Rapee, 2004). A parent acting in shy and inhibited ways can provide the child with information relevant to social threat or the value of avoidant coping. In an intriguing study, de Rosnay, Cooper, Tsigaras, and Murray (2006) trained mothers of 12- to 14-month-old infants to interact in both a shy and a nonshy fashion with two male strangers. Following observation of their mothers acting nervously in response to the stranger, infants responded with markedly greater fear and avoidance of the stranger on a subsequent encounter. Inhibited temperament interacted with the effects, such that more fearful infants showed a significantly greater effect of mothers' shy behaviors on their subsequent avoidance of the stranger. In a later study, Murray and colleagues (2008) showed that infants of mothers with social phobia showed increased avoidance in their interactions with an adult stranger over a 4-month period. Of perhaps greatest interest, the extent to which avoidance increased was a function of both the infant's inhibition and the extent to which the mother showed distress to the stranger and failed to encourage infant interaction.

These experimental observations with infants correspond with retrospective reports from adults with social phobia who recall their parents as less sociable, stressing the importance of other people's opinions, trying to isolate them from interpersonal interactions, and also using shame as a method of discipline (Bruch & Heimberg, 1994; Rapee & Melville, 1997). Despite the obvious limitations of retrospective recall, there is some evidence that mothers of adults with social phobia report some similar effects (Rapee & Melville, 1997). Some research has also shown that the degree of shyness in adopted infants is significantly related to the sociability of their adoptive mothers (Daniels & Plomin, 1985), pointing to a nongenetic pathway for this relationship.

Broader conditioning experiences associated with social phobia later in life have been supported by retrospective questionnaire studies indicating that people with social phobia recall a large number of direct, vicarious, and verbal conditioning episodes connected with the onset of their disorder (e.g., Hofmann, Ehlers, & Roth, 1995; Mulkens & Bögels, 1999). Of course, retrospective reports of presumably subtle conditioning effects need to be accepted with considerable caution, especially since there has been some failure to replicate these findings in people with generalized social phobia (Townsley Stemberger, Turner, Beidel, & Calhoun, 1995). Perhaps more importantly, aversive social experiences also occur with considerable frequency in people without social phobia (Mulkens & Bögels, 1999), and the events often reported as triggering onset of social fears in these studies appear to involve a degree of preexisting anxiety (Hofmann et al., 1995). Hence, if conditioning experiences are involved in the onset of social phobia, it is likely that they would be more likely to do so within the background of a preexisting inhibited temperament (Rapee & Spence, 2004).

LIFE EVENTS

According to theory, negative life events should interact with preexisting temperamental vulnerability to trigger disorders of anxiety (Chorpita & Barlow, 1998; Hudson & Rapee, 2004; Rapee & Spence, 2004). Hence, negative life events reflect one risk that may help to elucidate the relation between shyness and social phobia.

Although research into the role of life events and adverse circumstances in anxiety is not as extensive as it is for many other disorders, some evidence suggests that the onset of anxiety disorders (including social phobia) in childhood may be preceded by chronic adversities (Allen, Rapee, & Sandberg, 2008; Phillips, Hammen, Brennan, Najman, & Bor, 2005). These data are supported by epidemiological studies that indicate an association between childhood anxiety disorders and low family socioeconomic status (Cronk, Slutske, Madden, Bucholz, & Heath, 2004; Xue, Leventhal, Brooks-Gunn, & Earls, 2005), although the data on this relation are not entirely consistent (Ford et al., 2003).

More acute negative life events in childhood have been shown to increase the risk of social phobia and a range of other psychopathology. Compared with nonclinical controls, children with anxiety disorders report both a greater number and impact of negative life events (e.g., Rapee & Szollos, 2003; Tiet et al., 2001). Causal relations are difficult to demonstrate, and many of the events reported in these studies include events that are said to be "dependent" on the child's behavior. Hence, it is very likely that either features of the disorder or preexisting temperament may be responsible for producing negative life events. This does not mean, however, that these events are not involved in the development of the disorder. As is the case for several other risk factors, life events may be associated with anxiety in a cyclical relationship, such that inhibition may increase the risk for negative experiences, which in turn may increase the experience of inhibition. Alternatively, inhibition may lead to negative life events, which may facilitate the transition to social phobia. Not all life events associated with anxiety are dependent. At least some research has demonstrated a greater incidence of independent life events experienced by anxious children (Allen et al., 2008; Eley & Stevenson, 2000). Thus, negative life events may represent both temperament–environment correlations and independent environmental risk factors for social phobia.

A key role for temperament in the relationship of adverse experiences and social phobia may lie in the impact of the events. It is very likely that children who score high on inhibition will experience greater distress and interference following a stressor. In a particularly innovative study, family support assessed when the child was age 4 predicted the child's inhibition at age 7, but only for children with short alleles on the serotonin transporter (5-HTT) gene (possibly associated with shyness) (Fox, Nichols, et al., 2005).

OVERALL MODEL

Building on previous models of the development of anxiety disorders (e.g., Chorpita & Barlow, 1998; Manassis & Bradley, 1994), Rapee and Spence (2004) proposed a model of the development of social phobia. They argued that people characteristically lie along a continuum of social fearfulness (referred to as "social anxiety"), and that this characteristic has both trait and state aspects. The trait aspects act like a "set point," guiding the individual back to his or her characteristic level of social anxiety following minor changes. Minor (state) alterations in expressed social anxiety can occur for a variety of reasons and can in some cases dramatically alter the person's level of social anxiety for a finite period of time. The trait aspects of social anxiety have heavier genetic and temperamental input, while the state aspects have more influence from environmental factors. Hence, a deviation in social anxiety from the characteristic set point is likely to last as long as the environmental influence is current.

The model identified a number of factors that contribute to the risk for social anxiety as described throughout this chapter. Thus, for example, the level of characteristic social anxiety is predicted by genetic factors interacting with longer-term or especially salient environmental influences, such as chronic parental overprotection, chronic environmental adversity, or poor social skills. Similar factors may also affect the current expression of social anxiety. For example, if a parent loses his or her job and has a depressive episode, the child may increase his or her level of social anxiety while the parent is depressed, and while he or she is significantly under the parent's influence.

A key aspect of the model is that social anxiety and social phobia are distinct (although highly related) constructs. It is argued that social phobia requires a degree of life interference to be produced by the social anxiety behaviors. The extent of life interference is influenced by other risk factors, including age, gender, life goals, and so on. A potentially important factor that has not been extensively discussed here due to space limitations is the influence of culture. According to Rapee and Spence (2004), cultural factors may influence the development of social phobia at most levels of the model. The set point might be affected by the fundamental ways in which social anxiety is experienced and expressed across different cultures (Kim, Rapee, & Gaston, 2008). Shorter-term expressions of social anxiety may also be culturally influenced, especially given individual changes in subculture at various life stages. Finally, culture is likely to have a marked influence on a diagnosis of social phobia through its influence on life interference. Cultures vary in the extent to which they accept expression of social anxiety (Heinrichs et al., 2006) and may affect the point at which social anxiousness moves into a clinical disorder.

CLINICAL IMPLICATIONS
AND FUTURE DIRECTIONS

Models of the etiology and development of a disorder will have their greatest applied influence on prevention and early intervention efforts, although they will also hold relevance for treatment of clinical social phobia. The current review has identified several factors that may hold promise in prevention of the development of social phobia. For example, targeted programs can be aimed at children who score high on measures of shyness (and perhaps low on effortful control), have highly protective and/or anxious parents, or are rejected by peers. To be effective, prevention programs would need to reduce levels of risk (change expression of temperament, reduce parental overprotection, etc.). To provide a recent example, we selected preschool children who scored especially high on observed inhibition and also had at least one parent with an anxiety disorder (Kennedy, Rapee, & Edwards, 2009). Parents of the children were allocated to receive either eight sessions of intervention or no intervention. Active intervention was aimed at reversing avoidant coping, managing parent anxiety, and reducing overprotection. At 6-month assessment, children whose parents were in the active intervention showed lower levels of observed inhibition, less life interference, and fewer anxiety disorders.

In addition to prevention, the patterns of cyclical interaction between existing symptoms and certain environmental factors point to the value of the model for treatment of established social phobia. For example, it has been reported that being socially anxious may elicit peer teasing, which may increase levels of current social anxiety (Rubin et al., 2009). Hence, effective treatment may need simultaneously to increase skills to manage social anxiety and deal with peer teasing. Our empirically validated treatment for childhood anxiety, *Cool Kids,* includes components for increasing social skills, reducing parent overprotection, and dealing with teasing (Hudson, Lyneham, & Rapee, 2008).

Our current summary of knowledge about risks for the development of social phobia, combined with models such as the one described here, provides a snapshot of the state of knowledge at the moment. It is almost certainly also incomplete. We are still a long way from knowing why one person develops social phobia, why another has high shyness but not social phobia, and why still another develops low levels of shyness. A continued interplay between basic and applied research will help lead to future innovations.

REFERENCES

Alden, L. E., & Taylor, C. T. (2004). Interpersonal processes in social phobia. *Clinical Psychology Review, 24,* 857–882.

Allen, J. L., Rapee, R. M., & Sandberg, S. (2008). Severe life events and chronic adversities as antecedents to anxiety in children: A matched control study. *Journal of Abnormal Child Psychology, 36,* 1047–1056.

American Psychiatric Association. (1994). *Diagnostic and statistical manual of mental disorders* (4th ed.). Washington, DC: Author.

Andrews, G. (1996). Comorbidity in neurotic disorders: The similarities are more important than the differences. In R. M. Rapee (Ed.), *Current controversies in the anxiety disorders* (pp. 3–20). New York: Guilford Press.

Beidel, D. C., Turner, S. M., & Jacob, R. G. (1989). Assessment of social phobia:

Reliability of an impromptu speech task. *Journal of Anxiety Disorders, 3,* 149–158.

Bienvenu, O. J., Hettema, J. M., Neale, M. C., Prescott, C. A., & Kendler, K. S. (2007). Low extraversion and high neuroticism as indices of genetic and environmental risk for social phobia, agoraphobia, and animal phobia. *American Journal of Psychiatry, 164,* 1714–1721.

Bögels, S. M., & Brechman-Toussaint, M. L. (2006). Family issues in child anxiety: Attachment, family functioning, parental rearing and beliefs. *Clinical Psychology Review, 26*(7), 834–856.

Bond, L., Carlin, J. B., Thomas, L., Rubin, K., & Patton, G. (2001). Does bullying cause emotional problems?: A prospective study of young teenagers. *British Medical Journal, 323*(7311), 480–484.

Brown, T. A., Chorpita, B. F., & Barlow, D. H. (1998). Structural relationships among dimensions of the DSM-IV anxiety and mood disorders and dimensions of negative affect, positive affect, and autonomic arousal. *Journal of Abnormal Psychology, 107*(2), 179–192.

Bruch, M. A., & Heimberg, R. G. (1994). Differences in perceptions of parental and personal characteristics between generalized and nongeneralized social phobics. *Journal of Anxiety Disorders, 8,* 155–168.

Canino, G., Shrout, P. E., Rubio-Stipec, M., Bird, H. R., Bravo, M., Ramirez, R., et al. (2004). The DSM-IV rates of child and adolescent disorders in Puerto Rico. *Archives of General Psychiatry, 61*(1), 85–93.

Caspi, A., Elder, G. H., Jr., & Bem, D. J. (1988). Moving away from the world: Life-course patterns of shy children. *Developmental psychology, 24,* 824–831.

Caspi, A., Moffitt, T. E., Newman, D. L., & Silva, P. A. (1996). Behavioral observations at age 3 years predict adult psychiatric disorders: Longitudinal evidence from a birth cohort. *Archives of General Psychiatry, 53,* 1033–1039.

Chavira, D. A., Stein, M. B., & Malcarne, V. L. (2002). Scrutinizing the relationship between shyness and social phobia. *Journal of Anxiety Disorders, 16,* 585–598.

Chorpita, B. F., & Barlow, D. H. (1998). The development of anxiety: The role of control in the early environment. *Psychological Bulletin, 124,* 3–21.

Clark, L. A. (2005). Temperament as a unifying basis for personality and psychopathology. *Journal of Abnormal Psychology, 114*(4), 505–521.

Coplan, R. J., Gavinski-Molina, M. H., Lagacé-Séguin, D. G., & Wichmann, C. (2001). When girls versus boys play alone: Nonsocial play and adjustment in kindergarten. *Developmental Psychology, 37*(4), 464–474.

Cronk, N. J., Slutske, W. S., Madden, P. A. F., Bucholz, K. K., & Heath, A. C. (2004). Risk for separation anxiety disorder among girls: Paternal absence, socioeconomic disadvantage, and genetic vulnerability. *Journal of Abnormal Psychology, 113*(2), 237–247.

Daniels, D., & Plomin, R. (1985). Origins of individual differences in infant shyness. *Developmental Psychology, 21,* 118–121.

de Rosnay, M., Cooper, P. J., Tsigaras, N., & Murray, L. (2006). Transmission of social anxiety from mother to infant: An experimental study using a social referencing paradigm. *Behaviour Research and Therapy, 44*(8), 1165–1175.

de Wilde, A., & Rapee, R. M. (2008). Do controlling maternal behaviours increase state anxiety in children's responses to a social threat?: A pilot study. *Journal of Behavior Therapy and Experimental Psychiatry, 39*, 526–537.

Edwards, S. L., Rapee, R. M., & Kennedy, S. (in press). Prediction of anxiety symptoms in preschool-aged children: Examination of maternal and paternal perspectives. *Journal of Child Psychology and Psychiatry.*

Eley, T. C. (1999). Behavioral genetics as a tool for developmental psychology: Anxiety and depression in children and adolescents. *Clinical Child and Family Psychology Review, 2*(1), 21–36.

Eley, T. C., Bolton, D., O'Connor, T. G., Perrin, S., Smith, P., & Plomin, R. (2003). A twin study of anxiety-related behaviours in pre-school children. *Journal of Child Psychology and Psychiatry, 44*(7), 945–960.

Eley, T. C., & Stevenson, J. (2000). Specific life events and chronic experiences differentially associated with depression and anxiety in young twins. *Journal of Abnormal Child Psychology, 28*(4), 383–394.

Essau, C. A., Conradt, J., & Peterman, F. (1999). Frequency and comorbidity of social phobia and social fears in adolescents. *Behaviour Research and Therapy, 37*, 831–843.

Feng, X., Shaw, D. S., & Silk, J. S. (2008). Developmental trajectories of anxiety symptoms among boys across early and middle childhood. *Journal of Abnormal Psychology, 117*(1), 32–47.

Ford, T., Goodman, R., & Meltzer, H. (2003). The British Child and Adolescent Mental Health Survey 1999: The prevalence of DSM-IV disorders. *Journal of the American Academy of Child and Adolescent Psychiatry, 42*(10), 1203–1211.

Fox, N. A., Henderson, H. A., Marshall, P. J., Nichols, K. E., & Ghera, M. M. (2005). Behavioral inhibition: Linking biology and behavior within a developmental framework. *Annual Review of Psychology, 56*, 235–262.

Fox, N. A., Nichols, K. E., Henderson, H. A., Rubin, K. H., Schmidt, L. A., Hamer, D., et al. (2005). Evidence for a gene–environment interaction in predicting behavioral inhibition in middle childhood. *Psychological Science, 16*(12), 921–926.

Fyer, A. J., Mannuzza, S., Chapman, T. F., Martin, L. Y., & Klein, D. F. (1995). Specificity in familial aggregation of phobic disorders. *Archives of General Psychiatry, 52*, 564–573.

Gazelle, H., & Ladd, G. W. (2003). Anxious solitude and peer exclusion: A diathesis–stress model of internalizing trajectories in childhood. *Child Development, 74*(1), 257–278.

Gladstone, G. L., & Parker, G. B. (2006). Is behavioral inhibition a risk factor for depression? *Journal of Affective Disorders, 95*(1–3), 85–94.

Greco, L. A., & Morris, T. L. (2005). Factors influencing the link between social anxiety and peer acceptance: Contributions of social skills and close friendships during middle childhood. *Behavior Therapy, 36*(2), 197–205.

Gregory, A. M., & Eley, T. C. (2007). Genetic influences on anxiety in children: What we've learned and where we're heading. *Clinical Child and Family Psychology Review, 10*(3), 199–212.

Hane, A. A., Cheah, C. S. L., Rubin, K. H., & Fox, N. A. (2008). The role of maternal behavior in the relation between shyness and social withdrawal in early childhood and social withdrawal in middle childhood. *Social Development,* *17,* 795–811.

Hawker, D. S. J., & Boulton, M. J. (2000). Twenty years' research on peer victimization and psychosocial maladjustment: A meta-analytic review of cross-sectional studies. *Journal of Child Psychology and Psychiatry, 41*(4), 441–455.

Hayward, C., Killen, J. D., Kraemer, H. C., & Taylor, C. B. (1998). Linking self-reported childhood behavioural inhibition to adolescent social phobia. *Journal of American Academy of Child and Adolescent Psychiatry, 37*(12), 1308–1318.

Heimberg, R. G., Holt, C. S., Schneier, F. R., Spitzer, R. L., & Leibowitz, M. R. (1993). The issue of subtypes in the diagnosis of social phobia. *Journal of Anxiety Disorders, 7,* 249–269.

Heinrichs, N., Rapee, R. M., Alden, L. A., Bögels, S. M., Hofmann, S. G., Oh, K. J., et al. (2006). Cultural differences in perceived social norms and social anxiety. *Behaviour Research and Therapy, 44,* 1187–1197.

Heiser, N. A., Turner, S. M., & Beidel, D. C. (2003). Shyness: Relationship to social phobia and other psychiatric disorders. *Behaviour Research and Therapy, 41*(2), 209–221.

Hettema, J. M., Neale, M. C., & Kendler, K. S. (2001). A review and meta-analysis of the genetic epidemiology of anxiety disorders. *American Journal of Psychiatry, 158*(10), 1568–1578.

Hettema, J. M., Prescott, C. A., Myers, J. M., Neale, M. C., & Kendler, K. S. (2005). The structure of genetic and environmental risk factors for anxiety disorders in men and women. *Archives of General Psychiatry, 62,* 182–189.

Hirshfeld-Becker, D. R., Biederman, J., Faraone, S. V., Segool, N., Buchwald, J., & Rosenbaum, J. F. (2004). Lack of association between behavioral inhibition and psychosocial adversity factors in children at risk for anxiety disorders. *American Journal of Psychiatry, 161*(3), 547–555.

Hofmann, S. G., Ehlers, A., & Roth, W. T. (1995). Conditioning theory: A model for the etiology of public speaking anxiety. *Behaviour Research and Therapy, 33,* 567–572.

Hofmann, S. G., Heinrichs, N., & Moscovitch, D. A. (2004). The nature and expression of social phobia: Toward a new classification. *Clinical Psychology Review, 24*(7), 769–797.

Hook, J. N., & Valentiner, D. P. (2002). Are specific and generalized social phobias qualitatively distinct? *Clinical Psychology: Science and Practice, 9*(4), 379–395.

Hudson, J. L., Lyneham, H. J., & Rapee, R. M. (2008). Social anxiety. In A. R. Eisen (Ed.), *Treating childhood behavioral and emotional problems: A step-by-step, evidence-based approach* (pp. 53–102). New York: Guilford Press.

Hudson, J. L., & Rapee, R. M. (2004). From anxious temperament to disorder: An etiological model of generalized anxiety disorder. In R. G. Heimberg, C. L. Turk, & D. S. Mennin (Eds.), *Generalized anxiety disorder: Advances in research and practice* (pp. 51–76). New York: Guilford Press.

Inderbitzen, H. M., Walters, K. S., & Bukowski, A. L. (1997). The role of social anxiety in adolescent peer relations: Differences among sociometric status groups and rejected subgroups. *Journal of Clinical Child Psychology, 26*(4), 338–348.

Kendler, K. S., Karkowski, L. M., & Prescott, C. A. (1999). Fears and phobias: Reliability and heritability. *Psychological Medicine, 29*(3), 539–553.

Kendler, K. S., Myers, J., Prescott, C. A., & Neale, M. C. (2001). The genetic epidemiology of irrational fears and phobias in men. *Archives of General Psychiatry, 58,* 257–265.

Kendler, K. S., Neale, M. C., Kessler, R. C., Heath, A. C., & Eaves, L. J. (1992). The genetic epidemiology of phobias in women: The interrelationship of agoraphobia, social phobia, situational phobia, and simple phobia. *Archives of General Psychiatry, 49,* 273–281.

Kendler, K. S., Walters, E. E., Neale, M. C., Kessler, R. C., Heath, A. C., & Eaves, L. J. (1995). The structure of the genetic and environmental risk factors for six major psychiatric disorders in women: Phobia, generalized anxiety disorder, panic disorder, bulimia, major depression, and alcoholism. *Archives of General Psychiatry, 52,* 374–383.

Kennedy, S. J., Rapee, R. M., & Edwards, S. L. (2009). A selective intervention program for inhibited preschool-aged children of parents with an anxiety disorder: Effects on current anxiety disorders and temperament. *Journal of the American Academy of Child and Adolescent Psychiatry, 48,* 602–609.

Kessler, R., Berglund, P., Demler, O., Jin, R., & Walters, E. E. (2005). Lifetime prevalence and age-of-onset distributions of DSM-IV disorders in the National Comorbidity Survey Replication. *Archives of General Psychiatry, 62,* 593–602.

Kessler, R. C., Chiu, W. T., Demler, O., & Walters, E. E. (2005). Prevalence, severity, and comorbidity of 12-month DSM-IV disorders in the National Comorbidity Survey Replication. *Archives of General Psychiatry, 62,* 617–627.

Kim, J., Rapee, R. M., & Gaston, J. E. (2008). Symptoms of offensive type Taijin-Kyofusho among Australian social phobics. *Depression and Anxiety, 25,* 601–608.

La Greca, A. M., & Lopez, N. (1998). Social anxiety among adolescents: Linkages with peer relations and friendships. *Journal of Abnormal Child Psychology, 26*(2), 83–94.

La Greca, A. M., & Moore, H. H. (2005). Adolescent peer relations, friendships, and romantic relationships: Do they predict social anxiety and depression? *Journal of Clinical Child and Adolescent Psychology, 34*(1), 49–61.

Lampe, L., Slade, T., Issakidis, C., & Andrews, G. (2003). Social phobia in the Australian National Survey of Mental Health and Well-Being (NSMHWB). *Psychological Medicine, 33,* 637–646.

Lau, J. Y., Eley, T. C., & Stevenson, J. (2006). Examining the state–trait anxiety relationship: A behavioural genetic approach. *Journal of Abnormal Child Psychology, 34*(1), 19–27.

Lieb, R., Wittchen, H.-U., Hofler, M., Fuetsch, M., Stein, M. B., & Merikangas, K. R. (2000). Parental psychopathology, parenting styles, and the risk of social phobia in offspring: A prospective–longitudinal community study. *Archives of General Psychiatry, 57*(9), 859–866.

Magee, W. J., Eaton, W. W., Wittchen, H.-U., McGonagle, K. A., & Kessler, R. C. (1996). Agoraphobia, simple phobia, and social phobia in the National Comorbidity Survey. *Archives of General Psychiatry, 53,* 159–168.

Manassis, K., & Bradley, S. J. (1994). The development of childhood anxiety disorders: Toward an integrated model. *Journal of Applied Developmental Psychology, 15,* 345–366.

Massion, A. O., Dyck, I. R., Shea, M. T., Phillips, K. A., Warshaw, M. G., & Keller, M. B. (2002). Personality disorders and time to remission in generalized anxiety disorder, social phobia, and panic disorder. *Archives of General Psychiatry, 59*(5), 434–440.

McCabe, R. E., Antony, M. M., Summerfelt, L. J., Liss, A., & Swinson, R. P. (2003). Preliminary examination of the relationship between anxiety disorders in adults and self-reported history of teasing or bullying experiences. *Cognitive Behaviour Therapy, 32*(4), 187–193.

McLeod, B. D., Wood, J. J., & Weisz, J. R. (2007). Examining the association between parenting and childhood anxiety: A meta-analysis. *Clinical Psychology Review, 27,* 155–172.

McNeil, D. W. (2001). Terminology and evolution of constructs in social anxiety and social phobia. In S. G. Hofmann & P. DiBartolo Marten (Eds.), *From social anxiety to social phobia: Multiple perspectives* (Vol. 11, pp. 8–19). Boston: Allyn & Bacon.

Merikangas, K. R., Avenevoli, S., Acharyya, S., Zhang, H., & Angst, J. (2002). The spectrum of social phobia in the Zurich Cohort Study of young adults. *Biological Psychiatry, 51,* 81–91.

Mulkens, S., & Bögels, S. M. (1999). Learning history in fear of blushing. *Behaviour Research and Therapy, 37,* 1159–1167.

Muris, P., Meesters, C., & Blijlevens, P. (2007). Self-reported reactive and regulative temperament in early adolescence: Relations to internalizing and externalizing problem behavior and "Big Three" personality factors. *Journal of Adolescence, 30*(6), 1035–1049.

Muris, P., Meesters, C., & Rompelberg, L. (2007). Attention control in middle childhood: Relations to psychopathological symptoms and threat perception distortions. *Behaviour Research and Therapy, 45*(5), 997–1010.

Murray, L., de Rosnay, M., Pearson, J., Sack, C., Schofield, E., Royal-Lawson, M., et al. (2008). Intergenerational transmission of social anxiety: The role of social referencing processes in infancy. *Child Development, 79*(4), 1049–1064.

Neal, J. A., Edelmann, R. J., & Glachan, M. (2002). Behavioural inhibition and symptoms of anxiety and depression: Is there a specific relationship with social phobia? *British Journal of Clinical Psychology, 41*(4), 361–374.

Nelson, E. C., Grant, J. D., Bucholz, K. K., Glowinski, A., Madden, P. A. F., Reich, W., et al. (2000). Social phobia in a population-based female adolescent twin sample: Co-morbidity and associated suicide-related symptoms. *Psychological Medicine, 30*(4), 797–804.

Pedlow, R., Sanson, A., Prior, M., & Oberklaid, F. (1993). Stability of maternally reported temperament from infancy to 8 years. *Developmental Psychology, 29*(6), 998–1007.

Phillips, N. K., Hammen, C. L., Brennan, P. A., Najman, J. M., & Bor, W. (2005). Early adversity and the prospective prediction of depressive and anxiety disorders in adolescents. *Journal of Abnormal Child Psychology, 33*(1), 13–24.

Pine, D. S., Cohen, P., Gurley, D., Brook, J., & Ma, Y. (1998). The risk for early-adulthood anxiety and depressive disorders in adolescents with anxiety and depressive disorders. *Archives of General Psychiatry, 55, 56–64.*

Prior, M., Smart, D., Sanson, A., & Oberklaid, F. (2000). Does shy–inhibited temperament in childhood lead to anxiety problems in adolescence? *Journal of the American Academy of Child and Adolescent Psychiatry, 39*(4), 461–468.

Rapee, R. M. (1995). Descriptive psychopathology of social phobia. In R. G. Heimberg, M. R. Liebowitz, D. A. Hope, & F. R. Schneier (Eds.), *Social phobia: Diagnosis, assessment, and treatment* (pp. 41–66). New York: Guilford Press.

Rapee, R. M. (1997). Potential role of childrearing practices in the development of anxiety and depression. *Clinical Psychology Review, 17,* 47–67.

Rapee, R. M., & Melville, L. F. (1997). Recall of family factors in social phobia and panic disorder: Comparison of mother and offspring reports. *Depression and Anxiety, 5,* 7–11.

Rapee, R. M., & Spence, S. H. (2004). The etiology of social phobia: Empirical evidence and an initial model. *Clinical Psychology Review, 24,* 737–767.

Rapee, R. M., & Szollos, A. A. (2003). Developmental antecedents of clinical anxiety in childhood. *Behaviour Change, 19*(3), 146–157.

Rettew, D. C. (2000). Avoidant personality disorder, generalized social phobia, and shyness: Putting the personality back into personality disorders. *Harvard Review of Psychiatry, 8*(6), 283–297.

Robinson, J. L., Kagan, J., Reznick, J. S., & Corley, R. (1992). The heritability of inhibited and uninhibited behavior: A twin study. *Developmental Psychology, 28,* 1030–1037.

Rodebaugh, T. L., & Heimberg, R. G. (2008). Emotion regulation and the anxiety disorders: Adopting a self-regulation perspective. In A. Vingerhoets, I. Nyklicek, & J. Denollet (Eds.), *Emotion regulation: Conceptual and clinical issues* (pp. 140–149). New York: Springer Science + Business Media.

Roza, S. J., Hofstra, M. B., van der Ende, J., & Verhulst, F. C. (2003). Stable prediction of mood and anxiety disorders based on behavioral and emotional problems in childhood: A 14-year follow-up during childhood, adolescence, and young adulthood. *American Journal of Psychiatry, 160*(12), 2116–2121.

Rubin, K. H., & Burgess, K. (2002). Parents of aggressive and withdrawn children. In M. Bornstein (Ed.), *Handbook of parenting* (2nd ed., Vol. 1, pp. 383–418). Hillsdale, NJ: Erlbaum.

Rubin, K. H., Burgess, K. B., & Hastings, P. D. (2002). Stability and social-behavioral consequences of toddlers' inhibited temperament and parenting behaviors. *Child Development, 73*(2), 483–495.

Rubin, K. H., Coplan, R. J., & Bowker, J. C. (2009). Social withdrawal and shyness in childhood and adolescence. *Annual Review of Psychology, 60,* 141–171.

Rubin, K. H., Hastings, P. D., Stewart, S., Henderson, H. A., & Chen, X. (1997). The consistency and concomitants of inhibition: Some of the children, all of the time. *Child Development, 68,* 467–483.

Rubin, K. H., Nelson, L. J., Hastings, P., & Asendorpf, J. (1999). The transaction between parents' perceptions of their children's shyness and their parenting styles. *International Journal of Behavioral Development, 23*(4), 937–957.

Rubin, K. H., Wojslawowicz, J. C., Rose-Krasnor, L., Booth-LaForce, C., & Burgess, K. B. (2006). The best friendships of shy/withdrawn children: Prevalence, stability, and relationship quality. *Journal of Abnormal Child Psychology, 34*(2), 143–158.

Schwartz, C. E., Snidman, N., & Kagan, J. (1999). Adolescent social anxiety as an outcome of inhibited temperament in childhood. *Journal of the American Academy of Child and Adolescent Psychiatry, 38*(8), 1008–1015.

Shamir-Essakow, G., Ungerer, J. A., & Rapee, R. M. (2005). Attachment, behavioral inhibition, and anxiety in preschool children. *Journal of Abnormal Child Psychology, 33*(2), 131–143.

Simonian, S. J., Beidel, D. C., Turner, S. M., Berkes, J. L., & Long, J. H. (2001). Recognition of facial affect by children and adolescents diagnosed with social phobia. *Child Psychiatry and Human Development, 32*(2), 137–145.

Simpson, A. E., & Stevenson-Hinde, J. (1985). Temperamental characteristics of three- to four-year-old boys and girls and child–family interactions. *Journal of Child Psychology and Psychiatry, 26,* 43–53.

Spence, S. H., Donovan, C., & Brechman-Toussaint, M. (1999). Social skills, social outcomes, and cognitive features of childhood social phobia. *Journal of Abnormal Psychology, 108*(2), 211–221.

Stein, M. B., Chartier, M. J., Hazen, A. L., Kozak, M. V., Tancer, M. E., Lander, S., et al. (1998). A direct-interview family study of Generalized Social Phobia. *American Journal of Psychiatry, 155*(1), 90–97.

Stein, M. B., & Deutsch, R. (2003). In search of social phobia subtypes: Similarity of feared social situations. *Depression and Anxiety, 17,* 94–97.

Stein, M. B., Jang, K. L., & Livesley, W. J. (2002). Heritability of social anxiety-related concerns and personality characteristics: A twin study. *Journal of Nervous and Mental Disease, 190*(4), 219–224.

Stevenson-Hinde, J., & Glover, A. (1996). Shy girls and boys: A new look. *Journal of Child Psychology and Psychiatry, 37,* 181–187.

Stewart, S. L., & Rubin, K. H. (1995). The social problem solving skills of anxious–withdrawn children. *Development and Psychopathology, 7,* 323–336.

Storch, E. A., & Masia-Warner, C. (2004). The relationship of peer victimization to social anxiety and loneliness in adolescent females. *Journal of Adolescence, 27*(3), 351–362.

Sundet, J. M., Skre, I., Okkenhaug, J. J., & Tambs, K. (2003). Genetic and environmental causes of the interrelationships between self-reported fears. A study of a non-clinical sample of Norwegian identical twins and their families. *Scandinavian Journal of Psychology, 44*(2), 97–106.

Thomas, A., & Chess, S. (1977). *Temperament and development.* New York: Brunner/Mazel.

Thompson, S., & Rapee, R. M. (2002). The effect of situational structure on the social performance of socially anxious and non-anxious participants. *Journal of Behavior Therapy and Experimental Psychiatry, 33,* 91–102.

Tiet, Q. Q., Bird, H. R., Hoven, C. W., Moore, R., Wu, P., Wicks, J., et al. (2001). Relationship between specific adverse life events and psychiatric disorders. *Journal of Abnormal Child Psychology, 29*(2), 153–164.

Townsley Stemberger, R., Turner, S. M., Beidel, D. C., & Calhoun, K. S. (1995). Social phobia: An analysis of possible developmental factors. *Journal of Abnormal Psychology, 104*(3), 526–531.

Tran, G. Q., & Chambless, D. L. (1995). Psychopathology of social phobia: Effects of subtype and of avoidant personality disorder. *Journal of Anxiety Disorders, 9*(6), 489–501.

Turner, S. M., Beidel, D. C., & Townsley, R. M. (1990). Social phobia: Relationship to shyness. *Behaviour Research and Therapy, 28,* 497–505.

van Velzen, C. J., Emmelkamp, P. M., & Scholing, A. (2000). Generalized social phobia versus avoidant personality disorder: Differences in psychopathology, personality traits, and social and occupational functioning. *Journal of Anxiety Disorders, 14*(4), 395–411.

Warren, S. L., Huston, L., Egeland, B., & Sroufe, L. A. (1997). Child and adolescent anxiety disorders and early attachment. *Journal of the American Academy of Child and Adolescent Psychiatry, 36*(5), 637–644.

Weinstock, L. M., & Whisman, M. A. (2006). Neuroticism as a common feature of the depressive and anxiety disorders: A test of the revised integrative hierarchical model in a national sample. *Journal of Abnormal Psychology, 115*(1), 68–74.

Whisman, M. A., Sheldon, C. T., & Goering, P. (2000). Psychiatric disorders and dissatisfaction with social relationships: Does type of relationship matter? *Journal of Abnormal Psychology, 109*(4), 803–808.

Wood, J. J., McLeod, B. D., Sigman, M., Hwang, W., & Chu, B. C. (2003). Parenting and childhood anxiety: Theory, empirical findings, and future directions. *Journal of Child Psychology and Psychiatry, 44*(1), 134–151.

Xue, Y., Leventhal, T., Brooks-Gunn, J., & Earls, F. J. (2005). Neighborhood residence and mental health problems of 5- to 11-year-olds. *Archives of General Psychiatry, 62*(5), 554–563.

Yonkers, K. A., Dyck, I. R., & Keller, M. B. (2001). An eight-year longitudinal comparison of clinical course and characteristics of social phobia among men and women. *Psychiatric Services, 52*(5), 637–643.

14

Treating Social Anxiety in Youth

MATTHEW P. MYCHAILYSZYN
JEREMY S. COHEN
JULIE M. EDMUNDS
SARAH A. CRAWLEY
PHILIP C. KENDALL

Anxiety disorders are among the most prevalent type of psychopathology seen in children and adolescents (Costello, Egger, & Angold, 2004). With specific regard to social anxiety disorder (SAD),[1] epidemiological research suggests a typical onset in middle adolescence (Schneier, Johnson, Hornig, Liebowitz, & Weissman, 1992), though it has been diagnosed in children as young as 7 and 8 years old as well (Beidel & Turner, 1988). Despite generally favorable parental attitudes toward various treatments (Chavira, Stein, Bailey, & Stein, 2003), SAD is one of the emotional difficulties in children for which treatment is least often sought. Because socially anxious youth do not usually display behavior that leads teachers to complain or parents to be angered, they often suffer in silence (Beidel, Turner, & Morris, 1999; Rubin, Coplan, & Bowker, 2009). Compared to those with attention-deficit/hyperactivity disorder (ADHD) or depression, socially anxious youth are less often referred for treatment (Kashdan & Herbert, 2001). Only a small minority has ever received any kind of counseling, and fewer still have received pharmacological intervention (Chavira, Stein, Bailey, &

---

[1]The terms "social anxiety disorder" (SAD) and "social phobia" (SP) refer to the same condition and are often used interchangeably in the literature. Current prevailing opinion seems to favor use of SAD to describe the disorder (see Kashdan & Herbert, 2001; Liebowitz, Heimberg, Fresco, Travers, & Stein, 2000), and as such, this designation is used throughout this chapter.

Stein, 2004; Essau, 2005; Schneier et al., 1992; Wittchen, Stein, & Kessler, 1999).

Shyness and SAD are related constructs. Efforts to define "shyness" have offered descriptions that emphasize the appearance of nervousness and discomfort about, and hesitancy to engage in, social situations (Pilkonis, 1977; Buss, 1980; Jones, Briggs, & Smith, 1986). Such descriptions are equally applicable to SAD. Moreover, shy individuals and those with SAD exhibit social skills deficits, a range of somatic responses associated with autonomic arousal, and consequent behavioral avoidance (Chavira, Stein, & Malcarne, 2002). What *does* seem to differentiate between shyness and SAD is the degree of impairment in social and occupational functioning (Turner, Beidel, & Townsley, 1990). The greater level of interference linked to SAD may explain differences in prevalence compared to shyness, with the former ranging from 3 to16% in the general population (Furmark et al., 1999), and the latter closer to 30–40% (Lazarus, 1982; Caspi, Elder, & Bem, 1988; Zimbardo, 1977).

Despite being considered less severe, shyness is associated with a wide range of impairments, as these children and adolescents often suffer substantial distress and interference across a variety of life domains. Shyness in youth has been found to be linked with deficits in academic competence (Coplan, Gavinsky-Molina, Lagacé-Séguin, & Wichmann, 2001; Crozier & Hostettler, 2003), as well as a number of social difficulties (Rubin et al., 2009). Specifically, shyness is connected with being perceived as a less attractive playmate (Nelson, Rubin, & Fox, 2005) and can therefore lead to neglect, rejection, and exclusion by peers (Coplan et al., 2001; Coplan, Girardi, Findlay, & Frohlick, 2007). An increased propensity for loneliness, elevated trait anxiety, and low self-ratings of global self-worth often results from an absence of quality friendships (Fordham & Stevenson-Hinde, 1999; Rubin, Wojslawowicz, Rose-Krasnor, Booth-LaForce, & Burgess, 2006). Similarly, SAD is associated with deficits in social skills (Spence, Donovan, & Brechman-Toussaint, 1999), fewer friends, and dislike and avoidance of school and school-related activities that lead to impairments in school functioning (Beidel et al., 1999; Turner, Beidel, Dancu, & Keys, 1986).

Unlike fears of specific stimuli or situations (phobias), which are more common in earlier childhood, fears with social-evaluative bases increase in prevalence as youth become older (Achenbach, 1985; Beidel & Turner, 2007; Kashani & Orvaschel, 1990). Shyness in early childhood has been found to be relatively stable and to persist into adolescence and beyond (Fordham & Stevenson-Hinde, 1999; Prior, Smart, Sanson, & Oberklaid, 2000). The natural course of SAD appears to be chronic and unremitting (Beidel, Fink, & Turner, 1996; Reich, Goldenberg, Vasile, Goisman, & Keller, 1994), and individuals are unlikely to experience any tangible amelioration of this condition without some type of intervention (Juster & Heimberg, 1995).

SAD often continues into adulthood, with the National Comorbidity Survey (Kessler et al., 1994) finding lifetime prevalence rates over 13%, making it the third most common of all mental health disorders behind only major depression and alcohol dependence. Interestingly, and importantly with regard to intervention, SAD often temporally precedes other comorbidities (Schneier et al., 1992). Youth who go untreated or who do not exhibit a favorable response to treatment are at increased risk for the later development of additional problems, including other anxiety disorders, depression, substance abuse and dependence, and suicidal behavior (Kendall, Safford, Flannery-Schroeder, & Webb, 2004; Woodward & Fergusson, 2001).

Our descriptions of treatments for SAD are guided by the research evaluations that have been reported. Standards have been established for the determination of empirically supported treatments based on the extent of their demonstrated and replicated efficacy (American Psychological Association Task Force, 1995; Chambless & Hollon, 1998). Based on reviews of the literature (Kazdin & Weisz, 1998; Ollendick & King, 1998; Ollendick, King, & Chorpita, 2006), cognitive-behavioral therapy (CBT) has earned the classification of being deemed an efficacious intervention for the treatment of anxiety in youth. As such, CBT has been recommended as the first-line treatment (Compton et al., 2004; National Institute for Health and Clinical Excellence, 2004).

DEVELOPMENTAL CONSIDERATIONS

Developmental differences require therapists' consideration when treating youth with SAD, with treatment implemented in a developmentally appropriate manner. Particularly noteworthy developmental domains include (1) age-appropriate delivery; (2) cognitive, affective, and social development; and (3) social context.

Age-Appropriate Delivery

Preferred psychological treatments for shyness involve a collaborative relationship between therapist and child/adolescent. To engage youth best, the therapist's manner of interacting is playful and involving (Kendall, Chu, Gifford, Hayes, & Nauta, 1998). The therapist benefits when he or she can identify the youth's developmental level and skillfully choose engaging and enjoyable therapy activities. Three objectives are accomplished by the choice of developmentally appropriate treatment activities (Crawley, Podell, Beidas, Braswell, & Kendall, in press): (1) They facilitate development of the therapeutic relationship; (2) they provide the therapist with optimal opportunities to observe the youth's beliefs and expectations; and (3) they foster adaptive behavior and constructive thinking. Examples of activities that effectively accomplish these objectives include role plays, charades, art projects, computer activities, and board games. With young children, puppets, dolls, and superheroes may be employed, whereas interaction with older adolescents is benefitted by a more direct and respectful conversational style and fewer "play" activities.

Cognitive, Affective, and Social Development

It is also important to consider factors such as memory, attention capacity, verbal fluency/comprehension, and conceptual reasoning, all of which play significant roles in the youth's ability to understand and apply treatment strategies. For example, children with attention difficulties may have difficulty sitting through 1 hour of conversation and/or direct instruction. Furthermore, whereas some children are aware of and able to identify affective and cognitive responses to anxiety, others have more difficulty with this task. Therapy tasks that challenge a youth's beliefs, such as challenging negative thinking, may be experienced by very young children as punitive, and not be experienced as the intended "alternative views" until they are more cognitively developed.

Understanding psychosocial development aids the implementation of treatment. For example, adolescents often face different social stressors than younger children, such as dating, increased academic concerns, and autonomy from parents. These issues commonly emerge during therapy, and treatments for adolescents with SAD are best received when they address these issues in a sensitive and supportive manner.

Social Context

Children and adolescents live in a complex social context that includes parents, peers, and close friends. Given the powerful role of each of these social groups, it is valuable to incorporate social context into treatment. Indeed, youth may display socially anxious behavior in any or all of their available social contexts, and therapy is therefore more likely to be most effective when the therapist capitalizes on the strengths of the child's current social interactions. The quantity and quality of social relationships are thus considered when developing treatment goals.

Parents play an important role, whether they serve as consultants (by providing treatment information), collaborators (by working with the therapist and helping the child implement the treatment program), or coclients (when their behavior is contributing to or maintaining the child's anxious behavior) in treatment (Barmish & Kendall, 2005). Indeed, there is some evidence that children's adjustment and symptoms may improve when parenting issues are addressed (Barmish & Kendall, 2005). However, child characteristics may moderate the relationship between parental involvement and the degree of benefit experienced: For example, a very young child may benefit from more parental participation, whereas adolescents may do better when granted autonomy and parents are less involved. Additional research is needed to better determine the optimal role for parents in the treatment of SAD in youth.

TREATMENT COMPONENTS

A number of different strategies are commonly used in the treatment of child and adolescent SAD. These techniques that target the various behavioral and cognitive problems commonly believed to be at the root of the disorder include (1) social skills training; (2) psychoeducation; (3) cognitive restructuring; (4) relaxation; and (5) exposure tasks.

Social Skills Training

Shyness and social anxiety are linked with poor social skills, which often translate into difficulties with making introductions, starting or joining in conversations, effective cooperation, and appropriate display of affect in a given context (Kearney, 2005; Rubin et al., 2009). It has been suggested that the fear and anxiety of social situations predate these problems and are therefore key obstacles to the development of social competence (Beidel et al., 1999; Rubin, Burgess, Kennedy, & Stewart, 2003). Along these lines, therapists often use social skills training to remediate these deficits by teaching socially anxious youth adaptive modes of behavior, then allowing them to practice in a controlled environment, with a primary focus on skills building rather than anxiety reduction (Beidel & Turner, 2007).

Psychoeducation

A central component of CBT for anxious youth involves providing education about the anxious arousal and emotional distress with which they struggle. Children and adolescents are provided opportunities to learn about the interconnected nature of their thoughts, feelings, and behavior, with an emphasis on the multidirectional influences among them. Youth are also taught self-monitoring to identify the patterns of physiological symptoms, thoughts, and behavioral avoidance commonly associated with social anxiety. Such psychoeducation thus helps to kick-start children's understanding of the triggers and the outcomes of their social anxiety.

Psychoeducation may be useful for parents of anxious youth. Recent research suggests that parents may play a pivotal role in the maintenance of shyness and social anxiety. Anxious parents (Shamir-Essakow, Ungerer, & Rapee, 2005) who are controlling and who model poor coping strategies, such as catastrophizing and avoidance (Wood, McLeod, Sigman, Hwang, & Chu, 2003), or who engage in a fretful (Coplan, Arbeau, & Armer, 2008) parenting style or exhibit a biased pattern of elevated threat interpretation (Creswell, Schniering, & Rapee, 2005) may contribute to a greater likelihood of anxiety among their children. Whether these factors play a causative role is not yet known. Emerging evidence indicates that interventions involving psychoeducation for parents about anxiety and child management skills training (Creswell et al., 2005) may help to reduce both child- and parent-reported anxiety.

Cognitive Restructuring

Following an understanding of the role of self-talk (cognitive processing) in anxious distress, youth are better able to identify the facets of their own anxious experience. They are sensitized to recognize both (1) the automatic and distorted nature of irrational thinking and (2) its capacity to exacerbate negative emotions. Cognitive restructuring is a strategy to challenge the youth's mistaken processing about the anxiety-provoking context, with the goal of modifying and replacing such perceptions and interpretations with more rational alternatives. This cognitive change may be accomplished through reflection, examination of evidence for a thought's accuracy, decatastrophizing, and reframing (Friedberg & McClure, 2002; Kearney, 2005). Behavioral experiments (e.g., in exposure tasks; see below) also provide opportunities to challenge and correct misguided thinking.

Relaxation

Tension and other somatic symptoms can occur as physical manifestations of shyness and social anxiety. Relaxation training may help to reduce the distress that people frequently experience when confronted with an anxiety-producing social situation. Commonly utilized relaxation techniques include deep breathing exercises and progressive relaxation of various muscular groups (Koeppen, 1974; Ollendick & Cerny, 1981). Once youth have been taught to better identify the presence of anxious arousal, relaxation can help to decrease bodily discomfort and effectively lower overall anxiety (Koeppen, 1974). Practicing relaxation can also be particularly useful for youth whose anxiety reaches such heights that they feel "overwhelmed." Relaxation may allow a child to regain a sense of control and subsequently engage in coping self-talk. Despite its utility, relaxation may not be a *necessary* component of effective treatment. Some research has found that the removal of relaxation training from treatment protocols was not associated with a decrement to treatment outcome (Hudson, 2005; Rapee, 2000).

Exposure Tasks

It is often after youth have completed some skills-building sessions and acquired tools for coping with anxiety that optimal treatment then provides opportunities for them to face their fears. "Exposure tasks" in therapy refer to strategies that bring the client into close/direct contact with the very situations/stimuli that produce anxious distress. Exposure tasks have been employed for almost a century, with different terminology referring to subtle variations in implementation, such as "counterconditioning" (Jones, 1924), "systematic desensitization" (Wolpe, 1958), "extinction," and "habituation." The central feature is that anxiety-eliciting stimuli lose their fear-producing and arousing/distressing potential over time, often as a person engages in behavior incompatible with anxiety. The individual ceases to be negatively reinforced through avoidance and thus experiences a progressive diminution of arousal (Kendall et al., 2005). As individuals engage in exposure tasks, new learning opportunities emerge which lead to outcomes that are contradictory to the catastrophic beliefs about what will happen in a situation, and thus reinforce more adaptive and rational alternative beliefs.

It is generally agreed upon that exposure tasks represent an active element for effective treatment of shyness and social anxiety (Kazdin & Weisz, 1998). However, results are mixed as to whether exposure tasks alone are a sufficiently effective intervention: Some studies indicate that exposure tasks combined with cognitive change strategies are superior to exposure tasks alone (Kendall et al., 1997), whereas others have found no differences (see Juster & Heimberg, 1995, for a review).

INTERVENTION PROGRAMS FOR SOCIAL ANXIETY IN YOUTH

The treatment components described earlier are often combined in a variety of ways. The resulting intervention programs differ with regard to target ages, mode of treatment delivery, and variations in beliefs about the core deficit/problem in shyness and social anxiety. Five illustrative programs are described. Following each program description, we summarize relevant research on treatment outcomes.

The Coping Cat

One manual-based treatment for anxious youth is the Coping Cat program (third edition, Kendall & Hedtke, 2006a). Appropriate for SAD, the program is applied flexibly and is suitable for treating separation anxiety disorder and generalized anxiety disorder as well. [*Note.* Similar anxiety reduction treatments, modeled on the Coping Cat program, include the FRIENDS program; Barrett & Turner, 2001.] The Coping Cat program includes a child workbook (Kendall & Hedtke, 2006b), integrates family and emotional factors within a cognitive-behavioral framework, and is delivered in an individualized fashion over 16 sessions. The goal is to help youth learn to recognize the signs of their anxious arousal and to use these as cues to engage in anxiety management strategies.

The Coping Cat program has two parts. The first eight sessions are psychoeducational, during which skills are introduced in a sequential fashion. Learning is enhanced through assignment of "Show That I Can" (STIC) tasks to be completed outside of therapy to reinforce session content. Role-play procedures are used, with the therapist acting as a "coach" for the child and demonstrating "coping modeling" that acknowledges the challenges of situations and the possible approaches to overcome difficulties. Four main concepts are communicated during the psychoeducation portion of treatment: (1) the identification of physical reactions as a signal for the presence of anxiety; (2) the recognition of expectations and fears about what will happen in a given situation, and how these are reflected in anxious "self-talk" (Kendall & MacDonald, 1993; Ronan, Kendall, & Rowe, 1994; Treadwell & Kendall, 1996); (3) the modification of anxious self-talk into coping self-talk, as well as problem solving to develop plans for coping; and (4) the notion of rating one's own performance and being rewarded for effort. Together, these concepts constitute the FEAR plan—an acronym to help youth remember to utilize the plan for coping with anxiety:

F—Feeling Frightened?
E—Expecting bad things to happen?
A—Attitudes and Actions that can help
R—Results and Rewards

The second segment of treatment is devoted to practice. The use of exposure tasks, including imagined and real-life (*in vivo*) exposures, permit youth to face their fears and worries, ultimately allowing the development of mastery over anxiety. The exposure tasks are designed to be of gradually increasing anxiety provocation, to be developmentally appropriate for the youth, and to address specifically identified difficulties for the individual child/adolescent.

A series of randomized controlled trials (RCTs) provides support for the efficacy of the Coping Cat program. Given that the protocol was designed to treat various childhood anxiety disorders, samples included participants with separation anxiety disorder and generalized anxiety disorder, as well as SAD. In the first RCT (Kendall, 1994), 64% of children who received the treatment no longer met DSM-III-R diagnostic criteria for a disorder at posttreatment compared to 5% in the wait-list condition. Similarly, results from a second RCT found significantly greater improvements among children receiving treatment as compared to wait-list controls (Kendall et al., 1997). The study also found that maintenance of gains at 1-year follow-up did not differ across principal diagnoses (i.e., overanxious disorder, separation anxiety disorder, avoidant disorder). These diagnostic categories are comparable to DSM-IV diagnoses of generalized anxiety disorder, separation anxiety disorder, and SAD, respectively (Kendall & Warman, 1996). A third RCT (Kendall, Hudson, Gosch, Flannery-Schroeder, & Suveg, 2008) demonstrated the efficacy of individual cognitive-behavioral therapy (ICBT) for children and family cognitive-behavioral therapy (FCBT) compared to an active family-based education/support/attention (FESA) condition (Kendall et al., 2008). Of the 161 children included in the sample, 37% received a primary diagnosis of SAD prior to randomization. At posttreatment, 57, 55, and 37% of principal diagnoses in the ICBT, FCBT, and FESA conditions, respectively, were no longer present. Proportions of children who no longer met criteria for their principal diagnosis were significantly greater in both CBT conditions compared to the active control condition.

Cognitive–Behavioral Group Therapy for Adolescents

A program designed specifically for treatment of SAD in youth is cognitive-behavioral group therapy for adolescents (CBGT-A). Albano, DiBartolo, Heimberg, and Barlow (1995) describe CBGT-A as an integration of procedures found to be successful for the treatment of adult SAD (Heimberg et al., 1990; Heimberg, Salzman, Holt, & Blendall, 1993) combined with fundamental behavioral skills that are essential for effective social functioning (Christoff et al., 1985). Like the Coping Cat program, this intervention was crafted to be attentive and sensitive to developmental issues relevant to adolescents and to not treat youth as "little adults." The goals of CBGT-A are to help adolescents learn to control excessive anxiety and to cope with normal levels of anxiety, and in so doing, to master their social fears and break the pattern of associated avoidance of social situations (Albano, Marten, Holt, Heimberg, & Barlow, 1995).

The CBGT-A program is delivered in group format, with four to six participants per group. Treatment is led by cotherapists and conducted over 16 sessions, each lasting 1.5 hours (Albano, DiBartolo, et al., 1995).

The intervention has two phases. The first eight sessions provide psycho-education, during which time participants are provided information about the nature of social anxiety. Skills-building modules are then implemented to teach social skills, problem-solving skills, assertiveness, and cognitive restructuring. Therapists illustrate coping strategies through modeling, role play, feedback, and correction. Sessions 9–16 constitute the second phase and include exposure tasks. Participants create individualized fear and avoidance hierarchies at the beginning of treatment and review them at each session. They systematically face these feared situations during the exposure tasks, using the previously learned skills. Adolescents also experience vicarious exposure through serving as role players for the exposure tasks of fellow group members.

A preliminary examination provided initial support for the efficacy of the CBGT-A program (Albano, Marten, et al., 1995). Three months after completion of the intervention, four of the five adolescents who received treatment no longer met criteria for SAD. At 12-month follow-up, none of the participants met criteria for SAD. Hayward and colleagues (2000) conducted an RCT of CBGT-A with a sample of adolescent girls with SAD. At posttreatment 45% of girls in the treatment group no longer met criteria for SAD compared to 4% of girls in the wait-list control group. Although there were significant reductions in social anxiety symptoms, girls in the treatment group still evidenced elevated scores relative to non-socially-anxious controls. Generalizability of the study, however, is limited given the small sample size ($N = 35$), restricted age range, and exclusion of males.

Social Skills Training

Working from a social skills deficit model of social anxiety, Spence (1995) developed a program called social skills training (SST) for treating SAD in youth. Appropriate for children and adolescents, SST is a CBT program that combines a focus on social skills building with instruction on cognitive restructuring.

SST is conducted in group format, with six to eight individuals per group, and led by cotherapists. Treatment is delivered over 12 weekly 1-hour sessions, each of which ends with time devoted to relaxation, followed by 30 minutes for "games" (participants practice social skills while being guided by group leaders). SST begins by teaching basic skills (e.g., eye contact, facial expression, voice quality), as well as conversational and prosocial skills (e.g., listening, sharing, offering compliments) that lead to successful interactions. Participants also receive training in problem solving. Individuals are taught to approach social difficulties as "detectives," to identify the problem, brainstorm, choose the best option from various possible solutions, and develop a plan for implementation. Cognitive elements are interwoven throughout. Homework assignments require individuals to practice learned skills and face increasingly challenging social tasks.

In an evaluation of this protocol (Spence et al., 2000), 50 youth with SAD between the ages of 7 and 14 were randomly assigned to standard SST, SST with parent involvement, or wait-list control groups. The program content delivered to youth for the active treatment groups was the same, though involved parents received training on how to selectively encourage targeted social behaviors, while ignoring and not reinforcing anxious avoidance. At posttreatment, those in the treatment groups exhibited significantly greater reductions of anxiety and had significantly fewer youth continuing to meet criteria for a clinical diagnosis of SAD compared to those on the wait list. Treated youth demonstrated maintenance of gains at 12-month follow-up, with findings suggesting some evidence for greater improvement among youth whose parents were involved in treatment.

Social Effectiveness Therapy for Children

Social effectiveness therapy for children (SET-C; Beidel et al., 1998, as cited in Beidel, Turner, & Morris, 2000) was developed as a behavioral approach adapted from the adult-oriented SET program (Turner, Beidel, & Cooley, 1994; Turner, Beidel, Cooley, Woody, & Messer, 1994) by removing its cognitive components. SET-C is designed to address the various dimensions of impairment that exist for youth with SAD, including reduction of social anxiety, improvement of social skills and corresponding interpersonal functioning, and increased social participation (Beidel et al., 2000).

SET-C has both individual and group sessions lasting between 60 and 90 minutes, twice per week (one of each per week), and delivered over the course of 12 weeks. A child and parent education component allows families to become acclimated to the program, providing information about SAD and the opportunity to ask questions. An SST component teaches the use of one skill (starting conversations, listening and remembering, etc.) per week through instruction, modeling, rehearsal, and feedback. Peer generalization experiences come next, in which participants engage in weekly, youth-specific group activities (bowling, parties, etc.) with a group of nonanxious peers. These activities provide the opportunity to practice acquired skills in a natural setting with children without SAD. The final component is *in vivo* exposure, with sessions designed to address each child's own specific pattern of social fears, and to face one situation per week.

SET-C has also received empirical support for the treatment of socially anxious youth. In an initial study, children between the ages of 8 and 12 who met criteria for SAD were randomly assigned either to SET-C or to an active control group (Beidel et al., 2000). Both groups met twice weekly (once for individual therapy and once for group) for 12 weeks. At the end of treatment, 67% of children in the SET-C group no longer met criteria for SAD, compared to only 5% in the control group. Results from 6-month follow-up showed that these gains were maintained. Furthermore, at 3-year follow-up, 72% of children who received SET-C no longer met criteria for SAD, which was not significantly different than the percentage found at posttreatment (Beidel, Turner, Young, & Paulson, 2005). Eighty percent of children no longer met criteria for SAD at 5-year follow-up, which was a significantly greater percentage than that evidenced at posttreatment for this sample (Beidel, Turner, & Young, 2006).

Another RCT examined the efficacy of SET-C compared to fluoxetine in the treatment of SAD in youth (Beidel et al., 2007). Children between the ages of 7 and 17 were randomly assigned to one of three conditions: SET-C, fluoxetine, or pill placebo. Dosage of fluoxetine was fixed each week, starting at 10 mg per day for the first week and reaching 40 mg per day from Week 7 to the completion of the trial. At posttreatment, 53.0% of the SET-C group, 21.2% of the fluoxetine group, and 3.1% of the placebo group no longer met diagnostic criteria for SAD. Between-group differences were all statistically significant. In addition, both active treatments demonstrated significantly greater improvements than the placebo condition in SAD severity, although there were no significant differences in change of severity between the two active controls.

Skills for Academic and Social Success

The Skills for Academic and Social Success (SASS; Masia et al., 1999) program, based on the belief that social skills deficits are the major problem for anxious youth, incorporates SST with cognitive-behavioral components. SASS was derived primarily from the SET-C protocol, with adaptations for appropriateness with an adolescent population and the intention of creating a feasible treatment for delivery in high schools (Fisher, Masia-Warner, & Klein, 2004). To transport a clinic-based treatment successfully to the school setting, the program was designed to fit within a preexisting school structure, while taking advantage of the resources inherently available in schools.

The SASS intervention is delivered over the course of 3 months, with flexibility for accommodating school calendars. Twelve weekly sessions are conducted in group format within the school, typically lasting 40 minutes (one class period). Groups are led by a psychologist and a graduate student, and may have up to six students.

The program has five parts:

1. The first session is devoted to *Psychoeducation,* covering the nature and maintenance of social anxiety.

2. the second session focuses on *Realistic Thinking,* as participants are taught to identify their tendency to overestimate the likelihood of negative outcomes and to challenge such expectations.

3. *Social Skills for Success* (e.g., initiating conversations, maintaining conversations, listening and remembering, assertiveness) are reviewed over the next four sessions. Participants first observe group leaders demonstrating these skills through role plays, then participate in role plays themselves, receiving feedback and suggestions from the group.

4. Five sessions are dedicated to *Facing Your Fear,* during which participants progressively encounter typically avoided situations through exposure tasks. Because schools often represent the setting of greatest impairment for adolescents with SAD (Hoffman et al., 1999), the SASS program benefits from the availability of school personnel and peers who can be readily recruited to aid in exposures.

5. *Relapse Prevention* is the topic for the final session as participants are prepared for potential setbacks and how to handle future difficulties.

In addition to the main group sessions, participants have at least two brief individual meetings with group leaders to discuss specific treatment goals, identify obstacles, and strengthen rapport. Teacher- and administrator-nominated prosocial peers also join in four scheduled social events (e.g., going to the mall) with participants, providing opportunities for adolescents to practice their skills in realistic social settings. Two parent group meetings are held to provide education about social anxiety, to discuss common parental reactions to children's struggles, and to provide suggestions about how parents can support positive coping. Finally, two monthly booster sessions are conducted after completion, during which progress is monitored (see also Fisher et al., 2004).

Examination of the SASS protocol has yielded additional support for the efficacy of group therapy for the treatment of adolescents with SAD (Masia, Klein, Storch, & Corda, 2001; Masia-Warner et al., 2005). Results from an RCT indicated that following completion of treatment, 67% of children in the SASS group no longer met criteria for SAD compared to only 6% of participants in the wait-list control condition (Masia-Warner et al., 2005). SAD symptoms significantly decreased in the treatment condition compared to the wait-list condition, although no significant differences were found for measures of depression and loneliness. Reduction in anxiety was maintained at 9-month follow-up. Such findings provide encouraging support for the successful transportability of treatments for SAD into the school setting.

Cross-Protocol Comparison

Limited research has directly compared different protocols. However, one team of researchers has compared three protocols, including Social Effectiveness Therapy for Adolescents–Spanish Version (SET-A$_{SV}$), CBGT-A, and *Intervención en Adolescentes con Fobia Social Generalizada* (IAFSG; Garcia-Lopez et al., 2002; Olivares et al., 2002). Findings suggested that all treatments were more effective than a control group for reducing social anxiety symptoms. SET-A$_{SV}$ and IAFSG showed better maintenance of long-term gains at 1-year follow-up than did CBGT-A; however, these group differences were no longer significant at 5-year follow-up (Garcia-Lopez et al., 2006).

In summary, research evaluating the efficacy of various treatments protocols for SAD in youth has provided substantial support for CBT as an effective treatment (for reviews, see Cartwright-Hatton, Roberts, Chitsabesan, Fothergill, & Harrington, 2004; Kazdin & Weisz, 1998; Ollendick & King, 1998; Ollendick et al., 2006). The combination of cognitive and behavioral strategies has been shown to significantly reduce symptoms of social anxiety regardless of the format of the intervention (e.g., individual, family, group, school-based). In addition, interventions developed specifically for SAD in youth and those developed for a range of childhood anxiety disorders have both been found to significantly reduce anxiety symptoms for youth with SAD.

FUTURE DIRECTIONS

The passage of time has coincided with several advances in the treatment of SAD in youth. Nevertheless, the knowledge base surrounding this disorder is far from complete, as the available treatments produce response rates that are favorable but less than optimal. First, improved treatment outcomes will likely result from two distinct, yet equally important, endeavors: theory-driven research and practice-driven research.

The development of optimal treatments requires developmental research. Theory-driven developmental research will inform treatment by providing an improved understanding of the natural course of the development and the maintenance of social anxiety, as well as its absence, in youth. For example, prospective, longitudinal research on the role of parenting factors in the development of SAD may inform treatment about the family systems variables that need to be targeted in treatment (Kashdan & Herbert, 2001). Additionally, treatments may benefit from an advanced understanding of normal development of nonanxious social interactions, especially among adolescents (Kendall & Ollendick, 2004). Contrasting the development of social anxiety and normal development has allowed researchers to identify risk and protective factors, such as expressive language skills (Coplan & Armer, 2005), peer friendships (Rubin et al., 2006), peer exclusion (Gazelle & Ladd, 2003), and classroom climate (Gazelle, 2006). Such influences serve as potential targets for treatment and can help to better inform the optimal timing for prevention and intervention efforts.

Second, improved treatment for social anxiety requires research on optimal treatment practice. Kashdan and Herbert (2001) offer many future directions for social anxiety treatment research. For example, they address the importance of targeting specific populations in treatment studies. Some of the treatment evaluations reviewed herein target anxious youth generally, with the samples including a subset of socially anxious youth. To help determine the degree to which social anxiety is distinct from other childhood anxieties in terms of treatment response, future treatment outcome evaluations should include sufficient numbers of socially anxious youth, so that outcomes can be examined for this specific population. Subsequently, research can then examine the treatment processes and mechanisms of action associated with beneficial change for socially anxious youth.

Research examining the effectiveness of select and individual treatment components such as exposure tasks, cognitive restructuring, social skills training, and parental involvement, will also assist in the creation of optimal treatments. When exploring the treatment process, researchers should also focus on the relationship between the child and therapist (Kendall & Ollendick, 2004). Additionally, the creation of optimal treatment packages will profit from research on treatment delivery, such as the optimal format of delivery (group vs. individual vs. family) and the optimal number of sessions. Last, research on moderators of treatment responsivity, such as age, comorbidities, character traits, and self-regulatory competencies, will assist researchers and clinicians in appropriately adapting treatments.

The transportability of empirically supported treatments (ESTs) is a current concern. "Transportability" refers to the dissemination and implementation of a treatment in community settings. ESTs satisfy the Chambless and Hollon (1998) criteria: CTs with real patients, using proper measurements and analyses, that are found in more than one setting to produce meaningful outcomes. However, the majority of the RCTs have been conducted in controlled research settings to assess efficacy. It is now important to focus on transporting these programs to clinical settings out in the community to assess their effectiveness in these locations (Kazdin & Kendall, 1998; Weisz & Jensen, 2001). Research is also needed to inform the preferred ways to train service-providing clinicians and to determine how best to sustain adherence over time.

Cultural factors are critical but often understudied. Research on cross-cultural differences in social anxiety will inform clinicians in applying/

adapting treatments. Such research results may highlight differences in the development and presentation of social anxiety, as well as response to treatment across cultural groups (Ginsburg & Silverman, 1996). The promotion of research on the efficacy and effectiveness of ESTs across cultural groups is enhanced by the translation of treatments into different languages. For example, one treatment program, the Coping Cat, has been translated into numerous languages and is currently being evaluated in different countries (e.g., Norway, China).

In the pursuit of improved treatments, we should embrace burgeoning technology. Computers may be a useful tool when training community- and school-based clinicians, as well as primary care physicians (Lambert & Meier, 1992). In addition to aiding in dissemination (e.g., computer-based training for CBT [CBT4CBT]; Kendall & Khanna, 2008b), computer technology may also assist in interventions. Research with adults found a decline in anxiety symptoms following participation in a computer-based intervention (Cukrowicz & Joiner, 2007), as may a computer-assisted program for youth (e.g., Camp Cope-A-Lot; Kendall & Khanna, 2008a). Research can evaluate the feasibility and effectiveness of Internet- and/or computer-assisted interventions for anxious youth (Khanna, Aschenbrand, & Kendall, 2007; see also *Cool Teens*; Cunningham, Rapee, & Lyneham, 2007). Evaluations of the role of computer technology as a supplement to, or replacement for, individual or group treatments will likely guide the format for the provision of future psychological services.

To reach youth in need, we must consider multiple service-providing settings. A majority of youth with anxiety disorders fails to receive treatment (Chavira et al., 2004). The dissemination and implementation of treatments in community mental health clinics is laudable but may only be beneficial to the extent that these treatments are accessed. The dissemination of ESTs for use in schools (e.g., Masia et al., 2001; Masia-Warner et al., 2005) has the potential for reaching a large number of children in need. The school setting offers a platform for multiple types of intervention (both treatment and prevention programs, e.g., FRIENDS; Barrett & Pahl, 2006).

To expand optimal mental health care, we encourage researchers to partner with public health and policy advocates. Investigators should capitalize on current policy in favor of further development, examination, and dissemination of ESTs. Government policymakers desire to improve mental health care for youth. For example, the New Freedom Commission on Mental Health (2003) promotes ongoing dialogue among researchers, providers, consumers, and families to inform research and the dissemination of findings. It also recognizes the underutilization of technology and supports the use of telehealth—the "[use] of electronic information and telecommunications technologies to provide long distance clinical care and consultation [and] patient and professional health-related education" (p. 55). Similarly, the Surgeon General's Report (U.S. Public Health Service, 2000) recognizes the importance of treatment research and recommends improving the infrastructure for child and adolescent mental health services to approve scientifically supported interventions. The Surgeon General's Report also promotes the use of school-based resources and urges the training of school personnel to identify better the need for mental health care. Such developments reflect increasing public awareness concerning child and adolescent mental health issues, and represent a major opportunity for researchers to tackle these important issues.

CONCLUSION

Shy and socially anxious youth experience a wide range of hardships, with problems enduring into adulthood if left untreated. For those with SAD, a number of strategies hold promise for improvement, with the greatest evidence supporting the combined use of cognitive and behavioral interventions. However, with outcome research still in its relative infancy, much work remains to maximize treatment response. Those involved in the care of youth at all levels must heed the mandates of federal policy and work to mobilize and integrate resources. Only then can opportunities be provided for youth to overcome their social anxiety and have the optimum chance for future success.

REFERENCES

Achenbach, T. M. (1985). Assessment of anxiety in children. In A. H. Tuma & J. D. Master (Eds.), *Anxiety and the anxiety disorders* (pp. 707–734). Hillsdale, NJ: Erlbaum.

Albano, A. M., DiBartolo, P. M., Heimberg, R. G., & Barlow, D. H. (1995). Children and adolescents: Assessment and treatment. In R. G. Heimberg, M. R. Liebowitz, D. A. Hope, & F. R. Schneier (Eds.), *Social phobia: Diagnosis, assessment and treatment* (pp. 387–425). New York: Guilford Press.

Albano, A. M., Marten, P. A., Holt, C. S., Heimberg, R. G., & Barlow, D. H. (1995). Cognitive-behavioral group treatment for social phobia in adolescents. *Journal of Nervous and Mental Disease, 183,* 649–656.

American Psychological Association Task Force on Psychology Intervention Guidelines. (1995). *Template for developing guidelines: Interventions for mental disorders and psychological aspects of physical disorders.* Washington, DC: American Psychological Association.

Barmish, A. J., & Kendall, P. C. (2005). Should parents be co-clients in cognitive-behavioral therapy for anxious youth? *Journal of Clinical Child and Adolescent Psychology, 34,* 569–581.

Barrett, P., & Turner, C. (2001). Prevention of anxiety symptoms in primary school children: Preliminary results from a universal school-based trial. *British Journal of Clinical Psychology, 40,* 399–410.

Barrett, P. M., & Pahl, K. M. (2006). School-based intervention: Examining a universal approach to anxiety management. *Australian Journal of Guidance and Counseling, 16*(1), 55–75.

Beidel, D. C., Fink, C. M., & Turner, S. M. (1996). Stability of anxious symptomatology in children. *Journal of Abnormal Child Psychology, 24,* 257–269.

Beidel, D. C., & Turner, S. M. (1988). Comorbidity of test anxiety and other anxiety disorders in children. *Journal of Abnormal Child Psychology, 16,* 275–287.

Beidel, D. C., & Turner, S. M. (2007). Prevalence of social anxiety disorder. In *Shy children, phobic adults: Nature and assessment of social anxiety disorder* (pp. 81–89). Washington, DC: American Psychological Association.

Beidel, D. C., Turner, S. M., & Morris, T. L. (1998). *Social effectiveness therapy for children: A treatment manual.* Unpublished manuscript, Charleston: Medical University of South Carolina.

Beidel, D. C., Turner, S. M., & Morris, T. L. (1999). Psychopathology of childhood social phobia. *Journal of the American Academy of Child and Adolescent Psychiatry, 38,* 643–650.

Beidel, D. C., Turner, S. M., & Morris, T. L. (2000). Behavioral treatment of childhood social phobia. *Journal of Consulting and Clinical Psychology, 68,* 1072–1080.

Beidel, D. C., Turner, S. M., Sallee, F. R., Ammerman, R. T., Crosby, L. A., & Pathak, S. (2007). SET-C versus fluoxetine in the treatment of childhood social phobia. *Journal of the American Academy of Child and Adolescent Psychiatry, 46,* 1622–1632.

Beidel, D. C., Turner, S. M., & Young, B. J. (2006). Social effectiveness therapy: Five years later. *Behavior Therapy, 37,* 416–425.

Beidel, D. C., Turner, S. M., Young, B., & Paulson, A. (2005). Social effectiveness therapy for children: Three-year follow-up. *Journal of Consulting and Clinical Psychology, 73,* 721–725.

Buss, A. H. (1980). *Self-consciousness and social anxiety.* San Francisco: Freeman.

Cartwright-Hatton, S., Roberts, C., Chitsabesan, P., Fothergill, C., & Harrington, R. (2004). Systematic review of the efficacy of cognitive behaviour therapies for childhood and adolescent anxiety disorders. *British Journal of Clinical Psychology, 43,* 421–436.

Caspi, A., Elder, G. H., Jr., & Bem, D. J. (1988). Moving away from the world: Life course patterns of shy children. *Developmental Psychology, 24,* 824–831.

Chambless, D. L., & Hollon, S. D. (1998). Defining empirically supported treatments. *Journal of Consulting and Clinical Psychology, 66,* 7–18.

Chavira, D. A., Stein, M. B., Bailey, K., & Stein, M. T. (2003). Parental opinions regarding treatment for social anxiety disorder in youth. *Journal of Developmental and Behavioral Pediatrics, 24,* 315–322.

Chavira, D. A., Stein, M. B., Bailey, K., & Stein, M. T. (2004). Child anxiety in primary care: Prevalent but untreated. *Depression and Anxiety, 20,* 155–164.

Chavira, D. A., Stein, M. B., & Malcarne, V. L. (2002). Scrutinizing the relationship between shyness and social phobia. *Anxiety Disorders, 16,* 585–598.

Christoff, K. A., Scott, W. O. N., Kelley, M. L., Schlundt, D., Baer, G., & Kelly, J. A. (1985). Social skills and social problem-solving training for shy young adolescents. *Behavior Therapy, 16,* 468–477.

Compton, S. N., March, J. S., Brent, D., Albano, A. M., Weersing, V. R., & Curry, J. (2004). Cognitive-behavioral psychotherapy for anxiety and depressive disorders in children and adolescents: An evidence-based medicine review. *Journal of the American Academy of Child and Adolescent Psychiatry, 43,* 930–959.

Coplan, R. J., Arbeau, K. A., & Armer, M. (2008). Don't fret, be supportive!: Maternal characteristics linking child shyness to psychosocial and school adjustment in kindergarten. *Journal of Abnormal Child Psychology, 36,* 359–371.

Coplan, R. J., & Armer, M. (2005). Talking yourself out of being shy: Shyness, expressive vocabulary, and socioemotional adjustment in preschool. *Merrill–Palmer Quarterly, 51,* 20–41.

Coplan, R. J., Gavinsky-Molina, M. H., Lagacé-Séguin, D., & Wichmann, C. (2001). When girls versus boys play alone: Gender differences in the associates of nonsocial play in kindergarten, *Developmental Psychology, 37,* 464–474.

Coplan, R. J., Girardi, A., Findlay, L. C., & Frohlick, S. L. (2007). Understanding solitude: Young children's attitudes and responses towards hypothetically socially withdrawn peers. *Social Development, 16,* 390–409.

Costello, J. E., Egger, H. L., & Angold, A. (2004). Developmental epidemiology of anxiety disorders. In T. H. Ollendick & March, J. S. (Eds.), *Phobic and anxiety disorders in children and adolescents: A clinician's guide to effective psychosocial and pharmacological interventions* (pp. 61–91). New York: Oxford University Press.

Crawley, S. A., Podell, J. L., Beidas, R. S., Braswell, L., & Kendall, P. C. (in press). Cognitive-behavioral therapy with youth. In K. Dobson (Ed.), *Handbook of cognitive-behavioral therapies.* New York: Guilford Press.

Creswell, C., Schniering, C. A., & Rapee, R. M. (2005). Threat interpretation in anxious children and their mothers: Comparison with nonclinical children and the effects of treatment. *Behaviour Research and Therapy, 43,* 1375–1381.

Crozier, W. R., & Hostettler, K. (2003). The influence of shyness on children's test performance. *British Journal of Educational Psychology, 73,* 317–328.

Cukrowicz, K. C., & Joiner, T. E., Jr. (2007). Computer-based intervention for anxious and depressive symptoms in a non-clinical population. *Cognitive Therapy and Research, 31,* 677–693.

Cunningham, M., Rapee, R., & Lyneham, H. (2007). Overview of the *Cool Teens CD-ROM* for anxiety disorders in adolescents. *Behavior Therapist, 30,* 15–19.

Essau, C. A. (2005). Frequency and patterns of mental health services utilization among adolescents with anxiety and depressive disorders. *Depression and Anxiety, 22,* 130–137.

Fisher, P. H., Masia-Warner, C., & Klein, R. G. (2004). Skills for social and academic success: A school-based intervention for social anxiety disorder in adolescents. *Clinical Child and Family Psychology Review, 7,* 241–249.

Fordham, K., & Stevenson-Hinde, J. (1999). Shyness, friendship quality, and adjustment during middle childhood. *Journal of Child Psychology and Psychiatry, 40,* 757–768.

Friedberg, R. D., & McClure, J. M. (2002). *Clinical practice of cognitive therapy with children and adolescents: The nuts and bolts.* New York: Guilford Press.

Furmark, R., Tillfors, M., Everz, P., Marteinsdotir, I., Gefver, O., & Fredrikson, M. (1999). Social phobia in the general population: Prevalence and sociodemographic profile. *Social Psychiatry Psychiatric Epidemiology, 34,* 416–424.

Garcia-Lopez, L. J., Olivares, J., Beidel, D., Albano, A. M., Turner, S., & Rosa, A. I. (2006). Efficacy of three treatment protocols for adolescents with social anxiety disorder: A 5-year follow-up assessment. *Anxiety Disorders, 20,* 175–191.

Garcia-Lopez, L. J., Olivares, J., Turner, S. M., Beidel, D. C., Albano, A. M., & Sanchez-Meca, J. (2002). Results at long-term among three psychological treatment for adolescents with generalized social phobia (II): Clinical significance and effect size. *Psicología Conductual Revista Internacional de Psicología Clínica de la Salud, 10,* 165–179.

Gazelle, H. (2006). Class climate moderates peer relations and emotional adjustment in children with an early history of anxious solitude: A child × environment model. *Developmental Psychology, 42,* 1179–1192.

Gazelle, H., & Ladd, G. W. (2003). Anxious solitude and peer exclusion: A diathesis–stress model of internalizing trajectories in childhood. *Child Development, 74,* 257–278.

Ginsburg, G. S., & Silverman, W. K. (1996). Phobic and anxiety disorders in Hispanic and Caucasian youth. *Journal of Anxiety Disorders, 10,* 517–528.

Hayward, C., Varady, S., Albano, A., Thienemann, M., Henderson, L., & Schatzberg, A. F. (2000). Cognitive-behavioral group therapy for social phobia in female adolescents: Results of a pilot study. *Journal of the American Academy of Child and Adolescent Psychiatry, 39,* 721–726.

Heimberg, R. G., Dodge, C. S., Hope, D. A., Kennedy, C. R., Zollo, L. J., & Becker, R. E. (1990). Cognitive behavioral group treatment for social phobia: Comparison with a credible placebo control. *Cognitive Therapy and Research, 14,* 1–23.

Heimberg, R. G., Salzman, D. G., Holt, C. S., & Blendall, K. A. (1993). Cognitive-behavioral group treatment for social phobia: Effectiveness at five year follow-up. *Cognitive Therapy and Research, 17,* 325–339.

Hoffman, S. G., Albano, A. M., Heimberg, R. G., Tracey, S., Chorpita, B. F., & Barlow, D. H. (1999). Subtypes of social phobia in adolescents. *Depression and Anxiety, 9,* 15–18.

Hudson, J. A. (2005). Mechanisms of change in cognitive behavioral therapy for anxious youth. *Clinical Psychology: Science and Practice, 12,* 161–165.

Jones, M. C. (1924). A laboratory study of fear: The case of Peter. *Pedagogical Seminary, 31,* 308–315.

Jones, W. H., Briggs, S. R., & Smith, T. G. (1986). Shyness: Conceptualization and measurement. *Journal of Personality and Social Psychology, 51,* 629–639.

Juster, H. R., & Heimberg, R. G. (1995). Social phobia: Longitudinal course and long-term outcome of cognitive-behavioral treatment. *Psychiatric Clinics of North America, 18,* 821–842.

Kashani, J. H., & Orvaschel, H. (1990). A community study of anxiety in children and adolescents. *American Journal of Psychiatry, 147,* 313–318.

Kashdan, T. B., & Herbert, J. D. (2001). Social anxiety disorder in childhood and adolescence: Current status and future directions. *Clinical Child and Family Psychology Review, 4*(1), 37–61.

Kazdin, A. E., & Kendall, P. C. (1998). Current progress and future plans for developing effective treatments: Comments and perspectives. *Journal of Clinical Child Psychology, 27*(2), 217–226.

Kazdin, A. E., & Weisz, J. R. (1998). Identifying and developing empirically supported treatments for children and adolescents. *Journal of Consulting and Clinical Psychology, 66,* 19–36.

Kearney, C. A. (2005). The treatment of social anxiety and social phobia in youths. In M. A. Anthony (Ed.), *Social anxiety and social phobia in youth: Characteristics, assessment, and psychological treatment* (pp. 109–124). New York: Springer Publishing Co.

Kendall, P. C. (1992). *The Coping Cat workbook.* Ardmore, PA: Workbook Publishing. Available online at *www.workbookpublishing.com.*

Kendall, P. C. (1994). Treating anxiety disorders in children: Results of a randomized clinical trial. *Journal of Consulting and Clinical Psychology, 62,* 100–110.

Kendall, P. C., Chu, B., Gifford, A., Hayes, C., & Nauta, M. (1998). Breathing life into a manual: Flexibility and creativity with manual-based treatments. *Cognitive and Behavioral Practice, 5,* 177–198.

Kendall, P. C., Flannery-Schroeder, E., Panichelli-Mindel, S. M., Southam-Gerow, M., Henin, A., & Warman, M. (1997). Therapy for youths with anxiety disorders: A second randomized clinical trial. *Journal of Consulting and Clinical Psychology, 65,* 366–380.

Kendall, P. C., & Hedtke, K.A. (2006a). *Cognitive-behavioral therapy for anxious children: Therapist manual* (3rd ed.). Ardmore, PA: Workbook Publishing. Available online at *www.workbookpublishing.com.*

Kendall, P. C., & Hedtke, K.A. (2006b) *The Coping Cat workbook* (2nd ed.). Ardmore, PA: Workbook Publishing. Available online at *www.workbookpublishing.com.*

Kendall, P. C., Hudson, J. L., Gosch, E., Flannery-Schroeder, E., & Suveg, C. (2008). Cognitive-behavioral therapy for anxiety disordered youth: A randomized clinical trial evaluating child and family modalities. *Journal of Consulting and Clinical Psychology, 76,* 282–297.

Kendall, P. C., & Khanna, M. (2008a). *Camp Cope-A-Lot (The Coping Cat CD).* Ardmore, PA: Workbook Publishing. Available online at *www.workbookpublishing.com.*

Kendall, P. C., & Khanna, M. (2008b). *CBT4CBT: Computer-Based Training to be a Cognitive Behavioral Therapist (for anxiety in youth).* Ardmore, PA: Workbook Publishing. Available online at *www.workbookpublishing.com.*

Kendall, P. C., & MacDonald, J. P. (1993). Cognition in the psychopathology of youth, and implications for treatment. In K. S. Dobson & P. C. Kendall (Eds.), *Psychopathology and cognition* (pp. 387–427). San Diego: Academic Press.

Kendall, P. C., & Ollendick, T. H. (2004). Setting the research and practice agenda for anxiety in children and adolescence: A topic comes of age. *Cognitive and Behavioral Practice, 11,* 65–74.

Kendall, P. C., Robin, J. A., Hedtke, K. A., Suvegm, C., Flannery-Schroeder, E., &

Gosch, E. (2005). Considering CBT with anxious youth?: Think exposures. *Cognitive and Behavioral Practice, 12,* 136–148.

Kendall, P. C., Safford, S., Flannery-Schroeder, E., & Webb, A. (2004). Child anxiety treatment: Outcomes in adolescence and impact on substance use and depression at 7.4-year follow-up. *Journal of Consulting and Clinical Psychology, 72,* 276–287.

Kendall, P. C., & Warman, M. J. (1996). Anxiety disorders in youth: Consistency across DSM-III-R and DSM-IV. *Journal of Anxiety Disorders, 10,* 453–463.

Kessler, R. C., McGonagle, K. A., Zhao, S., Nelson, C. B., Hughes, M., Eshelman, S., et al. (1994). Lifetime and 12-month prevalence of DSM-III-R psychiatric disorders in the United States: Results from the National Comorbidity Study. *Archives of General Psychiatry, 51,* 8–19.

Khanna, M., Aschenbrand, S. G., & Kendall, P. C. (2007). New frontiers: Computer technology in the treatment of anxious youth. *Behavior Therapist, 30,* 22–25.

Koeppen, A. S. (1974). Relaxation training in children. *School Guidance and Counseling, 9,* 521–528.

Lambert, M. E., & Meier, S. T. (1992). Utility of computerized case simulations in therapist training and evaluation. *Journal of Behavioral Education, 2,* 73–84.

Lazarus, P. J. (1982). Incidence of shyness in elementary-school age children. *Psychological Reports, 51,* 904–906.

Liebowitz, M. R., Heimberg, R. G., Fresco, D. M., Travers, J., & Stein, M. B. (2000). Social phobia or social anxiety disorder: What's in a name? *Archives of General Psychiatry, 57,* 191–192.

Masia, C. L., Beidel, D. C., Albano, A. M., Rapee, R. M., Turner, S. M., Morris, T. L., et al. (1999). *Skills for academic and social success.* Available from Carrie Masia-Warner, PhD, New York University School of Medicine, Child Study Center, 215 Lexington Avenue, 13th floor, New York, NY 10016.

Masia, C. L., Klein, R. G., Storch, E. A., & Corda, B. (2001). School-based behavioral treatment for social anxiety disorder in adolescents: Results of a pilot study. *Journal of the American Academy of Child and Adolescent Psychiatry, 40,* 780–786.

Masia-Warner, C., Klein, R. G., Dent, H. C., Fisher, P. H., Alvir, J., Albano, A. M., et al. (2005). School-based intervention for adolescents with social anxiety disorder: Results of a controlled study. *Journal of Abnormal Child Psychology, 33,* 707–722.

National Institute for Health and Clinical Excellence. (2004). *Anxiety: Management of anxiety (panic disorder, with or without agoraphobia, and generalized anxiety disorder) in adults in primary, secondary and community care.* London: Author. Retrieved July 4, 2008, from *www.nice.org.uk/cg022quickrefguide.*

Nelson, L. J., Rubin, K. H., & Fox, N. A. (2005). Social withdrawal, observed peer acceptance, and the development of self-perceptions in children ages 4 to 7 years. *Early Childhood Research Quarterly, 20,* 185–200.

New Freedom Commission on Mental Health. (2003). *Achieving the promise: Transforming mental health care in America* [Final Report. DHHS Pub. No. SMA-03-3832]. Rockville, MD: Author.

Olivares, J., Garcia-Lopez, L. J., Beidel, D. C., Turner, S. M., Albano, A. M., & Hidalgo, M. D. (2002). Results at long-term among three psychological treatments for adolescents with generalized social phobia (I): Statistical significance. *Psicología Conductual Revista Internacional Psicología de Clínica de la salud, 10,* 147–164.

Ollendick, T. H., & Cerny, J. A. (1981). *Clinical behavior therapy with children.* New York: Plenum Press.

Ollendick, T. H., & King, N. J. (1998). Empirically supported treatments for children with phobic and anxiety disorders: Current status. *Journal of Clinical Child Psychology, 27,* 156–167.

Ollendick, T. H., King, N. J., & Chorpita, B. F. (2006). Empirically supported treatments for children and adolescents. In P. C. Kendall (Ed.), *Child and adolescent therapy: Cognitive-behavioral procedures* (3rd ed.). New York: Guilford Press.

Pilkonis, P. A. (1977). Shyness, public and private, and its relationship to other measures of social behavior. *Journal of Personality, 45,* 585–595.

Prior, M., Smart, D., Sanson, A., & Oberklaid, F. (2000). Does shy–inhibited temperament in childhood lead to anxiety problems in adolescence? *Journal of the American Academy of Child and Adolescent Psychiatry, 39,* 461–468.

Rapee, R. M. (2000). Group treatment of children with anxiety disorders: Outcome and predictors of treatment response. *Australian Journal of Psychology, 52,* 125–129.

Reich, J., Goldenberg, I., Vasile, R., Goisman, R., & Keller, M. (1994). A prospective follow-along study of the course of social phobia. *Psychiatry Research, 54,* 249–258.

Ronan, K., Kendall, P. C., & Rowe, M. (1994). Negative affectivity in children: Development and validation of a self-statement questionnaire. *Cognitive Therapy and Research, 18,* 509–528.

Rubin, K. H., Burgess, K., Kennedy, A. E., & Stewart, S. (2003). Social withdrawal and inhibition in childhood. In E. Mash & R. Barkley (Eds.), *Child psychopathology* (2nd ed., pp. 372–406). New York: Guilford Press.

Rubin, K. H., Coplan, R. J., & Bowker, J. C. (2009). Social withdrawal and shyness in childhood and adolescence. *Annual Review of Psychology, 60,* 141–171.

Rubin, K. H., Wojslawowicz, J. C., Rose-Krasnor, L., Booth-LaForce, C. L., & Burgess, K. B. (2006). The best friendships of shy/withdrawn children: Prevalence, stability, and relationship quality. *Journal of Abnormal Child Psychology, 34,* 139–153.

Schneier, F. R., Johnson, J., Hornig, C. D., Liebowitz, M. R., & Weissman, M. M. (1992). Social phobia: Comorbidity and morbidity in an epidemiologic sample. *Archives of General Psychiatry, 49,* 282–288.

Shamir-Essakow, G., Ungerer, J. A., & Rapee, R. M. (2005). Attachment, behavioral inhibition, and anxiety in preschool children. *Journal of Abnormal Child Psychology, 33,* 131–143.

Spence, S. H. (1995). *Social skills training: Enhancing social competence with children and adolescents.* Windsor, UK: NFER Nelson.

Spence, S. H., Donovan, C., & Brechman-Toussaint, M. (1999). Social skills, social outcomes, and cognitive features of childhood social phobia. *Journal of Abnormal Psychology, 108,* 211–221.

Spence, S. H., Donovan, C., & Brechman-Toussant, M. (2000). The treatment of childhood social phobia: The effectiveness of a social skills training-based, cognitive behavioural intervention, with and without parent involvement. *Journal of Child Psychology and Psychiatry, 41,* 713–726.

Treadwell, K. R. H., & Kendall, P. C. (1996). Self-talk in anxiety-disordered youth: States-of-mind, content specificity, and treatment outcome. *Journal of Consulting and Clinical Psychology, 64,* 941–950.

Turner, S. M., Beidel, D. C., & Cooley, M. R. (1994). *Social effectiveness therapy: A program for overcoming social anxiety and social phobia.* Toronto, Canada: Multi-Health Systems.

Turner, S. M., Beidel, D. C., Cooley, M. R., Woody, S. R., & Messer, S. C. (1994). A multicomponent behavioral treatment for social phobia: Social effectiveness therapy. *Behaviour Research and Therapy, 32,* 381–390.

Turner, S. M., Beidel, D. C., Dancu, C. V., & Keys, D. J. (1986). Psychopathology of social phobia and comparison to avoidant personality disorder. *Journal of Abnormal Psychology, 95,* 389–394.

Turner, S. M., Beidel, D. C., & Townsley, R. M. (1990). Social phobia: Relationship to shyness. *Behavioural Research and Therapy, 28,* 497–505.

U.S. Public Health Service. (2000) *Report on the surgeon general's conference on children's mental health: A national action agenda.* Washington, DC: U.S. Government Printing Office.

Weisz, J. R., & Jensen, A. L. (2001). Child and adolescent psychotherapy in research practice contexts: Review of the evidence and suggestions for improving the field. *European Child and Adolescent Psychiatry, 10,* 112–118.

Wittchen, H. U., Stein, M. B., & Kessler, R. C. (1999). Social fears and social phobia in a community sample of adolescents and young adults: Prevalence, risk factors and co-morbidity. *Psychological Medicine, 29,* 309–323.

Wolpe, J. (1958). *Psychotherapy by reciprocal inhibition.* Stanford, CA: Stanford University Press.

Wood, J. J., McLeod, B. D., Sigman, M., Hwang, W., & Chu, B. C. (2003). Parenting and child anxiety: Theory, empirical findings, and future directions. *Journal of Child Psychology and Psychiatry, 44,* 134–151.

Woodward, L. J., & Fergusson, D. M. (2001). Life course outcomes of young people with anxiety disorders in adolescence. *Journal of the American Academy of Child and Adolescent Psychiatry, 40,* 1086–1093.

Zimbardo, P. G. (1977). *Shyness: What is it, what to do about it.* Reading, MA: Addison-Wesley.

Index

Page numbers followed by *f* indicate figure; *n*, note; *t*, table